FEELING GOOD

STRENGTH TRAINING WITH YOUR SIGNIFICANT ELDER

By
John B. Payne and J. Jody Kelly

Bloomington, IN      Milton Keynes, UK

authorHOUSE™

AuthorHouse™
1663 Liberty Drive, Suite 200
Bloomington, IN 47403
www.authorhouse.com
Phone: 1-800-839-8640

AuthorHouse™ UK Ltd.
500 Avebury Boulevard
Central Milton Keynes, MK9 2BE
www.authorhouse.co.uk
Phone: 08001974150

First published by AuthorHouse 2/1/2006

ISBN: 1-4208-7627-9

Library of Congress Control Number: 2005907809

Printed in the United States of America
Bloomington, Indiana

This book is printed on acid-free paper.

Acknowledgements

We gratefully acknowledge the help and support of our mothers and our two additional case studies. This book would not have been possible without their generosity of time and spirit. Many thanks to Mother, Mama, Jack, and Lyn. On the front cover are Ann Payne, 91, performing the dead lift with 40 pounds and Faye Kelly, 90, performing the lateral pull with 45 pounds. Thanks to the Summit, the retirement community in Austin, TX, where our mothers live, as do several of John's other strength training clients over age 70.

John thanks his dear wife, Bernadette, for her love, encouragement, and patience. Jody thanks her mother, children, and grandchildren for their love and inspiration.

Thanks galore to Kelly Foster, who developed our Web site, www.significantelder.com, designed our logo, produced the T-shirts used in the video, and filmed and edited the Significant Elder video on the website. Many thanks also to Skye Kilaen for editing the book and to Gigi Harris for marketing ideas. Jody Kelly took all but three of the digital photographs and designed the page layout.

Thanks to Dave Goodin's Hyde Park Gym and to John's fellow trainers there, including Dave Goodin, Sean Endsley, Pattie Farley, Mark Heard, Lance Hooton, Amalia Litras, Andy Oliver, Marcus Reed, Kirby Sams, Trey Zepeda, and especially Marc "This may hurt a little" Frazier, who is also a massage therapist.

We are deeply indebted to Mary Holman, M.A., L.P.C., for reviewing Chapter 1; Jenifer Webb, M.O.T., former occupational therapist, for reviewing Chapters 1, 2, 3, 4, 9, and 10; Sonya Emery, R.M.T., for input on Chapter 9; and a licensed M.D., who requested anonymity, for reviewing Chapter 4. These reviewers provided valuable information and greatly improved the book. The remaining errors are our own. On that topic, we acknowledge with respect all previous authors of books containing strength training exercises. It's not as easy as it may sound to describe how to move the body and what safety precautions to take. We hope our explanations are clear, complete, and useful.

To all of John's older clients, current and past, we are deeply grateful. A few have moved away or discontinued strength training, but most have continued. Their ages range from 71 to 94. In addition to our case studies, his clients include Richard Alexander, Ann Carson, Louise Crawford, Pat Giddings, Tweet Gray, Bess Jones, Anne Jordan, Lois Leggett, Kathleen Lockhart, Lucille Lyons, Mary McDaniel, Esther Mallory, Lynn Miller, Mary Niendorff, Nancy Peoples, Anna Faye Peterson, Leonard Peikoff, Frank Schleicher, Helen Silverstone, Allyne Smith, Rex Spencer, Evelyn Taylor, Ruth Turbeville, Elizabeth Ware, and Frances Young. We are also grateful to the dozens of others who shared their stories.

Finally, we pay special tribute to the memory of John's clients who passed away in their 80s or 90s: Helen Arend, Minnie Ree Baccus, Mary Clark, John Crawford, Oma Gillis, George Ryan, Patricia Rush, Hardy Thompson, Dr. Harvey Thompson, Patty Thompson, Jack Turbeville, Edna Vacker, and Virginia Walker.

Foreword

This is *your* book if you're an adult who is worried about the health and strength of an older person in your life, your *Significant Elder* You will learn how to introduce strength training to improve the quality of life for your Significant Elder, even if he or she is 90 years old.

Your Significant Elder will need a doctor's approval to exercise, but the huge majority of older people can train for strength. They love working out because it makes them feel so good. Here's how you can help:

- Conduct the strength training sessions yourself if you have lifted weights with a certified personal trainer for some time. On the next page, see some examples of people over age 40 who could easily train a Significant Elder.

- If you haven't done strength training, take this book to a personal trainer and ask for at least four to six sessions so that you can learn the correct techniques to teach your Significant Elder. Then consult the personal trainer from time to time as needed.

- If you live too far away, use this book to find a personal trainer for your special older person. Then learn how to follow up to ensure success. Chapters 3 through 10 contain introductory notes just for you.

This is your book if you *are* a Significant Elder—age 65 or older. If you are in your 60s or early 70s, read the note below and schedule a dozen or so strength training sessions with a certified personal trainer. After that, you can probably continue strength training on your own. However, it's a good idea to find a workout partner so that the two of you can keep each other motivated and ensure each others' safety on some of the more challenging exercises.

If you are in your 70s, 80s, or 90s, congratulations! Please give this book to your favorite young person—a child, grandchild, niece, nephew, sibling, spouse, in-law, friend, or helper. Then surprise this person by asking for some assistance with strength training. It will do you both worlds of good. Another strategy is to give this book to a certified personal trainer and ask for the kind of strength training we recommend.

This is also your book if you are a *certified personal trainer* who wants some tips on working with older clients. It's the best job on earth if you really like to help people. Each chapter contains a special note near the end just for you.

Note: A physician's examination is recommended for all exercise participants with any restrictions and for those persons over 40 years of age. Fitness evaluation participants in these categories who have not had a physical examination in the past year must acknowledge that they have been informed of its importance and, therefore, accept full responsibility for their health and wellbeing. *Exercise participants must understand that no responsibility is assumed by a personal trainer or by the authors of this book.*

This Could Be You

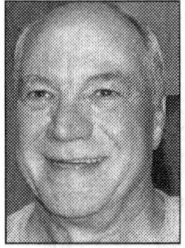 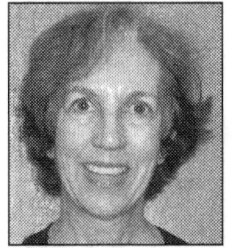 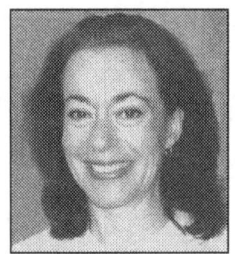 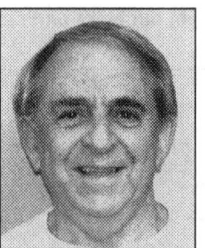

Ken, Mary, Bernadette, and Dave, in their 40s, 50s, or 60s, make their lifts look easy.

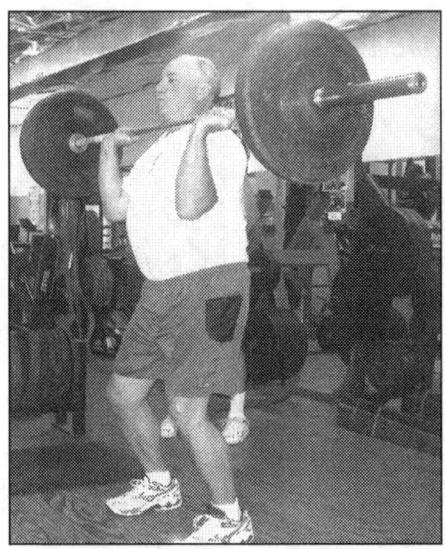

Ken power-cleans 90 pounds.

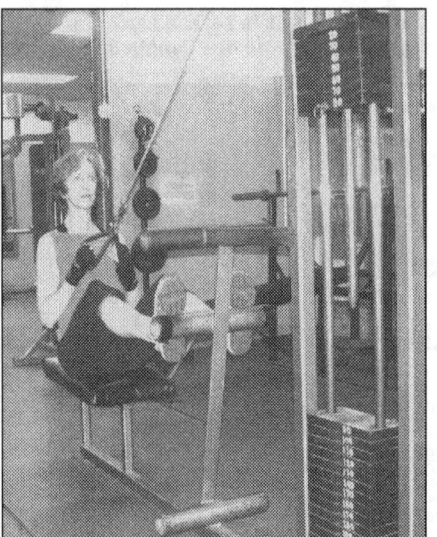

Mary pulls 80 pounds on the seated row.

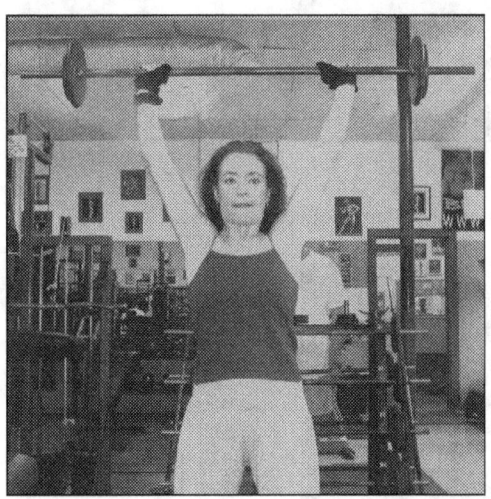

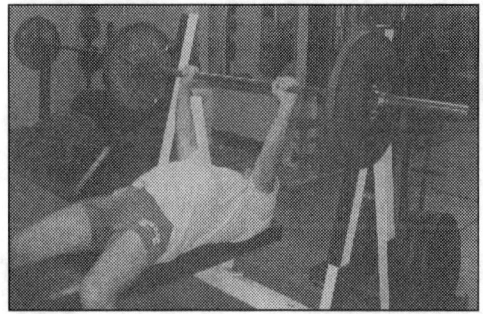

Above, Dave bench presses 110 pounds in a light workout. He set a world record at 275 pounds in his age group.

Left, Bernadette raises 45 pounds over head.

This Could Be Your Significant Elder

Meet our stars and case studies. See them in action in Chapters 5 and 6. Then read their stories in Chapter 8.

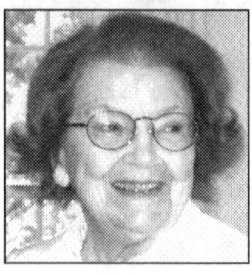 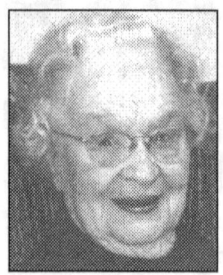 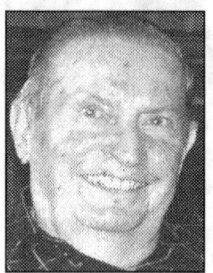 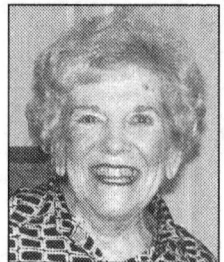

Ann is 91, Faye is 90, Jack is 74, and Lyn is 73.
Below, meet more stars who do strength training, and see them in action in Chapters 5 and 6.

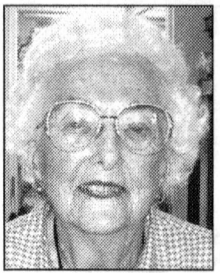 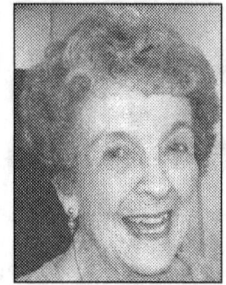 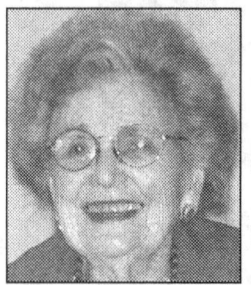 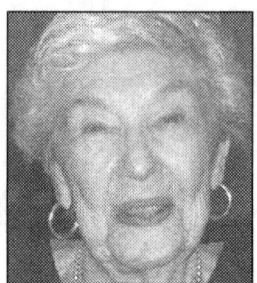

Anna Fay is 93, Virginia is 93, Esther is 92, and Mary is 91.

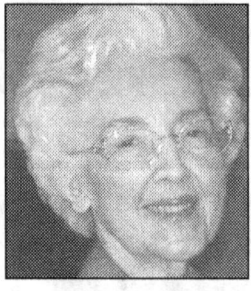 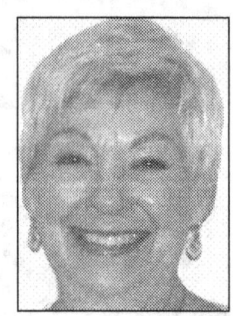 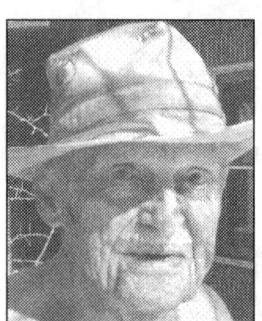 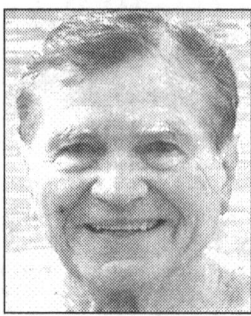

Frances is 84 and Kathleen is 77.
In Chapter 9, look for Weldon, 92, and Carl, 86, above, as well as Kathy and John, both 81, and Rae, 80, below.

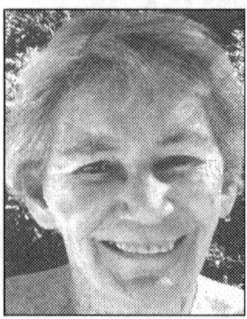 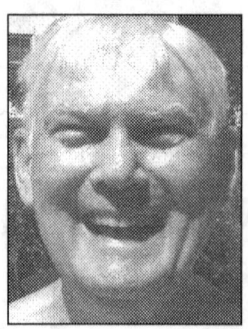 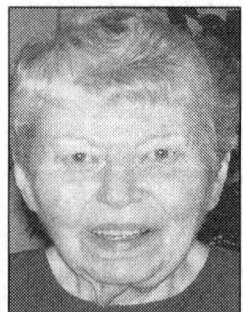

Table of Contents

List of Figures and Tables

PART I. GETTING READY

"Move or die is the language of our Maker in the constitution of our bodies."
John Adams, second President of the United States[1]

Part I starts with your first thought about doing something, anything, to help an older person enjoy a higher quality of life. We call that person your Significant Elder.

Part I concludes with your being prepared to take the next step into real strength training with your Significant Elder. Along the way, you will learn that:

- Exercise benefits nearly *everybody*. Feeling good is available to *everybody*.

- Your role in your Significant Elder's life is supremely important.

- Strength training doesn't take much equipment, but it does take some know-how.

- You can keep your Significant Elder safe during strength training.

When you finish Part I, you will be ready to learn how to teach or discuss the exercises that will help your Significant Elder regain and maintain strength and health throughout life.

---

[1] Cited in David McCullough, *John Adams* (New York: Touchstone, 2001), p. 452.

Chapter 1. Feeling Good about Strength Training

Motivation and Assessment for You and Your Significant Elder

"I feel terrible. I know I'm 90, but I'm not that old. I need to work out."
Ann, now 91, stepping off the plane after a two-and-a-half-week trip

A Note on Pronouns: This chapter uses feminine pronouns to refer to your Significant Elder (SE) because women outnumber men late in life and because the authors' Significant Elders are their mothers. Hereafter, we alternate chapter by chapter. Thus, you will need to substitute the pronoun appropriate for your SE only 50% of the time.

Introduction

Welcome. Take a deep breath and relax. You're in the right place to find out what action *you* can take that will measurably improve the strength and health of an older person in your life—your Significant Elder. She might be a parent, grandparent, in-law, spouse, sibling, other kinsman, or close friend. As her strength diminishes year by year, your concern grows.

Isn't there something you can do? Yes, there is, and we will show you how every step of the way.

It's called strength training, resistance training, or weight training. It's the systematic practice of performing progressive exercises customized for regaining and maintaining strength. Strength training helps older people perform the activities of daily living.

No one, *no one,* is too old to start strength training.

There simply is nothing better for keeping frailty at bay and postponing or preventing the need for a cane, walker, wheelchair, or scooter. Even people already using assistive devices can increase their strength and lead active, vibrant lives.

What Does This Have to Do with Me?

Hello, Baby Boomer, member of the Sandwich Generation, any adult child of aging parents, or anyone else who cares about an older person. This book is about improving the physical strength and quality of life for your Significant Elder with strength training. You really can help your SE to become stronger, a lot stronger. This book is for you if:

- You feel responsible for someone who is over age 65 or younger but frail, out of shape, or chronically ill.

- You are beginning to worry about her strength and health as she ages.

- You want to help her regain as much of her strength and health as possible.

- You would like to assist her in retaining her independence as long as she can.

- You want to be proactive instead of reactive—you would prefer not to wait for a major medical crisis.

- You might not be sure of the best way to help her, but you want to learn.

- Either you know something about strength training or you are willing to learn a little.

- You want her to feel good, and you want to feel good, too.

> This is your Significant Elder. You care about her, and you want to help.

If this describes you, then welcome to the club. You are not alone. It's true that you really *can* help your SE feel good and help yourself feel good at the same time.

Can Our Oldest Americans Really Work Out?

Our mothers, Ann and Faye, and scores of other people we know can certainly work out—and vigorously. John trains significant numbers of people in their 70s, 80s, and 90s and has garnered over 6,000 hours of experience with this age group.

- *All* of his clients are highly significant to their families and friends. Your SE is too.

- *All* have enjoyed getting stronger. Your SE will too.

- *All* of their adult children are happy with the results. You will be too.

With enough assistance and motivation, your SE can probably work out just as successfully. To convince yourself of this idea, meet our star athletes, Ann, Faye, Jack, and Lyn. Be sure to read their inspiring case studies in Chapter 8.

Ann

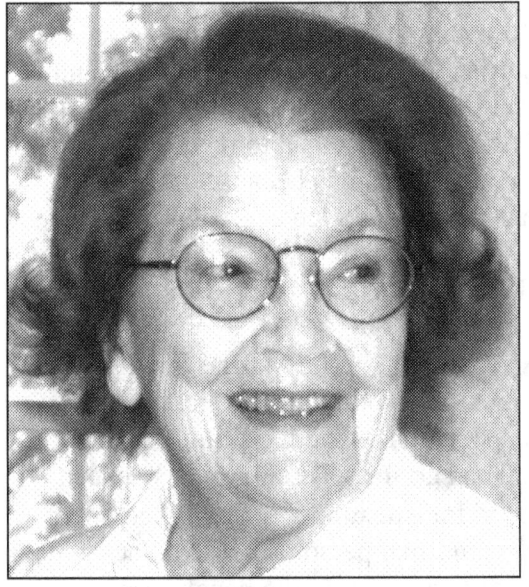

Figure 1-1. Ann Payne, 91

Do you have a potential star in your family like John's mother? Ann Payne, 91, started working out with her son, a certified personal trainer, after she had had back-to-back heart attacks at age 88. For a time, her five children were concerned that she might not survive.

Though Ann has never been an athlete before, she now feels strong and healthy and doesn't like to miss a training session, even for an enjoyable trip. "Working out probably saved my life, and of course I enjoy the time with my son," she says. Her favorite exercise is the chair squat, described in Chapter 5.

Faye

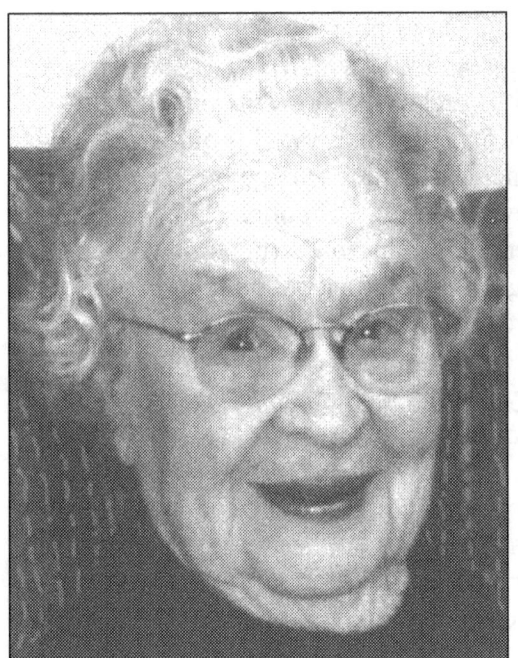

Figure 1-2. Faye Kelly, 90

Maybe your star athlete-in-waiting is someone like author Jody's mother. Faye Kelly, 90, used to take seven prescription drugs every day but is now down to half a pill daily. After a touch-and-go bout with pneumonia and a scary fall in a parking lot, she started strength training with John when Jody introduced her to him.

Faye had never participated in sports, but now she feels much stronger and healthier than she did 15 years ago when she was overcoming breast cancer—"I'm rarin' to go," she says. Her favorite exercise is the lat pull illustrated on the front cover. See Chapter 5 for an upper back pull that uses resistance tubing..

Jack

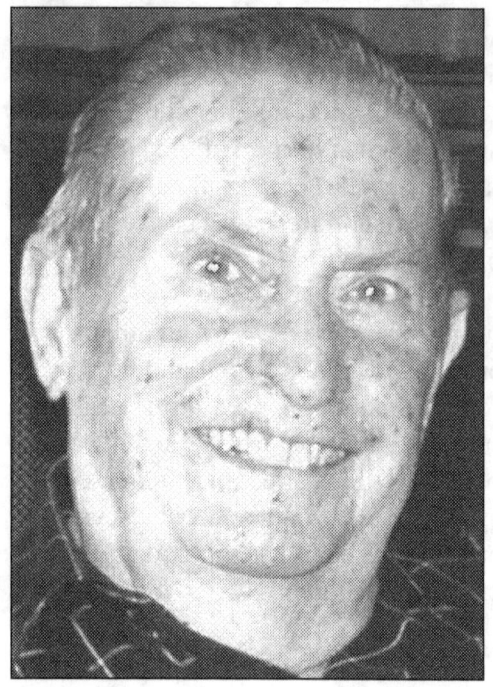

Figure 1-3. Jack Lewis, 74

Do you know a potential star like Jack Lewis, 74? He seemed quite young and healthy when he started working out at age 71 except that he had to receive monthly blood transfusions because of chronic gastrointestinal bleeding caused by inherited telangiectasia, a potentially fatal blood disorder.

After serving in the Marine Corps in the 1950s, Jack did relatively little to stay in shape. But now, he feels much stronger and can go for several months between blood transfusions—"I finally feel more like a normal person," he says. Jack's favorite exercise is the bench press, described in Chapter 6.

Lyn

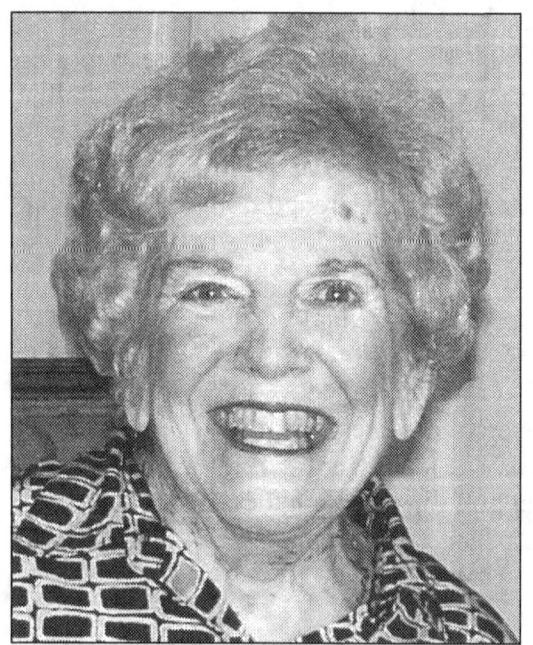

Figure 1-4. Lyn Byer, 73

Maybe your potential star athlete is someone like Lyn Byer, 73. She was born with cerebral palsy, which resulted in permanently dislocated shoulders among other difficulties. At age 69, she also developed severe scoliosis that pinched a nerve and caused excruciating pain in her legs. She couldn't walk and didn't have the strength to feed herself. After four years of strength training, "four horrible years," she says with a radiant smile, her pain is much diminished.

Now, on good days, she can walk short distances without her walker, and she can feed herself. She says, "I don't tell my age because I'm 73 going on 22." Her favorite exercise is the dead lift, described in Chapter 6.

What Can *You* Do to Help?

A lot, actually. Most of the people who start strength training after age 65 do so because their doctors or their grown children told them they needed to become stronger and pointed out the way. The older people featured here will convince you that *they* can do strength training, but aren't most people over 65 too old or weak to lift weights? No. Older people, even those who have been largely sedentary, can benefit dramatically from strength training, often doubling or tripling their strength within six months to a year.

Even frail older people can perform most of the strength training motions, sometimes with modified exercises at first and then with better technique as they become stronger. Rapid physical decline and frailty are not an inevitable part of the aging process, even in the very old.

In fact, frailty owes more to a sedentary lifestyle, poor nutrition, and fear and depression than it does to the passing of years. Most of the effects of frailty are preventable and even reversible to some extent.[2] As Mom's muscles improve, so will her mental and emotional powers. She may even gain a new purpose in life through strength training.

You will learn on page 18 how to administer a simple test to determine whether she can undertake strength training. Unless she has a medical condition listed on page 8, she will probably score high enough to begin working out with your help.

The best way to prevent extreme frailty is to help your SE become stronger. The quickest and most efficient way to do that is through strength training.

Here's how you can best help your SE become and remain stronger and healthier:

- **Recognize** the fact that you may be the only person in your SE's life who can help her begin exercising.

  "My granddaughter told me I needed to find a personal trainer to make me stronger, and I listened because she's also my doctor," said Minnie Ree, who began strength training at age 88. She enjoyed working out and greatly increased her strength.

- **Learn** enough about strength training to be your SE's Advocate and engage the right professional trainer. If you are willing and able, you can become the Spotter—a safety assistant during a training session—or the Strength Coach—an amateur but highly knowledgeable substitute for a professional trainer. Chapter 2 shows you how.

---

[2] Thomas T. Perls, Margery Hutter Silver, and John F. Lauerman, *Living to 100: Lessons in Living to Your Maximum Potential at Any Age* (New York: Basic Books, 2000).

"Mom and I have had our disagreements, but none of that stuff matters when we're celebrating her latest personal best," reports someone we will call Geri, 42. "I enjoy seeing what she's up to these days. She's a lot of fun."

- **Practice** motivational techniques to help your SE get through the inevitable rough spots that everyone encounters during an exercise program or any kind of major change.

   "I'm sympathetic about your rotator cuff strain," John told his mother, Ann, "but you gotta admit, it makes a great opportunity to get your legs super-strong."

What Do You Need to Know?

It's not a long list. You will need to know or learn something about:

- Strength training.

- Safety techniques.

- Your SE's current health and physical condition as well as her attitudes and outlook on life.

- Your own attitudes toward the aging process and toward your SE.

- A few motivational techniques.

- Optionally, a little about yoga, Tai Chi, or a similar practice because these are extremely useful for older people. See Chapter 9.

If you already work out regularly, congratulations! If not, you will find in this book everything you need to get started in strength training with your SE. Maybe you have already thought about exploring a way to strengthen her. But take a look at the books on strength training. You will notice that very few focus on people over 50, and those that do seldom address people over 70, much less those in their 80s and 90s.[3]

If you are already a caregiver, you have probably noticed that the resources on caregiving focus on how to help *after* your SE has become frail, bedridden, or in need of rehabilitative care. Wouldn't it be better to learn what to do *before* a crisis occurs, *before* the medical bills mount up? In fact, wouldn't you like to help prevent or postpone medical crises? We believe that it's possible to prevent some medical crises and either postpone or lessen the impact of others.

Become proactive in the life of your Significant Elder.

---

[3] *Strength Training past 50* by Wayne L. Westcott and Thomas R. Baeschle (Chicago: Human Kinetics, 1997) stops at 70. *Fitness over 50: An Exercise Guide from the National Institute on* Aging (New York: Norton, 2003) is very general and not challenging enough for many of the older people we know.

Both authors admit that they waited to take action in their mothers' lives until something traumatic occurred—heart attacks and pneumonia. Fortunately, both of our mothers are doing well now, but we wish we had known to get started earlier.

What's in It for Me, You Ask?

There are many benefits *for you* of helping your SE get stronger. You can:

- Reduce the number of medical crises in her life, probably lower her medical costs, and gain more control over your own life.

- Worry less about her and reduce your concern that she will have a medical crisis.

- Feel good about helping her and seeing her feel empowered.

- Improve communications. You may think there's an unbridgeable gap between the generations, but there really isn't.[4] We're all just human beings trying to get along. Talking about accomplishments in exercise is a lot more fun than talking about aches and pains.

- Learn how to improve and maintain your own health and strength as long as possible while you are still pre-elderly, before you become someone else's Significant Elder.

- Become part of the growing preventive medicine movement.

- Gain more control over your time and mental health. You can take comfort in doing the right thing—promoting a better quality of life for you and your SE.

Don't waste time worrying about your SE but not taking any action. Remove the stress by learning how to make life better for her and yourself. You can feel good, and so can she.

Another Reason to Get Strong

Being strong and fit not only feels good, it also enables people of any age to recover more rapidly after illness, injury, or surgery. The following examples illustrate the point.

Virginia

We call her the "Comeback Kid." Virginia, 93, is a testament to the advantages of being strong and fit. She bounced back from two surgeries for a pacemaker, one 15 years ago and one three years ago. She recovered from two cancer surgeries, a bad fall, and two shoulder injuries. In March of 2005, however, her health began to deteriorate, and everyone thought her heart was failing. Even Virginia thought "God was ready for me." When her condition was diagnosed as complications from a bleeding ulcer, she spent two and one-half months in and out of the hospital and hospice care. In June, she was able to resume light strength

---

[4] Mary Pipher, *Another Country: Navigating the Emotional Terrain of our Elders* (New York: Penguin, 1999).

training and was eager to do so. She trusts the process of coming back from illness and injury and wanted to work out, guessing that "God must have miscommunicated Himself to me."

Frances

When Frances, 84, had pacemaker surgery, her doctor advised her not to lift anything over five pounds during the first six weeks of recovery. She was able to walk regularly and resumed her workouts with John in the third week after surgery. She used only one-pound weights because, as she explains, "I couldn't raise my arms up to shoulder level." With her doctor's approval, she began adding more weight and, in her fourth week, she felt as strong as ever. She cut her recovery time by one-third.

Dave

A competitive power lifter, Dave, 69, "couldn't get out of the hospital bed" the day after he suffered a stroke. In two days, however, he was using a walker to get around. In three days he was walking alone, and the next day he went home. When he started rehab soon after, the physical therapist asked him to stand, bend his knees, and squat half way down. He was immediately able to do full squats. The therapist sent him home because Dave could do all of the rehab exercises already. He was soon back in the gym doing his regular lifts but with lighter weights at first. Soon, he built back up to the elite level at which he has set four world age-class records in power sports. He still holds one of them.

Kathy

For several months before a 44-year-old we will call Kathy scheduled tummy tuck surgery, she ate right, rested well, and built up her strength. She went to Pilates classes, ran on the treadmill, and did hundreds of ab crunches every week. Two days after surgery, she began alternating her high-powered pain prescription with an over-the-counter pain medication. The next day, she could do without the prescription, and one day later she didn't need any pain relief at all. A week after surgery, she felt "ready for salsa dancing."

Strength and fitness pay off handsomely at any age.

Is There Anyone Who Can't Work Out?

Strength training is not appropriate for people with a disease that causes muscle weakness, such as muscular dystrophy, multiple sclerosis, or amyotrophic lateral sclerosis (Lou Gehrig's disease). Infantile paralysis and its frequent follow-on, post-polio syndrome, may cause permanent muscle weakness, so the affected muscles can't develop further. However, muscles that weren't affected can grow stronger.

In addition, some glaucoma patients are told not to lift heavy weights, so consult a physician to find out how much weight your SE with glaucoma can lift. Since many women 80 and older have vertebral fractures, your SE may need to limit the amount of weight she lifts. Even if the muscles are strong enough, the bones may be susceptible to fractures. Again, consult your SE's physician for advice.

For everyone else, even those with health problems, strength training is wonderful. See "Handling Health Issues Safely" on page 87 for suggestions on working out safely with other diseases and conditions.

Feeling Good

What does *feeling good* mean in regard to strength training with your Significant Elder? Unless something feels good, at least occasionally, you won't stick with it and neither will your SE. Knowledgeable people tell us to exercise to improve our health, and we know we should, but here's the open secret that all regular exercisers know—the only thing that keeps us exercising week in and week out is that *exercise makes us feel good*.

Exercise produces *endorphins*, which are pain-killing chemicals the body creates naturally during physical activity. More important, endorphins yield feelings of mild euphoria. Exercise makes us feel better emotionally and mentally as well as physically. As you look and feel better, your body image improves and so does your self-esteem.

People who work out feel good. People who work out strenuously feel even better. As the body feels better, the mind follows and the mental processes seem sharper. A good workout seems to dissipate bad moods, lift depression, decrease stress, and diminish or lessen worries. What's not to like?

Don't I Already Know This Stuff?

Of course. We all know that the doorway to feeling good is within each of us. We know the simple secrets of the good life—eat right, sleep well, and exercise regularly. A sure-fire way for anyone to feel good is to produce large amounts of endorphins. One of the quickest and most efficient ways to produce endorphins is to do strength training.

What about running and the mystique of the runner's high? Yes, wind sprints, running, jogging, and even walking can make you feel good and produce endorphins, but running or even walking long distances are beyond the ability of most older people, especially those over 70 or 75. A couple of vigorous sets of well-performed chair squats will rev up your SE's endorphin production without ever making her lift her feet from the floor.

Strength training is one of the quickest, safest, most accessible ways to produce endorphins and feel good.

Endorphins last a long time. After a fairly taxing workout, the positive effects of endorphins that the body produces will last all day. Exercise is like a one-a-day vitamin, but even better—and it's either free or low in cost.

You do know a lot already. The one thing you may not be familiar with is how much time and effort it may take to help your SE change her sedentary lifestyle, start eating right, and begin exercising. It will take some of your time and energy to get this program up and running. But if you do a simple cost-benefit analysis, you will realize that you can't afford *not* to make the effort.

What Could Happen If I Don't Get Involved?

Maybe nothing—maybe something distressing or worse. Everyone will die, but no one wants to go through a long, lingering, painful, increasingly debilitated stage before death. And family members certainly don't want to see that happen to their loved ones. So what's it going to be for your SE and, later on, for yourself? Here are a few questions that may jump start your thinking:

- What are the top causes of death for people age 65 and over?

- Are any of these diseases preventable through strength training and other types of exercise?

- What disabilities and chronic conditions do I need to be worried about?

Table 1-1 below shows the top five causes of death among people age 65 and over, along with the number of deaths caused annually by these diseases. As a point of interest, we provide the total financial burden on the American health care system.

Top Five Causes of Death

Top Five Causes of Death at age 65+	Number of Deaths per Year at 65+	Total Cost per Year for All Ages	Can exercise prevent or postpone it?
Heart Disease	594,000	$300.6 billion	Yes
Cancer (All forms)	392,000	$202 billion	Indirectly
Stroke (Cerebrovascular Disease)	148,000	$51 billion	Yes
Chronic Obstructive Pulmonary Diseases	106,000	$32 billion	Yes
Influenza and Pneumonia	59,000	$14.3 to $21.7 billion See **Note 1** below.	Indirectly
Total	1,300,000	Averages $606 billion	3 out of 5. See **Note 2**.

Table 1-1. Top Five Causes of Death at Age 65+
(Source: http://www.cdc.gov for 2004)

Notes:

1. The exact figure for influenza and pneumonia during a specific year depends in part upon whether an epidemic occurs.

2. Three of the top causes of death can be prevented or postponed by a solid exercise program, which includes strength training. The other two may also be moderated because people who exercise tend to have stronger immune systems, to be of normal weight, and to enjoy better health in general.

In 2001, the national health expenditure per person (all ages) was $5,035. For people over 65, the figure is higher because they typically consume more of the health care resources. By 2003, the total annual cost of all health care for all ages was $1.4 trillion. By now, it is far more and growing.

> Poor health costs a lot. Strength training costs much less.
> Exercise improves your health and makes you feel good.

Table 1-2 helps you quantify the degree of concern that you and your SE might have about a particular cause of death. Circle *Yes* or *No* for family history of the specific disease, and then circle *High*, *Medium*, or *Low* for the level of concern that you and your SE may feel about it.

Concerns about the Top Five Causes of Death

Top Five Causes of Death at age 65+	Family History of the Disease?	Your SE's Level of Concern	Your Level of Concern
Heart Disease	Yes No	High Medium Low	High Medium Low
Cancer (All forms)	Yes No	High Medium Low	High Medium Low
Stroke (Cerebrovascular Disease)	Yes No	High Medium Low	High Medium Low
Chronic Obstructive Pulmonary Diseases	Yes No	High Medium Low	High Medium Low
Influenza and Pneumonia	Yes No	High Medium Low	High Medium Low

Table 1-2. How Concerned Are You and your SE?

There is often a high correlation between family history of a disease and the family's worry. However, note any discrepancies between your concerns and your SE's concerns.
For example, Mom may be more worried about breast cancer than about heart disease, but you can let her know that heart disease is the number one killer of both men and women. Since heart disease can definitely be postponed or prevented with an ongoing exercise program, this information might help motivate her to start working out.

If the top five causes of death seem unlikely for you or your SE, then Table 1-3 from the Administration on Aging might be more instructive. It shows five chronic medical conditions afflicting significant numbers of people over 65. Recall that heart disease and stroke, although not repeated below, can also cause chronic problems and major disability, and both can be postponed or prevented with exercise.

Five Chronic Conditions

Chronic Medical Conditions in People 65+	Percent of Those 65+ with the Condition	Can exercise prevent or postpone it?
Overweight, Obesity See **Note 1** below.	66-70% See **Note 2**.	Yes
Arthritis	48%	Yes
Hypertension	37%	Yes
Hearing and Balance Impairments	32%	Yes. See **Note 3**.
Depression	5-25%. See **Note 4**.	Yes
Total	See **Note 5**.	5 out of 5

Table 1-3. Chronic Conditions of People 65+ (Source: http://www.aoa.gov/ for 2004)

Notes:

1. The figures for overweight and obesity do not include diabetes and other related diseases.

2. The figure of 66-70% is for the general population, and the figure keeps rising. For people over 65, the percentage is likely to be higher[5] because they don't exercise as much as younger people do. Those over 75 are particularly inactive. *But they don't have to remain sedentary. Most are capable of exercising.*

3. Recent research shows that even the sense of hearing may improve somewhat with exercise.[6]

4. Although clinical depression is diagnosed in only 5 to 10% of people over age 65, many more suffer the garden variety, which they may attempt to disguise by calling it the blahs or by saying they are "just a little out of sorts."

5. The total adds up to more than 100% because 70% of people over age 65 have *more than one* chronic condition; 80% of people over age 55 have at least one chronic condition.

Table 1-4 below gives you a way to quantify concerns about these chronic conditions. Circle *Yes* or *No* for family history of the specific condition, and then circle *High*, *Medium*, or *Low* for the level of concern that you and your SE may feel about a particular disease or condition.

---

[5] However, see Chapter 7 for problems with underweight in a significant number of people 65 and over.
[6] Kathleen M. Hutchinson, et al. "Effects of Cardiovascular Fitness and Muscle Strength on Hearing Sensitivity," *Journal of Strength and Conditioning Research* (Vol 14, No. 3, pp. 301-309).

Concerns about Five Chronic Conditions

Chronic Medical Conditions in People 65+	Family History of the Condition?	Your SE's Level of Concern	Your Level of Concern
Overweight and Obesity	Yes No	High Medium Low	High Medium Low
Arthritis	Yes No	High Medium Low	High Medium Low
Hypertension	Yes No	High Medium Low	High Medium Low
Hearing Impairments	Yes No	High Medium Low	High Medium Low
Depression	Yes No	High Medium Low	High Medium Low

Table 1-4. How Concerned Are You and Your SE?

If you have no family history and no concerns about these chronic conditions, then you are to be congratulated. You probably lead very active lives. As with Table 1-2, however, look for discrepancies between your concerns and those of your SE.

For example, Dad may claim to feel okay even though he carries 60 extra pounds, but you know the strain those pounds are placing on his entire body, from arteries and heart valves to breathing difficulties and joint pains. Your concern for his health may be just the motivating force he needs to get started with an exercise program.

Again, some families experience none of the problems discussed here, but many do. Chances are good that your SE will need to deal with one or more of these diseases or chronic conditions between now and death unless you get involved. Your interest and support can make a very big difference in how your SE spends the last years of her life.

Okay, What's the Good News?

Feeling good is the good news. You can feel good by helping your SE get into strength training, and she will feel good when she incorporates exercise into her daily life. She will be much healthier than if she remained sedentary. Although it has not been proven that exercise makes us live longer, the real payoff is feeling *alive*, even at age 95, and not feeling half-dead at age 65 or younger.

Mittie Mae

Mittie Mae, 84, is fully alive. She goes to her small town's wellness center three times a week without fail. She lifts weights, takes exercise classes, and walks a mile on the treadmill in 20 minutes. Her watchword is, "Just keep moving."

When Mittie Mae retired from her job at a bank, she thought she would get to read all the books she hadn't had time to read and watch all the TV programs she hadn't had time to watch. She tolerated inactivity for six weeks before she started feeling terrible. Then she became active again through exercise and volunteer work.

Under five feet tall and weighing less than 100 pounds, Mittie Mae is strong, limber, and alert. Maybe it helped that she grew up on a dairy farm and got used to hard work. But the difference between Mittie Mae and many older people is that she kept right on being herself, working hard, and having fun. "Just move it!" she says.

Why Don't More Older People Exercise?

Good question. The reasons are many. One may be that Americans today receive too many negative messages. For example, nearly everything that we hear and read about old age seems discouraging, depressing, and death-oriented.

Even healthy older people buy into this mistaken assumption. Similarly, much of what we hear and read about exercise is presented as strident commands, as things we *must* do or *must not* do—or else it sounds like scare tactics.

For most people, these negative attitudes toward older people and toward exercise are a turn-off. However, there is no need for the negative approach because it's not the main point about older people nor is it the main point about exercise.

The main points are that older people are quite capable of strength training and that exercise makes you feel good, no matter your age.

These points are not new, but they are often overwhelmed by unflattering images of older people and uninspiring messages about working out. It's true that exercise helps people of all ages stay healthy. It slows or prevents the frailty common but *not* inevitable in old age, helps prevent falls and subsequent injuries, and promotes better oxygenation and circulation of the blood. However, there are many reasons why you may find it hard to use these benefits as the motivation to help your SE exercise:

- You're busy. No one has time to do everything.

- You may not be ready to make the connection between exercise and good health for your SE.

- You think there will be plenty of time to catch up on taking care of your SE later on when she really needs you.

- You feel your SE is in decent shape right now without much effort, and she can probably go on like this for years.

Maybe so, but attitudes like these although understandable and widespread will sooner or later lead to frailty, preventable illness, or both. The resulting medical crises may take a great deal of your time and energy, not to mention worry.

From your SE's point of view, exercise may be a dirty word. She probably was more active between the ages of 2 and 50 than you were or will be if you are under 50. After all, she grew up without the modern conveniences. She may not quite realize how her life has changed since she started using washing machines, prepared foods, and other labor-saving features. Admittedly, it's hard to overcome negativity, but there are ways to achieve a positive attitude.

A Positive Mind-Set

Two positive mind-sets, *altruism*—unselfish concern for the welfare of others—and *enlightened self-interest*—insightful regard for your own interests—can help you and your SE feel good about implementing a strength training program.

There are many negative motivators, such as fear and external force, but the best motivators over time seem to be those that come from a positive mind-set. Fear and force can last only so long, but a fixed, positive mental attitude—a mind-set—can last a lifetime. Altruism and enlightened self-interest work very well for the authors.

How Altruism Works for John

In John's words:

> Altruism works for me both personally and professionally. Personally, I got into training the same way most trainers do. I took up weightlifting in college and found, over a period of years, that it helped prevent injuries in other sports and made me feel good and look good. These characteristics made it an ideal activity for me.
>
> Then I realized that I was sitting on a secret. I felt that I had to tell someone. I wanted to get my friends as excited and interested as I was, so I started sharing the wealth and showing them how to lift.
>
> This practice led me, eventually and circuitously, to my profession as a certified personal trainer. In this field, I know I'm doing good things for people, the right things. Nearly all of my older clients have come to agree with me that strength training works and that they look and feel better.
>
> A few of them may gripe about exercise and give me a hard time by saying that they will do it but they "won't enjoy it." Pretty soon, they *do* enjoy it. Every single one of them.

John and His Mother

> Doing the right thing leads me to my mother, Ann Payne, 91, who calls up both the personal and professional aspects of my work. Everyone is someone else's child. All parents sacrifice for their children, and we can never really pay them back. We can

praise them and honor them and respect them, but all we can do is to pass down the good things they gave us to our own children.

In the case of my mother, when she was 88 years old and near death's door, I had the opportunity to make a big change in her life by helping her move to Austin so that I could look after her. I know that helping her is as close as I can come to repaying her.

Ann's Crisis

When she moved to Austin, she had already had back-to-back heart attacks. She lived alone in her large house in Shreveport, Louisiana, and none of her five children lived nearby. When she moved here to Austin, none of us knew whether she would recover. I told my siblings that as soon as her doctor allowed it, I would begin training her.

Three years later, she's been all the way through the usual behaviors that I've seen with most of my older clients—not knowing anything about strength training, not quite accepting my having any expertise, and training only because someone told her to. Now she's hooked.

The first thing that got her attention was the disappearance of a nagging hip pain that would sometimes confine her to her apartment for a day or two. Just as I thought would happen, she improved quickly as the direct result of doing chair squats. She also used to have a shoulder injury, but now when I inquire, she reports, "I never think about it except when I'm working out with you." Very subtle, my mama.

Ann's Improvement

Her real turning point, though, came after a two and one-half week trip when she got no exercise. Now, she knows that she *needs* to work out. She recognizes the connection between working out and feeling good.

Recently, she took a very hard spill on concrete, went down on her hands and knees, and rolled over onto her shoulder. She was with my sister, who was horrified as she watched helplessly. But my mother picked herself up, dusted herself off, and basically forgot about the fall within 24 hours. One of her friends now wants me to train her to "be a rubber ball like your mother."

How Enlightened Self-interest Works for Jody

In Jody's words:

My mother, Faye Kelly, 90, moved to an Austin retirement community in August of 1997 at the age of 82. I was really worried about her health and her chances for an active life. She was still recovering from a major bout of pneumonia earlier that year and was quite weak and pale.

It scared me to see her this way because she had always been a real dynamo. I spent as much time with her as I could on top of my 60-hour-a-week job, but still I worried.

Jody and Her Mother

My mother has always been a strong, powerful woman, and I hoped she could return to that core identity with just a little help from me. She needed to regain her independence in order to be who she is. I needed to see her as a strong person, too. I didn't want to be consumed with worrying about her frailty and just waiting helplessly for her next illness.

So I started talking to her about the weight lifting program I was doing with John, only I called it "strength training" because I didn't want her to think about intimidating gyms, huge muscular guys, and loud grunting. At first, she wasn't interested.

Faye's Crisis

We both experienced a turning point the night we went to hear an author we had both read who was in town to speak about his latest book. Walking through the parking lot, Mama tripped and fell, bumping her forehead on the asphalt. This was something she had never done before.

Without even thinking, I reached down, partially blocked her fall, and picked her up. This was something I had never done before; I didn't know I was that strong. She realized that she needed to work on becoming stronger, and I knew exactly how she could do it. She agreed to take one strength training session with John just for the experience. Almost immediately, she recognized the benefits because she started feeling better right away.

Faye's Improvement

Now she's much stronger and healthier—quite the athlete. She has worked out faithfully for six years, and I hope she will continue for many, many more. I will continue lifting, too. Now, whenever I sorta don't feel like working out, I think of her and remember the night that changed our lives.

Readiness Assessment Questionnaires

Before you consider starting a strength program with your SE, you need to make sure that both she and you are reasonably positive about it. Nearly everyone has enough physical strength to exercise.

At least one of you must have a positive attitude toward the program.

You will find that readiness is more a matter of attitude than it is of strength. Therefore, you need to get acquainted with your SE's current physical and emotional states quite well, unless you already know. Closely observe her physical abilities and attitudes, preferably on several occasions. Also, take a long, hard look at your own attitudes toward exercise, toward your SE, toward aging, and toward life. Then fill out at least three of the following questionnaires.

1. **The Physical Inventory for your Significant Elder.** Determine the range of motion in her joints and her general physical condition on page 19. If your SE is over 80, quite frail, or both, see the "Note on Diagnosing Frailty," page 21.

2. **The Attitudinal Inventory for your Significant Elder.** Size up her basic temperament and current emotional outlook, page 22.

3. **Optional: The Depression and Anxiety Inventory for your Significant Elder.** Check for these conditions in case her Attitudinal Inventories warrant a closer look that could lead to a professional assessment (see page 24). The American Psychiatric Association (APA) estimates that between 15 and 25% of people 65 and older experience a mental disorder, including depression and anxiety, but very few seek treatment. You might be the only person in your SE's life who can spot the symptoms and provide the help she needs. For more information, see the APA web site at http://www.psych.org/public_info/elderly.cfm.

4. **The Personal Inventory for you.** Find out on page 26 whether you are or could become the right kind of person to undertake the job of Advocate, Spotter, or Strength Coach, as defined in the next chapter.

After you complete the questionnaires, see "Combinations of Scores that Predict Success" on page 28 for information on putting all the scores together and interpreting them appropriately. We provide several combinations of scores that predict a high likelihood of success in strength training for your SE. If her scores and yours are initially too low for such a program, you can work to develop more positive attitudes. Chapters 8, 9, and 10 contain more on motivation.

Disclaimer

No set of questionnaires in a book can substitute for a professional evaluation. Use the scores on these questionnaires merely to guide you in deciding whether to obtain professional assessments for your SE, for yourself, or for both of you.

Declining mental abilities usually present little or no reason to avoid exercise, but see the "Note on Alzheimer's and Other Mental Impairments" on page 29.

The Physical Inventory for Your Significant Elder

Observe your SE for at least half an hour, preferably on more than one encounter, as you do some activity together—shopping, cooking, taking a walk, playing with a child or a pet, gardening, wrapping Christmas or birthday gifts, washing the car or the dog, trimming the hedges, and the like.

If you enjoy easy communications with your SE and have talked with her about strength training, tell her that you want to test her range of motion to see if she can perform certain actions. If you haven't talked with her or find it difficult to communicate, you can still estimate her physical abilities by watching how she moves each time you see her. If you don't live near your SE, make these observations on your next visit.

Questionnaire for the Physical Inventory

Circle *Yes* or *No* for each question. On multi-part questions, give her up to half a point if she can do some but not all of the motions or if she needs assistance:

1. Yes/No   Can she steadily maintain an upright posture without leaning forward at the lower back?

2. Yes/No   Can she look over both shoulders without turning her entire torso, and can she tilt her head forward and backward, looking at the ceiling overhead and touching her head to her chest, without shrugging her shoulders and without getting dizzy?

3. Yes/No   Can she crouch, pick up something from the floor, and then straighten up without hanging onto a walker or a piece of furniture?

4. Yes/No   Can she get up from a straight chair without using her arms and hands for assistance? From an easy chair, can she get up without rocking back and forth to launch herself upwards?

5. Yes/No   Can she walk without assistance for 20 to 30 feet in a straight line without veering off course?

6. Yes/No   Can she walk without a noticeable shuffle or dragging of the feet?

7. Yes/No   Can she stand on tiptoes for two seconds without losing balance?

8. Yes/No   Can she raise both arms overhead within a 15-degree angle from vertical?

9. Yes/No   Can she walk up five or six steps without gasping for breath?

10. Yes/No   Can she see, hear, and comprehend well enough to respond to a trainer's instructions?

Score Card for the Physical Inventory

The more *Yes* answers, the better. Use the following scores as a guide:

8-10   **Excellent**. Your SE definitely has the physical ability to begin the program, and you can probably conduct the workouts yourself if you have the desire and the knowledge to do so *and* if your Personal Inventory on page 26 produces a high enough score.

5-7   **Good**. Your SE probably has the physical ability to begin a strength program. She needs to start soon, preferably with a professional trainer at first.

2-6   **Fair**. Your SE must start a strength program right away. She can probably regain considerable strength and function by working with an experienced trainer or physical therapist.

0-1   **Poor**. You may feel that it's too late for your SE unless she has enough attitudinal strength, a highly experienced trainer or physical therapist, or both. However, exercising can be of benefit even to those who have been bedridden for a year or more.

If your SE is extremely frail, make sure that you and the personal trainer are aware of the principles discussed in *Exercise for Frail Elders.* [7]

Interpreting the Results

Note that the Physical Inventory includes no questions related to heart disease, cancer, stroke, other cardiovascular diseases, diabetes, chronic pain, chronic respiratory diseases, kidney disease, liver disease, and other illnesses that contribute to the top ten causes of death in the United States.

While older people suffering from these conditions may require special techniques and extra caution, *the mere presence of a disease* does not indicate that your SE will be unable to work out. Quite the contrary. Most physicians approve of strength and conditioning programs for many of their chronically or terminally ill patients, especially in the early and

---

[7] By Elizabeth Best-Martini and Kim A. Botenhagen-DiGenova (Chicago: Human Kinetics, 2003).

middle stages of a disease. Some physicians encourage their patients to remain active as long as they can because activity will improve their physical and mental health.

In short, few older people are unable to work out. Nearly everyone can benefit from an increase in activity, especially a customized strength and conditioning program. If your SE has a large number of physical problems, the only accommodations you will need to make are to engage a personal trainer or physical therapist who is highly experienced in working with the frail. Also, the more encouragement and support you provide for your SE, the better.

One of John's clients, Anna Fay, scored 2 on the physical inventory, but her attitude was so positive that John knew he could work with her. She is doing very well in strength training. See her perform the lat raise on page 132.

Diagnosing Frailty

Dr. Linda Fried, founder and director of the Center for Aging and Health at Johns Hopkins School of Medicine, suggests that the presence of any three of the following five conditions indicates the truly frail:

- Walking slowly and with difficulty—or not walking at all, according to the authors' experiences.

- Looking gaunt, especially after losing 10 pounds or 5% of body weight in a year without trying to lose weight.

- Displaying very little strength—unable to carry a small sack of groceries, for example.

- Admitting to feeling exhausted and weak most of the time.

- Living a wholly sedentary life.

Frailty puts elders at "higher risk for falls, disability, the inability to carry on activities of daily living, hospitalizations—and finally death."[8] If you have any doubts about your SE's frailty, a doctor, an occupational or physical therapist, or a nurse can make a frailty or fall risk assessment.

Getting Help for the Frail

If your SE is diagnosed as frail, then a medical clearance from her doctor is especially important. Everyone over 40 should get a checkup, but you need to be particularly careful if your SE is frail. Find a certified personal trainer who specializes in the frail or ask a doctor to write a prescription for a licensed physical therapist.

---

[8] Edelson, Mat, "The Face of Frailty," *Hopkins Medical News*. Spring/Summer 2002.

Attitudinal Inventory for Your Significant Elder

This inventory[9] has two parts. The first one relies on your life-long knowledge of your SE. You can probably answer these questions without having to think about them. The second part may require you to interview or spend time listening to your SE because she may be the only one who knows the current answers.

Part 1. Questionnaire for Your Significant Elder's Customary Attitudes

The purpose of this inventory is to determine how positive your SE's attitudes have been during most of her life. Circle *Yes* or *No* based on your lifetime of knowledge:

1. Yes/No   Is she usually self-confident, assertive, adventurous, gutsy, or feisty?

2. Yes/No   Is she usually optimistic and able to look on the bright side of things?

3. Yes/No   Is she usually serene, happy, non-judgmental, or easy-going?

4. Yes/No   Is she fairly open about her feelings, does she ask for help when she needs it, or does she admit it when things are not going well for her?

5. Yes/No   Has she usually accepted your earlier attempts to help her or to improve her life in some way?

Part 2. Questionnaire for Your Significant Elder's Current Attitudes

The purpose of this inventory is to determine whether there has been a major change in your SE's attitudes. Spend an hour or more chatting but mostly listening to her talk about her life. You may have a very close, day-to-day relationship with your SE and could answer the questions from your memory of recent conversations. If not, you probably shouldn't tell her that you are assessing her attitudes because she might consciously or unconsciously control her true feelings. You need to obtain the truth if you can.

Circle *Yes* or *No* based on recent observation:

1. Yes/No   Is she free of complaints about food, the weather, the economy, friends, family members, or the people who help her in her daily life?

2. Yes/No   Does she seem comfortable with her life and the abilities she still has?

---

[9] Parts of the Attitudinal Inventory and the Depression and Anxiety Inventory for your SE are adapted from Stanford University's Mood Scale and Geriatric Depression Scale, which are in the public domain and are available at http://www.stanford.edu/~yesavage.GDS.english.long.html.

3. Yes/No   Does she seem interested in resuming an activity she used to enjoy or seem interested in taking up a new activity?

4. Yes/No   Has she recovered from the death of a friend or relative?

5. Yes/No   Does she imply that she has things to live for, trips to take, tasks to accomplish, or similar optimistic plans to make?

Score Card for the Attitudinal Inventory

Add up the number of *Yes* answers for Part 1 and Part 2. Then use the following scores as a guide to her attitudinal readiness for a strength program:

0-2   **Excellent**. Your SE is a terrific candidate for beginning a strength and conditioning program right away. You can probably conduct the workouts yourself if you have the desire and the knowledge to do so *and* if your Personal Inventory on page 26 produces a high enough score.

3-6   **Good**. With a little encouragement, your SE might be willing to start in the near future if you keep talking about it. Engage a professional trainer for a while, but over time you can probably take over the training sessions yourself, especially if your Personal Inventory score is reasonably high.

2-4   **Fair**. Consider administering the Depression and Anxiety Inventory to determine whether your SE has a mental health situation that merits further consideration. If her score on the Depression and Anxiety Inventory does not indicate depression or anxiety, then be prepared to keep on providing information about the benefits of a strength program for some time. While your SE does not initially appear to be a good candidate, she may eventually change her mind, so keep talking it up. Start looking for an experienced personal trainer to introduce to her.

0-1   **Poor**. Administer the Depression and Anxiety Inventory right away. Your SE could be depressed or anxious. It's possible to have a generally negative attitude and not be depressed or anxious, but she could probably benefit from some psychological therapy. If she would agree to see a counselor, her attitude might improve enough that you could eventually interest her in trying a strength program, which would further improve her mental and emotional health. In the meantime, try to find some other activity, such as gardening or walking, to increase her production of endorphins.

Interpreting the Results

In short, your SE's attitudes are usually a stronger indicator than her physical abilities of whether she would be willing to try something new, such as strength training. Even with an initially discouraging score, your SE might eventually come around if you provide sufficient support and encouragement. The case studies and success stories in Chapter 8 might help to inspire her

Depression and Anxiety Inventory

If you feel unable or unwilling to take on the responsibility of assessing your SE's mental health, you certainly won't be the only caregiver who feels this way. However, someone needs to do it, so your job may be to find another person who can help you make the assessment—a spouse, a friend, a sibling, another relative, or a healthcare professional.

People over age 65 are as likely as teenagers to suffer from depression or anxiety, and suicide is a more common cause of death in this age group, especially men, than it is among teens. Depression and anxiety are a serious and growing problem in the U.S. today. If you suspect that your SE is depressed or anxious, arrange for her to receive professional help immediately, such as psychotherapy, medication prescribed by a physician, or both. An anti-depressant drug can lower her anxiety and improve her attitude.

Note that depression can sneak up on anyone. You might even begin to show signs of it yourself if you perform significant caregiving duties over an extended period of time. Up to 60% of caregivers suffer at least occasionally with depression.[10]

Questionnaire for the Depression and Anxiety Inventory

Circle *Yes* or *No* for the following questions. Use them as a very rough guide to determine whether you need to obtain a professional diagnosis and treatment:

1. Yes/No   Has she recently started saying that she feels useless or has no purpose in life, that the world would be better off without her, or that she would be better off if she were out of her misery? The misery can be physical, emotional, mental, or spiritual. If *Yes*, see the "Warning" on page 25.

2. Yes/No   After a low period, has she suddenly brightened and started giving away her possessions or arranging her affairs? If the answer is *Yes*, see the "Warning" on page 25.

3. Yes/No   Has she suffered a great loss recently, such as the death of a spouse or close friend, the diminishing of a physical ability, especially vision, hearing, or mobility? Has she had an unwelcome move from her home into your home or into a retirement community, the diagnosis of a chronic or terminal illness, or any loss that she seems unable to accept?

4. Yes/No   Has she been free of disease and disability but listless or fatigued for

---

[10] For more information, see "Recognizing and Treating Depression" at http://www.ec-online.net/Knowledge/Articles/depressionguide.html.

more than a month? Does she sleep and nap much more than usual? Has she recently developed a large number of digestive complaints, aches and pains, or tensions for which there is no obvious cause?

5. Yes/No   For more than a month, has she had trouble getting to sleep or staying asleep during the night?

6. Yes/No   Has she gained or lost a noticeable amount of weight over the last several months?

7. Yes/No   Does she seem more nervous, agitated, fearful, compulsive, or anxious than usual? Has she recently started crying or tearing up easily?

8. Yes/No   Does she express repeated, excessive guilt or remorse about mistakes in her past?

9. Yes/No   Has she seemed unable to focus, concentrate, or make decisions for more than a month?

10. Yes/No   Has she become more withdrawn, angry, hostile, or sarcastic than usual over the past several weeks?

Warning

If you answered Yes to either of the first two questions, then take immediate steps to protect the life of your SE, just as you would do for a friend or relative in his teens or twenties.

Your SE may be thinking of suicide or may be entering a careless state of mind in which a fatal accident could occur because her self-protective skills are diminished. For example, if she isn't walking as carefully as usual, she might trip and fall. The result could be a head trauma, a fractured hip, or a similar event. Medical crises like these can cause death or permanent disability. In frail older people, for example, a broken hip has a huge death rate—90% or more.

There is somewhat less urgency with the remaining eight questions. However, if you answered as many as three or four of them with *Yes*, begin looking for a mental health or medical professional who can either rule out or confirm a diagnosis of depression or anxiety and provide treatment if needed.

One thing you can do for your SE while you are looking for signs of depression or anxiety is to redouble your efforts to increase her activity level even if she is unable or unwilling to start a fitness program. It's well known that, for many people, a significant amount of exercise is almost as effective as medication in fighting mild depression or anxiety. Even a daily walk helps.

Since there seems to be a genetic component to depression and anxiety, you will do yourself a favor if you learn to spot the symptoms because one or both problems might happen to you. Research shows that people who have lower serotonin levels in the brain are pre-disposed to depression or anxiety. Casual observation indicates that these difficulties seem to run in families, but it's well known that exercise elevates serotonin levels.

Personal Inventory for You

Let's face it. Many of us have issues with our parents, and most of us have issues with time pressures and with our own aging process. In some families, older parents and their grown children haven't spoken in 30 years and don't plan to do so. Some caregivers work 60 or more hours a week, endure long commutes, have children of their own to support, carry a large mortgage, lead an active social life, take on important civic or volunteer responsibilities, and also make time to care for their aging parents.

Most people over 40 acknowledge that they are no longer young and express—sometimes by extreme behavior—a degree of fear about their own aging process. Clearly, it's no fun to watch your parents lose their strength and power, whether you feel emotionally close to them or not, in part because seeing their decline reminds you of your own inevitable aging process.

This final questionnaire will help you see whether *your* attitudes toward your SE and toward the aging process are positive. You also need to determine whether you have the time to help your SE.

Questionnaire for Your Personal Inventory

As honestly as you can, answer the following questions. Circle *Yes* if any part of the question is true or *No* if all parts of the question are false:

1. Yes/No   Do you use hair loss remedies, complexion restorers, hormone replacement therapy, erectile dysfunction medication, or any other youth-enhancing prescriptions? Do you regularly use over-the-counter products to help you look or feel younger? Have you had cosmetic surgery in order to look younger? Do you dye your hair?

2. Yes/No   Do you dress in clothing appropriate for teenagers? Do you avoid spending time with people over 65 and consciously choose friends who are much younger than you are? Do you listen to the same music that teenagers prefer? Do you go to all the teen movies? Do you speak the current teen slang?

3. Yes/No   Do you anticipate a large inheritance from your SE and hope she will die as soon as possible so that you can get your hands on all that money?

4. Yes/No   Are you angry that, in your opinion, your aging parents failed to take good

care of you when you were growing up? Do you feel that they abandoned neglected, or abused you in some way?

5. Yes/No   Is it emotionally painful to spend time with your SE? For example, do you cringe or get angry when she tells stories you have heard 50 times before? Are you ashamed of her? Do you let her make you feel like a child who is being judged or punished? When you are on your way to see your SE, do you sigh heavily, grumble, or wish you could get out of going?

6. Yes/No   Are you so busy with your own life, job, spouse, children, house, and other responsibilities that you don't see how you could possibly find time to work with your SE? If so, are you unwilling to check on her progress with phone calls and occasional visits?

7. Yes/No   Would you rather hire someone to work with your SE than spend time with her yourself? Do you have a sibling or other relative that you could interest in taking primary responsibility for your SE? Do you resent the time and effort you spend in caring for her?

8. Yes/No   Do you believe that your SE has little or no genetic or environmental influence over you?

9. Yes/No   Do you plan to hire people to take care of you in your old age instead of relying on your children, siblings, spouse, or nieces and nephews if you ever need a caregiver?

10. Yes/No   Do you avoid looking ahead to your own later years because the very thought is just too painful? Do you expect to remain pre-elderly forever?

Score Card for the Personal Inventory

Okay, some of these questions may seem silly or hit below the belt, but the more *Yes* answers you record, the less likelihood there is of successfully conducting a strength program for your SE and, therefore, of learning how to improve your own old age.

Count the number of *No* answers you gave. In general, use the following scores as guides:

10   You lie! Or else, congratulations, Mother Teresa, Jr. Hats off to you!

7-9   **Excellent**. Go for it. You and your SE have every chance of working together successfully, and you will position yourself optimally for success in your own later years. Altruism can work well for you and your SE. Even if you live at a considerable distance, you can help your SE by initiating the discussion about a strength and conditioning program, by helping to find the right personal trainer for her, and by checking regularly on her progress.

4-6   **Good**. Your attitudes toward the aging process and toward your SE are positive enough. You may be able to use the enlightened self-interest approach toward helping her and helping yourself in the future.

1-3   **Fair**. You have a great deal of work to do on your attitude before you can be of any use to your SE or to yourself when you reach your later years. It might be in your best interest to consider getting some counseling. You may have unacknowledged fears about aging or unresolved issues with your parents.

0   **Poor**. *Stay away from your SE* until you have undergone a significant amount of counseling to overcome your negative attitude toward your parents or toward the aging process. Your SE deserves better, and so do you. You could do more harm than good until you get your attitude adjusted, and *not* with alcohol, drugs, or chocolate.

Interpreting the Results

Your SE is only half of the equation. You must also have or be willing to develop a positive attitude in order to conduct a strength program for her or to engage the right certified personal trainer to work with her. The Readiness Assessment applies to you as well as to your SE. With enough work and determination, you can achieve a more positive attitude than you have now. Your SE's attitudes are more important than your own, but you still must be reasonably positive.

Scoring the Assessment Questionnaires

Table 1-5 provides a summary of the range of scores on the three recommended questionnaires. The ranges receive ratings of *Excellent*, *Good*, *Fair*, or *Poor* so that you can easily determine whether you and your SE can be successful in working together.

Table of Scoring Ranges

Physical Inventory for Your SE	Attitudinal Inventory for Your SE	Personal Inventory for You
8-10: Excellent	8-10: Excellent	7-10: Excellent
5-7: Good	5-7: Good	4-6: Good
2-4: Fair	2-4: Fair	1-3: Fair
0-1: Poor	0-1: Poor	0: Poor

Table 1-5. Summary of the Range of Scores on the Inventories

Predicting Success

The highest scores (10) for all three inventories are, of course, ideal for success. But you can also do well with combined scores lower than 30. Following are some guidelines:

- **Excellent** is a score of 23 or over. Go for it!

- **Good** is a score with a low point of 14. Go right ahead.

- **Fair** is a score with a low point of 5. Get started and work on improvements.

- **Poor** is a score of 4 or lower. Work on becoming more positive. Get going whenever you can and practice good safety techniques.

The Depression and Anxiety Inventory is missing from these combinations. If your SE is depressed, anxious, or both, then get some help for those conditions at the same time that you start the exercise program.

A Note on Alzheimer's and Other Mental Impairments

If your SE has received a medical diagnosis of memory loss, dementia, Alzheimer's, or some other disability that affects the mind, you might believe that there would be no use in helping her with a strength program. *You would be wrong.*

Physical activity benefits everyone, even those with mental or emotional problems. Many older people who are experiencing the early stages of some type of dementia realize what's happening to them and become depressed, anxious, or angry. Exercise can help ease the depression and relieve the stress of this realization. You may be able to help your SE keep on exercising until the late stages set in.

Working Out with Mental Impairments

In the early and middle stages of a disease, your SE can probably work out just as successfully as any other older person. You will need, however, to implement some extra safety measures because she may not remember to be careful. Even mentally strong older people require safety precautions.

You will need to repeat the purpose of the training session, the names of the exercises, the instructions, the reasons for the rest periods, and so on because your SE may not remember them. You may also need to use visual aids, including the safety watchwords on page 96.

Consider working on your own attitude as well because our culture seems to discriminate against mental disabilities more than physical disabilities. If your SE begins to lose mental faculties permanently, she is no longer herself, and it may become difficult to relate to her the way you always have. When you factor in our culture's age discrimination as well, you may need to work to stay positive. It can be done.

Recommendations

Continue the strength and conditioning program *as long as her doctor approves* and as long as the sessions provide some benefit, whether physical, emotional, or spiritual. Just being with her and doing an activity together can provide all the justification anyone needs for continuing the program.

In short, don't let anyone—a negative physician, your SE, yourself on a down day, or any person who knows you or your SE—talk you out of improving her quality of life through a customized strength and conditioning program.

Physical activity is beneficial to almost everyone. Physical inactivity is not.

A Note to Certified Personal Trainers

The main points to get from this chapter are to make sure that you are the right kind of person to work with people over 65. You need a big heart, a fairly outgoing personality, a positive attitude, and a high tolerance for the abilities of older people. Take the inventory on page 26 with your own parents or grandparents in mind and see if your attitude is positive enough.

You will need to exercise great patience with older people who haven't participated in many organized physical activities during their lives. Most women, especially those over 80, are in this category as well as many of the men. As younger people, however, they stayed fit by doing daily chores long before the invention of automatic washing machines, escalators, motorized lawn mowers, and so on.

Be prepared to teach and repeat the instructions many times for each exercise, but always maintain a positive attitude. John advises finding half a dozen different ways to explain the same motion if an older client doesn't seem to understand your first several attempts. If possible, relate the new exercise to something your client already knows how to do. The good morning exercise in Chapter 5, for example, is similar to the way a gentleman might bow to a lady.

Older people are usually just as intelligent as they ever were, barring the onset of dementia, but often they aren't accustomed to taking instructions from a younger person and having to learn something new. Remember:

- Big heart.

- Tons of patience.

- Excellent communication skills.

- Frequently repeated demonstrations.

Summary of the Main Points

Following are the main points to take away from this chapter on feeling good and getting ready:

- A strength and conditioning program makes your SE feel good.

- Helping your SE makes you feel good.

- Altruism and enlightened self-interest are excellent motivators.

- Readiness is important both physically and psychologically.

- If your SE is depressed or anxious, help her receive appropriate professional treatment and follow-up care.

- Either your or your SE must have or develop a positive attitude.

- All of us can improve our attitudes by working on them.

- Exercise benefits *everybody* except for those few with certain conditions.

- Feeling good is possible for *everybody*.

- **Doing the right thing is beyond price**.

What's Next?

These points sound pretty convincing, right? But strength training may also sound like a big commitment. If you are not sure whether to become the Spotter or Strength Coach for your Significant Elder or to take the role of Advocate and find a professional trainer to work with her, the next chapter will help you decide. You will also learn how to advocate for your SE, no matter what else you do or how far away you live.

Chapter 2. Finding Your Role

Advocate, Spotter, Strength Coach

"Who knew I'd ever be my mother's Advocate? She was always so vigorous I didn't think she would ever need my help. But at age 90, she does, and I'm glad to be here for her."
Jody, 67, Advocate for her mother—Significant Elder to her four children

Introduction

What role can you take in your Significant Elder's strength and conditioning sessions? Are you able to do the training yourself? The decision may be easy—a resounding yes or no. Or you may need to think about it for a while.

The chart on the next page shows the decision process. Even though you may find your role right away, you can take a look at what the others entail because your role may change over time. You may want to expand your role from Advocate to Spotter to Strength Coach.

The Advocate doesn't need to know much about strength training, but the Spotter and the Strength Coach do. Even if you live in the same city, you may start out as the Advocate but add the Spotter role later on if you start lifting weights. Later still, you might feel knowledgeable and enthusiastic enough to become the Strength Coach for your SE.

> Remember: There is no wrong role. Any role that you take will be very important in improving the health and strength of your SE.

Chart for Finding Your Role

The flowchart in Figure 2-1, also in color on the back cover of this book, clarifies the decision process. It helps you select the role that's right for you at the present time. Later, you may be able to expand your role if you and your SE would like the closer connection.

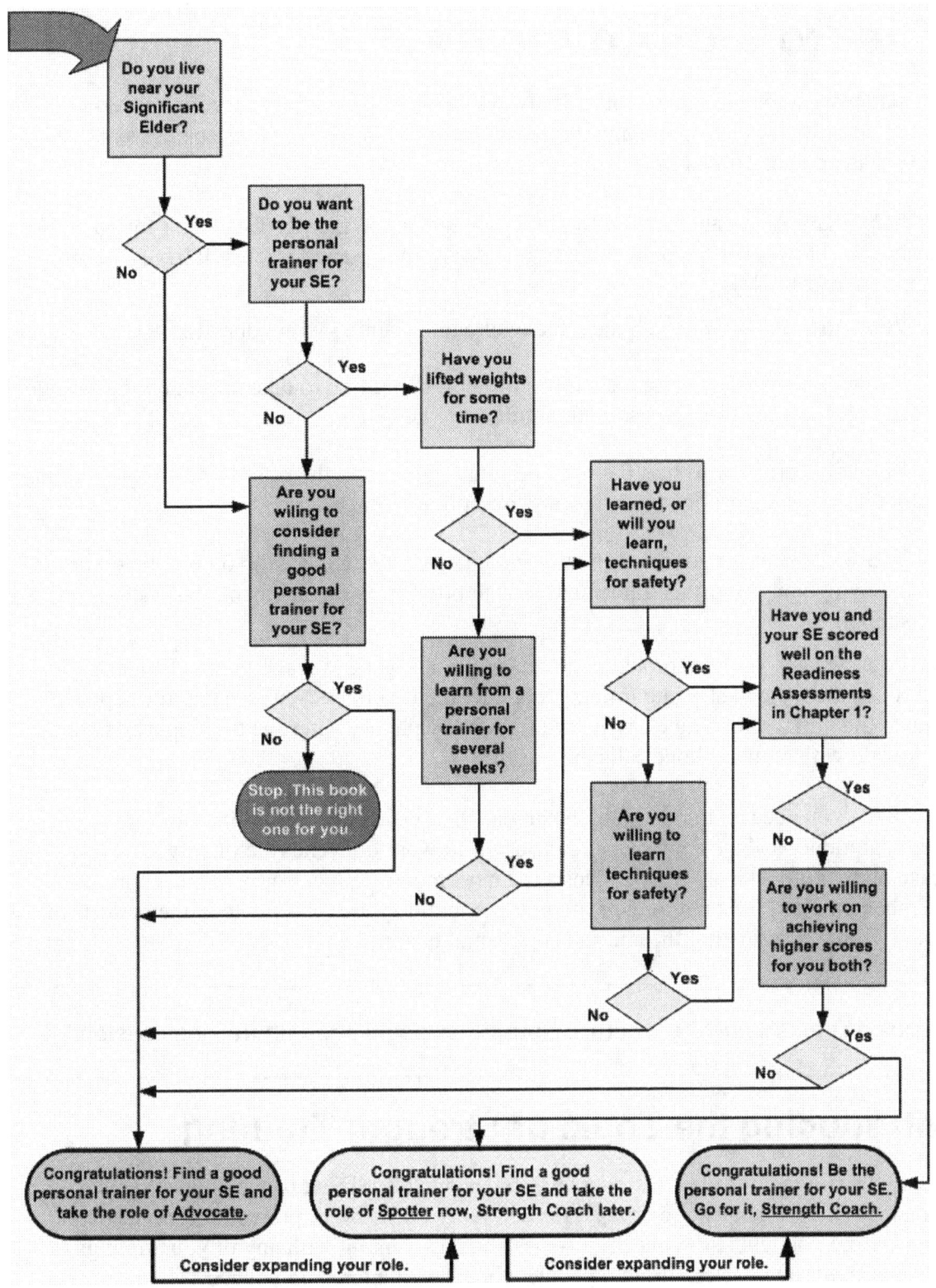

Figure 2-1. Finding Your Role—Advocate, Spotter, Strength Coach

The Role of Advocate

No matter what role you take, you will always be an advocate for your SE. Over 34 million Americans provide care for an aging relative. Over five million of those caregivers live more than an hour's travel time away.[11]

As the primary Advocate for your SE, you may live at too great a distance or for other reasons may be unable to conduct the training sessions yourself. You still have a very important role to play:

- You will see how to broach the topic of strength training with your SE.

- You will learn a few basic techniques for motivating him to take up something strange and new, especially if he has seldom or never exercised.

- You will learn how to find the right personal trainer and the right location for working out by using a thorough interview and observation process.

- You will also learn good follow-up techniques—how to check up on progress without annoying your SE or his trainer and how to provide encouragement, motivation, and support.

As the Advocate, you will probably do much of your work over the phone. You can introduce the topic of strength training, conduct the Readiness Assessment in Chapter 1, and do the initial screening of gyms and trainers by phone. After the training starts, you can follow up with regular phone calls to your SE.

However, you need to do one thing in person. On a visit, you need to find just the right personal trainer and the right place for your SE to work out. The role of Advocate takes the least amount of hands-on time but costs the most money, either yours or his. Gym memberships and personal trainers are not free, but they are reasonable in the budgets of many people, considering the enormous potential benefits.

You can't afford *not* to encourage your SE to begin strength training sessions.

Introducing the Topic of Strength Training

It's not usually a good idea to spring new things on your SE out of the blue, any more than it is to do this with other age groups. He will need a little bit of preparation, and so will you. Before you talk with your SE, discuss strength training with any of your siblings, cousins, aunts and uncles, or other people who take an interest in your SE.

---

[11] "Miles Away: The MetLife Study of Long-Distance Caregiving," available from www.maturemarketinstitute.com.

Your purpose is to build up a strong support group. Involve as many people as possible, especially any who live near your SE. The reason for a support group is to reinforce the idea that strength training is important, that it leads to better health, and that a large number of supporters can motivate, commiserate, and celebrate with him.

Using the Keys to Success

There are three keys to success in introducing the topic of strength training to your SE:

- **Listen** closely when he talks about his health and physical abilities, especially when he mentions skills that he's beginning to lose or activities that he can no longer do.

- **Observe** for yourself any activities of daily living he has lost or is having trouble with. Look for poor posture, a shuffling walk, wincing with pain, and other signs of incipient frailty.

- **Advocate** strength training as the quickest and most efficient way to regain enough strength to keep on doing the activities that he wants to continue doing.

For example, he might mention planning to take his beloved 30-pound dog to be groomed because it's getting too hard to lift Rover up into the laundry sink. You have the perfect opportunity to ask if he would like to regain enough strength to continue bathing the dog at home for as long as he wants to.

Similar opportunities may occur if he mentions losing the ability to carry groceries, place heavy items on a high shelf, go up a flight of stairs, get up from an easy chair without first having to rock back and forth, dance, garden, walk, swim, play golf, and so on. Listen for any activities that he wants to continue doing. If you pay attention and show your interest in his health and strength, you will hear the perfect chance to speak up with something like this:

"I know how much you love gardening, and I'm sorry you feel you may have to give it up soon. What if there were some way that you could get strong enough and stay strong enough to keep on gardening for the rest of your life? Would you go for that?"

Handling Negative Responses

Get whatever help you need in learning to talk with your SE.[12] Be prepared for him to reject strength training at first, perhaps for some time. Without badgering or nagging him, you can work into your regular phone calls some information about people close to his age who have doubled their arm strength or tripled their leg strength in a matter of months. See Chapter 8 for case studies of normal, regular, everyday older people who have accomplished these impressive feats of strength, and more.

---

[12] Though not dealing with strength training, "Ten Tips for Talking to Your Aging Parents" provides useful advice. It is available at www.maturemarketinstitute.com.

You can also ask members of the support group you have set up to listen for opportunities to talk about strength training as the best way to regain or maintain strength. If he hears the same thing from three our four sources, he's likelier to believe it and, eventually, to take action.

If nothing you say convinces him to start exercising, see Chapters 9 and 10 on motivation through the mind-body connection as well as empowerment and full engagement training. Enlist the aid of a doctor or nurse. In short, try to leave your SE with no excuses for sitting on the sofa.

Lou and Dan

Your SE may be like someone we will call Lou, 70, and it may be difficult to counteract her refusal to become active. Lou has never been interested in any kind of exercise. In fact, she confesses to "forging my mother's signature to get out of physical education class as often as I could get away with it."

Though much younger than many people who have shared their stories with us, she's already unsteady on her feet, afraid of falling, and on the verge of serious frailty.

The only one who might get Lou into strength training is the man she married less than a year ago, whom we will call Dan, 77. He plays golf several times a week, bicycles, and walks. Always active, he's encouraging his bride to become more active so she can keep up with him. Lou is Dan's Significant Elder, and he wants to do the right thing for her. Let's hope he succeeds.

Providing Motivation to Start and to Continue

John notes that the most common reasons why older people start strength training with him are these, in the order in which he hears them:

- "My doctor told me to." See "Orders from a Doctor" below.

- "My children made me." See "Suggestions from You" on page 37.

- "I saw how strong my friend was getting, so I thought I could do it, too." See "The Example of Friends" on page 38.

Find the motivation that will work best for your SE.

Orders from a Doctor

Probably the best motivator for your SE to begin strength training is orders from a doctor. Talk with his physician to find out whether he or she believes that your SE is healthy enough to exercise and believes that exercise is beneficial for people his age.

Sara

Get a second opinion or find another doctor if your SE tells you something resembling the report of a 91-year-old we will call Sara, who had had a heart attack. "My doctor said, 'Why would you want to exercise to get stronger at *your* age?'"

Some doctors may not yet realize that even people in their 80s can and should exercise, so you may need to find one who is up to date. Since you will need to get a medical clearance for your SE to work out, it's important to find a doctor who approves of exercise and knows the status of his health quite well.

Be suspicious if your SE tells you that a doctor has prohibited him from exercising. Listen to the doctor yourself because some older people have hearing, memory, or attention losses that cause them to get a little mixed up. Like all of us at any age, an older person can have selective hearing, memory, or attention span.

Rose

Rose, not her real name, was 86 when she fell and fractured her shoulder: "My doctor told me never to exercise again as long as I live," she said.

If your SE makes a similar statement, find out why (or if!) the doctor said this. You may discover that such an extreme prohibition was not the doctor's intent. Handle this situation gingerly because you don't want your SE to think you doubt his doctor, even though you may.

Suggestions from You

Running a close second to a doctor's prescription to exercise is *your* encouragement and support. Your interest in his health and the personal attention you will give him are crucially important. Your SE really will listen to you and, in many cases, will take your words seriously.

Although there are people over 65 who have been known to take the initiative in joining a gym and working out with a personal trainer, many older people need help because they have seldom or never exercised, feel that they're too old, find gyms intimidating, or don't see much use because they will die anyway.

Some older women who don't know anything about strength training fear that they will turn out looking like the body builders they may have seen on television. They have no idea how hard it is to develop a ripped body. If your Mom is like this, you can assure her that her outward appearance won't change much. She will be herself, only stronger and more compact.

Following are several things to try in motivating your SE to start exercising:

- Tell him that you love him and want him to live a long time in good health.

- Point out that physical strength is an important component of good health and that getting strong feels good.

- Tell him that you want to be actively involved in his progress.

- Assure him that you will find a great trainer on your next visit and that you will check on him often.

- Do everything you can to assure him that he will be successful with exercise and that he won't have to do the job all alone.

- Never let your suggestions sound as if you are criticizing his current lifestyle.

> Even the most constructive criticism can be hard to take, especially when it comes from a spouse, relative, friend, casual acquaintance, or complete stranger.

The Example of Friends

Peer pressure may not work on older people as well as it does on teenagers, but peer *comparison* does. Almost any older person, on seeing a friend shuffling along all humped over, will stand up straight, throw his or her shoulders back, and walk firmly.

John had worked with older people for some time, but Faye was his first client over age 80. She lives in one of the retirement communities in Austin, Texas, and has many friends there. After Faye started training with him, her friends could see her progress and several began training, too.

The Influence of Faye

When asked how she influenced so many people to start strength training, Faye provided some insight: "Well, for those who were ready, I didn't have to open my mouth. They could see what strength training was doing for me. I stood straighter, I walked better, I had more energy, I could carry my own groceries—things like that. I have no intention of going on a walker or one of those electric scooters. And I do *not* want to fall again. Once was enough."

When asked about those who weren't ready, she just shrugged and said, "People can find any excuse in the world if they don't want to do something. I knew a woman who said she never wanted to be challenged or stimulated again as long as she lived. And she was a lot younger than I am. I just don't understand an attitude like that. Some people seem to give up on life. They're content to sit and do nothing, but I don't see how they can be very happy."

Finding a Gym for Your SE

If your SE lives in a retirement community, glance through this section and focus on the information related to personal trainers. Then give closer attention to "Finding the Right Trainer" on page 42.

Look for a gym if your SE still:

- Still drives his own car.

- Lives in his own home, not a retirement facility, and has transportation.

- Has someone—spouse, sibling, friend—to go to the gym with him, if not for every session then at least occasionally.

Skip to "What about Special Cases?" on page 41 if one or more of these is not true, especially the first one. Also see "What about a Trainer Who Comes to your SE's Home?" on page 42.

If your SE lives in the town you grew up in, it may be relatively easy to get the names and phone numbers of several gyms that are reasonably close to his house or apartment. If he retired and moved to a place you are not familiar with, you can go to your computer or the local library to look for city maps and phone books or, better, make a preliminary trip to become more familiar with his new location.

Questions for the Gym Manager

Phone several gyms within easy driving distance of your SE and ask the manager or owner the following questions:

- How many members do you have who are over 65?

- What is the age of your oldest members?

- What time of day do your older members tend to come to the gym?

- How many of your members over age 65 work out with a personal trainer?

- Who among your staff trainers seems to enjoy working with older members?

- Do any of your staff trainers specialize in working with older clients?

- If not, do you know of anyone, perhaps an independent trainer or a staff member at another gym, who specializes in working with people over age 65?

- What is the shortest membership plan that you offer? A daily or weekly rate is best at first. If your efforts fail, who wants to be stuck with an unused long-term gym membership?

- Possibly negotiate a short-term membership by telling the gym manager about your SE, an older person who has never lifted weights before. The older population, especially those 65 to 75, could be a future gold mine for the gym.

- Ask about senior discounts or discounts for members of the American Association of Retired Persons (AARP).

If you can, get the names and phone numbers of several trainers who enjoy working with older clients. If you can't do this by phone, you can collect the information on another visit.

Checking out the Gym

During your trip home to get your SE set up with a trainer and a gym, be very open with him and discuss the reasons you want to help him and the things you will be investigating. Then take the following steps:

- Look for gyms and times of day that are quiet and not very crowded. Look for personnel and members who are friendly to everyone, including older people. Look for a women-only gym if Mom likes the idea.

- Select one or two gyms to examine more closely. Discover for yourself the ratio between older and younger members, looking for people near your SE's age and abilities.

- Ask to talk with several trainers and use the interview questions in "Finding the Right Trainer" on page 42.

- When you have found the gym and a couple of trainers that you think may be right for your SE, ask them, separately, if they are willing to meet in your SE's home, perhaps over coffee, lunch, or dinner. Treat this occasion as a social visit, but closely observe how the trainer and your SE interact and whether they warm up to one another.

- Interview several trainers and ask them for their rates and terms:

    - How much can we expect to pay per session or per month and what are the terms of payment? Hourly rates range from $40.00 or less to $150.00 or more.

    - Is there a discount for the purchase of longer blocks of time?

    - Are you available for one, two, or three sessions per week?

    - What is your procedure for handling missed sessions?

    - Do you have to train clients at the gym, or can you also work in other locations?

- When you have found a trainer your SE seems to like, arrange for a couple of training sessions with him or her.

- Attend these sessions and observe the interaction. The trainer should treat your SE with warmth and respect, of course, and should go easy on him at first. During the testing and assessment period, the trainer may need to swaddle him in cotton. But later on, the trainer can push him just a little. The trainer can't be intimidated or fearful that your SE will break or suddenly drop dead. The trainer will need to talk him through the times when he feels tired or discouraged so that he will continue to make progress with his health and strength.

- Watch for the ways in which the trainer tests your SE for strength, level of function, and range of motion in his joints. Listen to what he or she asks your SE to do. Are these tests and actions similar to the tests in Chapter 1 and the Appendix of this book?

- If no one has any objections, take pictures or videos of these early sessions so that you can help your SE boast about his greater strength later on. There's nothing better than taking justified pride in one's accomplishments.

- Talk with your SE afterwards and find out what he liked and didn't like about the trainer and about working out. You may want to mention any negative comments to the trainer so that he or she can attempt to make the suggested corrections.

If everything went well and your SE seems happy with the trainer or trainers, then arrange for a short-term membership and weekly or twice-a-week training sessions. If you can afford this expense, it's a very nice gesture to write the check yourself. If your SE has a lot more money than you do, then you might consider offering to pay a small percentage of the cost if you are able.

Your time, interest, and encouragement will be much
more valuable to your SE than your dollars.

What about Strength Training for Two Significant Elders?

When you have two SEs, find out by observing and asking them whether they would feel more comfortable working out together or separately. If they want to work out together, many trainers will take them both in one session in which one does a set of exercises while the other rests. The trainer's fee will be higher than for one person but not double the fee. Another option is working out in two back-to-back sessions with the same trainer.

Mom and Dad may prefer to work out separately and at different times, and they may or may not want the same trainer. For example, if Dad wants a male trainer and Mom wants a female trainer, you will have more work to do. But welcome the chance to get them both into strength training. Do whatever it takes.

What about Special Cases?

If your SE doesn't drive, has already moved to a retirement facility, and is older than his mid to late 70s, then you shouldn't expect him to go to a gym for strength training. You need to find a trainer who will come to his residence. More and more trainers who work with older people are seeing the necessity of adding out-calls to their business plans. They may sometimes charge a little more for travel time or car expenses. By visiting the residence, a trainer can also learn more about the daily lives of his or her clients and design specialized programs if needed.

Many retirement facilities have exercise rooms, rehabilitation areas, or both, sometimes in the same place. A good trainer is adaptable and can work with any kind of equipment that may be available. The one catch is that some retirement communities prohibit outside trainers—someone not on the staff of the facility—from working in these areas. In this case, you can hope that one of the staff trainers or physical therapists will meet your requirements and those of your SE.

If the staff trainers don't seem suitable, you may still be able to hire your own. In your SE's apartment, you can store a small amount of equipment at a cost of $50.00 or less—see Chapter 3. The trainer can conduct the sessions there, provided your SE has no objections. The retirement center should have no say about the guests your SE invites into his home, provided they follow the rules of the facility

You would think this solution might make it easy for your SE to work out by himself on one or two additional days of the week, assuming that the trainer comes once a week. But listen to the voice of experience: "Most of my older clients," notes John, "won't do their exercises unless I'm right there or unless a family member helps them."

Therefore, the role of Spotter on page 46 will give you a very important job in motivating your SE to work out.

What about a Trainer Who Comes to Your SE's Home?

If your SE is still living in his own home, but either not driving or reluctant to go to a gym, then you or he can certainly provide a small amount of equipment. In this case, finding exactly the right trainer is of utmost importance because your SE may be on his own in the company of a much stronger person. You must find someone that you and he can trust completely.

Another possibility is to find a friend or relative who lives close by and will drop in occasionally to see that he is safe. Certified, experienced trainers are trustworthy, of course, but both you and your SE need a sense of security about *anyone* who comes into his home, regardless of a trainer's recommendations and good intentions. Elder abuse is all too common. There is nothing wrong with running a background check on a prospective trainer or at least asking for and talking with references.

Finding a Personal Trainer

It may be possible to find a good trainer from 3,000 miles away, especially if you grew up where your SE lives and can enlist the help of friends or relatives who still live there. But you will have much better success if you make the final selection in person. You will also have greater peace of mind and easier communications with the trainer after you have met him or her.

The best way to find a good trainer is the same way that you find anything good—by word of mouth. Ask everyone you know for candidates. Even if a trainer comes highly recommended, ask some important questions before you introduce him or her to your SE:

- *What organization certifies you?* Look for someone certified by the National Strength and Conditioning Association (NSCA), the American College of Sports Medicine (ACSM), or the American Council on Exercise (ACE). You should also follow up with the certification agency to ensure that the trainer is legitimate.

- *How long have you been certified?* Look for someone with several years of training experience.

- *Does your organization require that you take continuing education credits to keep up with improvements in the field?* Most organizations do, so expect a positive answer. Some certifying associations will tell you if a member takes continuing education courses regularly.

- *Do you keep your safety certifications up to date?* Again, expect a positive answer. For more on the all-important topic of safety, see Chapter 4.

- *Do you have to conduct all your sessions in the gym, or can you travel to your clients' homes?* If your SE is in the special cases category on page 41, this question is crucial.

- *What percentage of your clients is over 65?* If you can find someone who specializes in older people, give this person careful consideration.

- *How long have you been working with clients over age 65?* Look for someone with some experience in training older clients. You don't want your SE to be a guinea pig.

- *If applicable, how many clients over age 80 are you currently training?* Look for someone who has trained several clients over 80 for six months or more. If your SE is under age 80, you certainly hope that he will continue training well into his 80s and 90s, preferably with the same trainer.

- *What do you like and dislike about training older clients?* If the trainer implies that the work is easy, run for the nearest exit. It can be quite a bit more difficult to train an older client than to train a young person, mostly because of the safety factor. Since some older people have balance problems, the trainer must be constantly vigilant.

- *Would you mind if we watched you training a person who is about the age of my father?* Be suspicious of anyone who says no.

- *Do you think I could talk with a couple of your clients who are about the age of my father?* Again, be suspicious of anyone who can't or won't provide references.

Trust your instincts. If a trainer doesn't seem quite right to you, keep looking.

Following Up

You're back home, your SE is increasing his strength and feeling good, and all's well with the world. Your work is done, right? *Wrong*. Now comes the vitally important phase of following up with your SE. You are probably aware that it takes about three weeks of daily vigilance to change an old habit or form a new one, which explains the slew of books and articles on 21 days to a new whatever. You might start to relax after your SE has been working out for a month or so. Surely you can back off a little after three or four months, can't you?

No, you can't. It's so easy for people of any age to backslide or give up that you really have to continue checking up on your SE on a regular basis. If a problem develops, you must know about it right away in case you need to help solve it. You want to keep him strong and healthy—part of the job is the weekly follow-up. This doesn't need to be yet another chore in your busy life. It can be fun and uplifting if you approach it with a positive attitude. Here's how.

Phoning Your Significant Elder

Call your SE once a week. That's right, once a week. The ideal time to phone is about half an hour after his training session is over. He will be feeling good because the workout will have increased his endorphins, which gives him a boost in energy and an elevated mood. He will probably have something new to tell you—a personal best on the heel raise, a new exercise for the shoulders, a pain that's no longer troubling him. You may have to prompt him with questions: "How's that shoulder coming along?" or "Did you get to do dead lifts today?"

Every week, you can tell him how proud you are of his progress, how happy you are that he feels good, and how grateful you are that you will have him in your life for a long, long time. In short, give him all the praise, encouragement, and positive statements that you feel are appropriate.

Keep the lines of communication open—wide open.

Suppose you are always too busy at work to make the call right after your SE's workout sessions. Don't let this be an excuse for not phoning. Make the call at any time, even well into the evening, on the day he sees his trainer. The endorphins will still be circulating, he will still be feeling good, and he will still have new things to tell you. Also, if he knows you are going to call, he will be much less likely to skip a training session.

The call doesn't need to be long. You can cover a lot of ground in five to ten minutes. Dedicate this call entirely to his strength training. Use longer calls at other times for different topics. For the computer-literate SE, you can try keeping in touch by email, but you will miss his tone of voice when he tells you something. Watch out for sounds of discouragement and provide as much positive reinforcement as you can. The important point is to establish a routine that both you and he can come to rely on.

If You Don't Follow Up—Martha and Danielle

If you don't follow up, it's likely that your SE will stop working out. A mother and daughter, whom we will call Martha, late 50s, and Danielle, late 30s, provide a good example of why you need to follow up.

For years Danielle had worried about her mother's health because Martha steadily gained weight over the years and was becoming sedentary.

Living thousands of miles away, Danielle felt there was little she could do to encourage her mother to take better care of herself. Then she had a brainstorm. Danielle gave her mother a gym membership and three months of sessions with a personal trainer. Martha dutifully kept every appointment to work out. But after the three months were over, she stopped strength training regularly.

Danielle didn't realize that she had to follow up and didn't even know her mother had stopped exercising until several months later. Martha felt that she had learned the exercises, could do them on her own, and could save some money, too. "I don't work out with weights nearly as often as I should," said Martha. She hopes to exercise more regularly when she has more time.

Visiting during Workout Sessions

Another important aspect of following up is to observe parts of your SE's strength training sessions each time you come for a visit. Ask the trainer to tell you the best time to attend so you can see the most challenging part of the workout. If you took photographs or taped your SE's first few sessions, you can do the same on each visit. You and he will be amazed at the progress, and you will have an endless topic of conversation. Seeing is believing.

Jody as the Advocate

Jody learned a lot the first time she watched John conduct a session with her mother, Faye. Although she had trained with John for several years, Jody at first had no idea that she and her mother did basically the same exercises. The only difference was the amount of weight.

> I had looked in on an exercise class where older people just sat on chairs and moved their arms and legs a little bit. I guess I thought she would just do some similar, non-challenging motions. But no. She really lifts. She really sweats. She huffs and puffs with the best of them. My mom, the athlete! By the way, I think an athlete is anyone who works hard at a physical activity and intends to improve, and I know

that a triceps extension is a triceps extension whether the athlete is 25 or 85. My mom is just as much an athlete as anyone else who lifts weights. She and I are proud and supportive of each other and always have something positive to talk about. She's a real inspiration.

Following Up with the Trainer

One other person you need to check in with is the trainer. There is no need to phone every week, but you can check in with him or her every couple of months to see how things are going from the trainer's perspective. The trainer is an important part of the support group that you have set up for your SE.

If the trainer reports any problems, such as your SE's complaining of soreness more than usual, skipping training sessions, or threatening to quit working out, you need to talk with Dad, find out the nature of the problem, and make every effort to solve it. Make sure that you give the trainer your phone number so that he can reach you in case he spots a possible health problem. Also provide a back-up contact in case you can't be reached.

For example, the trainer might be the only person who can spot a series of silent strokes—those without the usual symptoms of paralysis, weakness, or loss of memory or language. These can add up over time to affect the walking gait, as well as some of the mental faculties. If the trainer notices a change in the way your SE walks, moves, or speaks, ask him to call you right away. Make sure your SE's physician diagnoses the problem as soon as possible.

As you will see in the next chapter, the trainer should be familiar with your SE's medical history. He or she may check your SE's pulse 10 seconds, 60 seconds, and possibly 120 seconds after a strenuous exercise to make sure that he works at a heart rate appropriate for his age and that he recovers in a timely manner.

The Role of Spotter

The Advocate has a big job, but the Spotter has a bigger one. As the Spotter, you will do everything the Advocate does but up close instead of from a distance. After all, 29 out of 34 million caregivers live within an hour's travel time of an aging parent. To be a Spotter, you also need to know a little about strength training because you will assist your SE with his exercise sessions when the trainer isn't there.

The Spotter has three important jobs to perform and an optional role to take if desired:

- The Spotter as attendance motivator—Meet your SE in the exercise room once or twice a week.

- The Spotter as safety supervisor—Keep him safe by setting up the equipment and watching him closely.

- The Spotter as record keeper—Write it down.

- The Spotter as workout partner—While your SE rests between exercises, do a light version of your own strength training workout if you like.

The Spotter as Attendance Motivator

John has found that many of his older clients won't go to the exercise room on their own. So you will attend training sessions with your SE. Your job is to get him to the exercise room by meeting him there for one or two workout sessions per week when the trainer is *not* present.

If your SE works out twice a week, he will receive more than two times the benefits of working out only once—it's more like three or four times the benefits. If he is able to work out three times a week, his health and strength will improve even faster.

How can you inspire your SE to meet you for a second and possibly a third workout per week? For many, if you just make the suggestion and show up faithfully, he will be motivated. If he seems reluctant or raises objections, here are several things to try:

- Tell him that you are just following the trainer's instructions and reinforcing the benefits—the trainer will want him to exercise more than once a week.

- Tell him you are saving money. It is less expensive for you to meet with him than to hire the trainer for the extra sessions.

- Ask him to name the best days of the week and the best times of day for these supplemental sessions, even if you would prefer other days or times. Make it easy for him to say yes, but also make sure he rests for one or two days between sessions.

- Tell him that it will be fun and you will both enjoy it. Joke with your SE, praise him for his successes, bring small gifts—a flower, a few juicy blackberries, a new picture of his grandchildren, an inspirational video, and so on—or share high-protein snacks afterwards. You might also be a little tired after a training session because you will have a lot of responsibility and some hands-on work.

- Quote the saying, "If not now, then when?" Do your best to get a commitment from him that he will increase the number of workout sessions per week.

- Give him a month or so with the trainer alone if he seems to need this time, but settle on a specific date for him to begin letting you help him as the Spotter.

- Since you probably took a "before" picture at the start of his training, take a series of "after" pictures to share with him. He may be surprised at his improved posture.

The Spotter as Safety Supervisor

Getting your SE to the workout room is the first job to complete, but your most important job as Spotter is to be the safety supervisor. Make sure that each training session is safe and that your SE doesn't hurt himself. Before he starts exercising, make sure that he has eaten a meal within the previous three hours, but not a heavy meal within an hour before working out. Help him warm up adequately using the recommended warm-up on page 72. You will also set up the equipment for each exercise and will make sure that each exercise is conducted safely.

As the Spotter, you will also watch each exercise carefully and provide a tiny bit of assistance if your SE needs help or becomes too tired to complete the last couple of inches of a lift. In strength training gyms, a person who provides this type of assistance is also called a Spotter, but you will be doing a lot more than spotting your SE.

To be a good safety supervisor, you need to have learned safety techniques by working with your own trainer, by lifting weights yourself for several months, by reading Chapters 3, 4, 5, and 6, or by observing several sessions between the trainer and your SE. Be sure you ask the trainer to tell you which exercises are the most likely to cause injuries and to demonstrate how to make them as safe as possible.

The Spotter as Record Keeper

Another important job for the Spotter is keeping careful records, if possible using the same workout form as the trainer. (See the Appendix for a sample workout form.) The act of writing down the specific exercises, the number of repetitions, and the amount of weight for each lift is another reinforcement of the concept that working out is important.

You can also record anything else that seems significant, such as his general health, an unusually high or low energy level, or specific complaints or pains.

John notes that occasionally clients have protested that they are "getting nowhere" or that "it's just not working for me." He brings in a workout sheet from the first month of exercising. He has the client perform one of the early workouts, and the effect is worth a thousand words.

Jack

When John showed Jack, then 72, a workout sheet from his first months of training, Jack said, "Now I warm up with weights heavier than these." Exactly. He made progress.

You can also use the records to inspire your SE to keep going during times of discouragement or minor illnesses by saying something like this: "I know you can do it. Six months ago, you started with 10 pounds, but three weeks ago, you lifted 15 pounds. That's a 50% increase. Rest for a couple of minutes, and I'm sure you will be able to lift 15 pounds again. You're the greatest!"

Maintain good records and good enthusiasm.

The Spotter as Workout Partner

There you are in the strength training area, so you might as well get in a workout yourself. If you are as busy as most caregivers, you may welcome the chance to do two things at once. Note the advantages and disadvantages of being your SE's workout partner.

Advantages

- Your SE can learn a lot just by watching you lift. Since you need to demonstrate every new exercise for him anyway, you can do a few reps with a weight appropriate for your strength. You will never get sloppy in your technique with your "student" watching you.

- If you don't have time to go the gym very often, serving as your SE's workout partner may be the only way you can squeeze in a workout.

- If he thinks you might not get to your own gym as often as you want to, he may take justifiable pride in helping you keep up your program. Give him all due thanks for his help and encouragement.

- It can be fun to work out with a buddy, even one a lot older than you are. You may find yourselves showing off for each other. That's fine as long as safety is paramount.

Disadvantages

- Since your SE's safety is *always* of utmost importance, your focus must always be on him, even when you are exercising. Don't take on the role of workout partner if you can't keep most of your attention on him at all times, even when he is resting.

- Unless he trains in a well-equipped workout area, you may not have access to your usual equipment. You may not be able to challenge yourself, but a maintenance routine is better than no routine.

- Your SE may feel neglected if he just sits there while you do your set. Over time, you may be able to show him how to be *your* spotter. Always keep him involved by connecting with him just as you would if you were not lifting. Maybe you can show him some exercises that he might perform later on.

- If your SE is highly competitive, he may chafe at your greater strength or at least at your relative youth. Give him plenty of praise for his excellent technique, and take joy in his increased strength as he gradually improves.

The Role of Strength Coach

The Advocate has a big job, the Spotter has a bigger one, and the Strength Coach has the biggest job of all. As Strength Coach, you replace the trainer. You may not be certified, but you know enough about strength training to do the entire job of training others, and you are willing to take on the responsibility with your SE.

To be a good Strength Coach, it's best to have had some kind of teaching experience, though not necessarily in a classroom. Maybe you have coached your kid's soccer team, taught your children how to ride a bike, given your fellow "gym rats" a few pointers on the more complicated lifts, taught someone to dance, and so on. These and similar experiences in showing people how to perform physical activities will come in handy with your SE.

There are two additional responsibilities for the Strength Coach:

- Test your SE's strength, level of function, and range of motion by using the information in the next chapter and the Appendix.

- Assess his needs and goals and design a program to develop his strength.

Reusing Your Knowledge

As the Strength Coach, you will put your knowledge of strength training to a whole new use that you probably didn't anticipate when you started lifting weights. It's a great idea to reuse your expertise by finding another purpose for all the time and money you have spent on your own health and fitness. It has paid off for you, and now it can pay off for your SE. You already know how beneficial strength training is and how great it makes you feel. Now you can share your wealth of knowledge with your SE.

Seeing your Significant Elder as an Athlete

The only change you may need to make in your thinking is to see your SE as an athlete, too. It may surprise you that he can make such huge gains in his strength and fitness levels, especially if he has adopted the largely inactive lifestyle of so many older people. But it shouldn't surprise you that he will feel great after he starts exercising.

Chapters 5 and 6 contain complete workouts that you can use with your SE. While it's always good to have a game plan in mind, it's equally important to remain flexible. Write out your plan for a specific training session in pencil, and don't decide on an exercise, an amount of weight, or a number of repetitions until you have observed how your SE feels on the day of the workout.

Use the warm-up to assess how he's doing *today*. If he's tired or didn't sleep well the night before, back off a little on the weights and repetitions (reps). If he's feeling terrific, challenge him a little with slightly heavier weights, more reps, shorter rest periods, or new exercises.

The Advantages of Being the Strength Coach

One of the main advantages of taking the role of Strength Coach is that it can lead to a much closer relationship between you and your SE. You will be spending quality time together, working toward a common goal, encouraging each other to stay strong and healthy, and taking pride in each other's accomplishments. You can also use your own experiences in the gym to share anecdotes with him, encourage him, and keep him interested in continuing the strength and conditioning program.

Another advantage is that training others always makes you safer, smarter, and more insightful about your own training. If your workouts have ever gotten a bit stale or perfunctory, you will regain your enthusiasm by seeing first hand how beneficial strength training is for your SE. Being the Strength Coach is a great win-win situation for both of you. Get ready to be amazed at what your SE can do.

Frances and Edna

You might share the story of Frances, 84 who works out with John twice a week. He asked her what she would have thought if, when she was only 65, someone had told her that she would be strenuously lifting weights in her 80s. She replied, "I'd have been shocked. I wouldn't have believed it. My mother was very active all her life and lived to be 94. But I never dreamed I'd live this long."

Frances also talked about her older sister, Edna. "Edna never had the stamina my mother had. She didn't. We always sort of favored Edna. I did the harder things because she couldn't. She wasn't up to it. She didn't have the strength."

And yet Edna also worked out with John for two and one-half years until her death in 2004 at age 85. When asked if she was surprised when Edna started a strength training program, Frances said: "Yes, I was surprised. Edna gained a lot more strength and much more ability to do things after she started exercising. I think that influenced me. I was always told that old people just don't have the energy to keep on doing the things they want to do. I was amazed at what Edna was able to do."

Being both Easy and Hard

An important thing to keep in mind in your role as Strength Coach is that you will need to be both easy and hard on your SE. You need to be easy in that you have to adapt any lift that you regularly perform because he won't be as strong as you are and won't have the knowledge that you have. He may also have limited body awareness.

For example, when you ask Dad to move his left foot forward and he moves his right foot, acknowledge that he's doing the best he can and simply lacks the close connection between mind and body that you have developed over the years and now take for granted. Instead of getting angry or chastising him, treat the mistake humorously: "I meant your *other* left foot. Let's try that again."

With your gentle encouragement and patience, he will get the hang of it. For more on body awareness and the mind-body connection, see Chapter 9.

Going Easy

In being "easy" on your SE, you will have to start him out with very little weight or just with his body weight. Teach him how to use his body to perform the correct motions before you introduce the weights. Chapters 5 and 6 show you the top exercises that will help your SE reclaim and retain his strength. There's a good starting point for him even if he has been inactive for years. You can start with the easier exercises and work up to the more challenging ones as you and he become ready.

Going Hard

Eventually, you will need to be a little tough with your SE. You won't want to baby him for long. You can't wrap him in a protective cocoon and never challenge him to work harder, lift more weight, or learn new exercises. Remember that the formal name of strength training is *progressive resistance exercise*. His technique will improve, the weights will get heavier, the repetitions will increase, and the rest intervals will get shorter. That's progress. That's the point of coming to the exercise room, and it's the same for everyone.

Come to the gym often—leave tired.

When your SE is coming down with something or recovering from an illness, he may not want to work out, and you shouldn't force him. But you can offer a light session instead of the usual workout. Unless he is in the hospital or his doctor temporarily prohibits exercise, try to come up with the courage, the humor, and the love to help him continue being active.

Sitting on the sofa all day isn't good for anyone, even older people who don't feel up to par. You know that your SE will feel better after a light workout or at least a short walk, and over time he will come to this realization, too.

Does He Want You as Strength Coach?

If you are qualified to be the Strength Coach—you have lifted for quite some time and have helped others with their techniques—and want the job, the chances are excellent that your SE will prefer to work out with you instead of with a personal trainer. After all, he has known you all your life and will certainly feel more comfortable with you than with a stranger. You will also save money. But talk with him and listen carefully before making any assumptions.

For many older clients, chatting with the trainer during rest periods provides a valuable social interaction. Further, if Dad prefers to take instructions from a male and you happen to be female, then it's a good idea to treat his preferences seriously. Remember that there is no wrong role. No role is any better than another. All roles are good, and all can get the job done.

Combining the Roles

If you have the time to spend three hours a week with your SE, even for only a few weeks or months, you will really get him off to a great start. You will see first hand the improvement in his health and strength. To make the maximum commitment, you would meet three times a week for 45-60 minutes, taking three different roles:

- In one session, you would be the Strength Coach, teaching new information, correcting technique, challenging him to work a little harder, and keeping him motivated. You would act as the personal trainer but without the formal certification.[13]

- In another session, you would be the Spotter, ensuring that the equipment is set up properly, watching for safety and correct technique, and keeping records.

- In the third session, you would be his workout partner, alternating between his exercises and your own but keeping the focus on his safety, enjoyment, and motivation.

John as the Advocate

John wanted to be her Advocate long before his mother, Ann, moved to Austin. He carefully designed a workout program for her when she was 82 and made clear diagrams of all the exercises he wanted her to do. He found a trainer who was willing to come to Ann's house in Shreveport for weekly training sessions. But the three of them never sat down together to discuss Ann's program, and he wasn't aware that he needed to follow up with the trainer.

John didn't know until his next trip home that the two of them hadn't hit it off and his mother had stopped the training sessions. He found his diagrams neatly taped to the wall by her breakfast table and asked his mother what happened with the exercises.

> "Yes," she smiled, "I see them there every time I drink my coffee."
> "Do you ever do them?" John asked.
> "No."
> "Why not?"

---

[13] If you have concerns about the legality of acting as a trainer, check the laws of your state. In Texas, there is no law requiring certification to give someone strength training sessions.

"Oh, I don't know," she said.

Now that Ann lives in Austin and John is her Strength Coach and trainer, she rarely misses a session.

John as the Strength Coach

As a professional trainer with ten years' experience and a recreational weightlifter for over 35 years, John is in the unique position of being the trainer, the Advocate, and the Strength Coach for his mother. Here's how he feels about his many roles:

> The thing with my mother personally is that I know the way she moves and walks very well, and I could see that she was starting to lose her strength after her heart attacks two years ago. She also had a hip that was trying to go bad, mostly through inactivity. I was pretty confident that I could get her over the hip problem with some simple but rigorous exercises, which has happened. She is a genetic athlete too, my mother is. She has excellent posture for someone of 91. She has good muscle tone. She can do things pretty well. I'm proud of her.

> The difference in our lives now is that I see her twice a week for anywhere from 45 minutes to an hour. We have a great talking relationship. She doesn't rely on me too much, but she loves to see me. She feels secure that I'm there in a pinch and that my family is too. Also, my mother walks very well. She takes long daily walks. She has a good long stride, keeps her head up, and swings her arms naturally.

> It's been fascinating for me to watch my mother's physical strength, agility, and endurance increase since she's been working out. At the same time, I see that slowly her hearing and balance are getting even worse, and her eyesight is failing her rapidly. And she's more and more prone to forgetfulness. So that makes me reflective and thoughtful about her, about myself, about life and death.

A Note to Certified Personal Trainers

Forming a support group for your older clients is as important for you as it is for the grown children. Enlist the aid of the grown children and make practical use of their influence on their parents. Consider them as partners in improving the health and strength of their parents or other SE. Involve them as much as you can so that your older clients will have a good support system for their motivational needs and for any training setbacks they may encounter.

Training older people is quite rewarding because of the huge gains they can make in strength, health, and optimism, especially if they have been sedentary for a while. However, you need to be prepared for them to sustain various physical and mental losses, including death.

John trained Edna, 85, for two and one-half years and grew very fond of her. Their last training session was on a Thursday in the spring of 2004. Three days later, she died suddenly of a massive, undetected intestinal infection.

It always hits John hard to lose a client to death, but he knows he has to be prepared because very few of his ongoing older clients stop training with him except for hospitalization or death. As a trainer, you will have to content yourself with the knowledge that you are doing great things for your clients, who all have to die at some point. But it's never easy to lose a client. Remember:

- Consider your older clients' grown children as your partners.

- Recognize that it's always hard when a client dies.

- Take care of yourself.

Summary of the Main Points

Use the chart on page 33 to decide which role to take:

- Be the **Advocate** if you live too far away or don't have the knowledge or the time to train your SE—page 34.

- Be the **Spotter** if you live near your SE and know something about strength training but don't have the expertise to design his training program—page 46.

- Be the **Strength Coach** if you live near your SE, have the expertise because you learned from long experience or a good trainer, want to train him, and know that he wants you to train him—page 49.

- Combine the roles if you can possibly manage to find the time. Be the Strength Coach, the Spotter, and the workout partner in three sessions per week. And always serve as your SE's Advocate, no matter what else you do.

What's Next?

The next chapter gives you the vocabulary of strength training so that you can be an effective Advocate. It also explains the importance of getting medical clearance for your SE before he starts an exercise program, shows you the equipment you might need as Strength Coach, and discusses the elements of a typical training session, starting with the all-important warm-up.

Chapter 3. Laying the Foundations for Success

Preparing to Train Your Significant Elder

"My son tried to get us into strength training 25 years ago. But he didn't suggest a personal trainer. He just got us a bench with some dumbbells and said, 'Here, go at it.' That's not the best way to start. We didn't know what to do."
   Faye, age 90

Important Points for Advocates: Learn some of the terminology in this chapter so you can talk with your SE in your weekly follow-up phone calls. Ask your SE to make sure the trainer completes the necessary forms and the tests starting on page 63. It's also a good idea to ask about the warm-up and the cool-down/calm-down to make sure these important parts of the workout are covered.

Introduction

Now that you are motivated and have found your role, you may feel ready to start the actual training sessions. Not so fast! Even if you are an experienced lifter and often help others in the gym with their lifts, you will need to review some basics so you can make the training successful for your Significant Elder over the long term. Working with older people can be a little different from working with people your own age and younger.

No matter what role you take with your SE, you need to lay the foundations for success by translating concepts, vocabulary, and activities into terms that your SE will appreciate, understand, and adopt. Anyone who takes up a new activity can feel a little intimidated by the new ideas and the new jargon, so you will need to take some care in smoothing your SE's way into strength training.

You may also need to convince yourself of the importance of the warm-up because chances are good that you have occasionally skipped it in your own workouts. You really can't let your SE work out unless she's had a good warm-up.

The Basics

First, a word about science. In strength training, you can easily apply the principles of good science—observation, recording, prediction, and control—for your benefit as well as your SE's. Even if you are an Advocate who knows little about strength training, you can rapidly master its principles. You need to know the terminology so that you can communicate effectively with the trainer occasionally and with your SE every week.

For Spotters and Strength Coaches, this review will remind you of how to control the variables and how and why to keep careful records of your SE's progress. Setting goals may or may not have been important to you when you started lifting weights, but it's very important to encourage your SE to set some realistic goals and to anticipate and celebrate improvements in her strength and health.

Definitions

Progressive resistance exercise, discussed in greater detail on page 59, is the technical name of a set of activities also known as strength training, resistance training, and weight training.[14] Resistance exercise can include resistance against gravity, against another person, against elastic or rubber bands, against a wall or chair, against rocks or stones, or against lifted weights in the form of dumbbells, barbells, and various specialized machines.

In the section on equipment on page 67, we show you how to coach your SE with little or no equipment or with homemade equipment. Many of the exercises in Chapters 5 and 6 require only a couple of sturdy straight chairs with arms. You will use your SE's body weight or your own strength to provide the necessary resistance.

The basic terminology of strength training is very simple. You can start out with just a few terms:

- An *exercise*, also called a *lift*, is the specific motion from start to finish that your SE will perform for a specific muscle group. Each exercise has a descriptive name, such as the *bench press*. Chapters 5 and 6 show the top exercises to reclaim and maintain strength and provide methods of teaching them to your SE. If you are an Advocate, you will learn how to discuss these exercises with the trainer occasionally and with your SE in your weekly follow-up phone calls.

- The *weight* is the number of pounds that your SE lifts for each exercise. As Mom gets stronger, she will lift heavier weights, but she starts with very light weights, such as a one-pound dumbbell, or sometimes just the weight of her limbs or body. When you are providing the resistance yourself, it will be harder to gauge the effort, but you will know she's getting stronger when you have to resist with more of your strength. Develop your own scale of measurement for your effort, such as the following:

  1 = Very Light, 2 = Light, 3 = Medium, 4 = Heavy, and 5 = Very Heavy

  Record the approximate resistance it takes for each exercise. For more on record keeping, see page 61.

---

[14] The term *weightlifting* refers to the Olympic sport in which participants lift, pull, or push huge weights. The term *bodybuilding* refers to improving the appearance of the body with weight training, diet, and other techniques. In competition, bodybuilders strike muscle-popping poses instead of lifting weights. Most gym members do *recreational weightlifting*, but we prefer the term *strength training* because it best describes our goals.

- A *rep*, which stands for *repetition*, means performing the motion of an exercise one time from start to finish.

- For our purposes, a *set* is a group of reps for one exercise. A set typically contains 8 to 15 reps. You will typically ask your SE to do one to three sets for each exercise.

- A *rest interval* is the time between sets in which your SE will rest and recover from the preceding set before moving on to the next set or the next exercise.

- A *training session* comprises the warm-up, the sets of exercises, the rest intervals, and the cool-down/calm-down. A typical training session for your SE will run between 45 minutes and an hour. Chapters 5 and 6 provide two complete training sessions.

If you prefer to use a different term than *training* then substitute *teaching* or *instructing*. Call a training session a *workout* if you like. Do whatever it takes to convince yourself and your SE that strength training is terrific and will make both of you feel good.

For most older people, the exercises, sets, reps, and training sessions are similar to those for younger lifters. The main differences are that the weight will be much less and the rest intervals may be slightly longer. Another difference is *never* to skip the warm-up on page 72 and cool-down/calm-down on page 135. Also, some of the exercises may need to be modified to accommodate physical problems.

Rest Intervals

Although the term *rest interval* may seem self-explanatory, the concept is a very important part of strength training. Many people who start strength training are impatient with the rest periods—see the story of J. C. on page 93. For our purposes, there should be about 30-60 seconds of rest between sets. If the exercise is especially hard, such as chair squats and dead lifts, increase the rest period to a minute and a half, perhaps two minutes or more.

The focus of the training sessions is on strength, not on aerobic capacity. Therefore, you need to provide adequate rest for your SE. At a later date, if you want to build her endurance and stamina, you can shorten the rest interval in order to increase the aerobic aspects of the training session. But at the beginning, from the strength standpoint, provide her with adequate rest. Chapter 7 contains more information on rest, relaxation, and sleep because these are important components of any exercise program.

Sets

In the general case, an older person undertaking a specific exercise can perform two or three sets of 8-15 reps with 30-120 seconds of rest between sets. A training session will contain six to twelve exercises and, including the warm-up and the cool-down/calm-down, should last 45 minutes to an hour, depending upon your SE's energy level during a specific training session.

If this plan sounds familiar, it should, because younger weight lifters often follow exactly the same plan. In the bench press, for example, the young male recreational weightlifter might lift 175 pounds in three sets of eight reps. The older female lifter might start with as little as five pounds in two sets of eight reps. Over time, she can probably work up to 30 or 35 pounds in two or three sets of 12-15 reps.

Progressive Resistance

In strength training, the key word is *progressive*. It means that something is going to change over time. If you are doing your job right, your SE will always be tired at the end of the training session. As she gets stronger, the workout stays challenging because you will make adaptations to match her increased strength.

The concept of progression is the most crucial key to success. The weight must slowly get heavier. The number of repetitions must systematically increase. Later on, the rest intervals may need to be shortened in a way that taxes the system. Just as with younger people, she grows accustomed to the strength training as her body adapts.

When people begin strength training, after learning the correct technique and the breathing, they will progress rapidly. Everyone does, especially older people, who can increase their strength exceptionally rapidly. This progress is very heartening. At first, the progress may be more a case of neurological adaptation than muscle growth, but the reason doesn't matter. Progress is progress. You can measure it, and you will both see it.

This initial period is followed by a period of steady progress that lasts anywhere from two to six months. However, with every older person and with every younger weight lifter as well, you will find a point past which progress is slow. Somewhere in that span of time, your SE will reach a point at which she is working a lot harder for minimal increases. Be prepared when you reach a *plateau*. At this point, you can either solidify her gains by adopting a maintenance routine or start instituting systematic variations in the training sessions.

Maintenance Routine

When your SE begins functioning substantially better than she did before she started training, do your best to prevent her from quitting. If she were to stop, she would lose these good effects. Use it or lose it. Keeping on at the maintenance level will enable your SE to continue enjoying the benefits of strength training for the rest of her life or as long as she's capable of performing the exercises.

Oma

Oma, 92, worked out faithfully for several months and got rid of a pesky shoulder pain from an old fracture. Then she discontinued the training sessions, thinking she was cured. But the pain returned. After four months of increasing misery, she started working out again, the pain disappeared, and she finally understood that she should keep on working out for as long as she could. "I didn't know what I was getting into," she confessed. "I had no idea I'd have to do this forever, but now I'm convinced."

Variations during the Maintenance Phase

Most of John's clients settle into a maintenance routine with few variations. There seems to be something comforting about doing the same near-and-dear exercises at each workout. Get to know your SE's preferences quite well. If she's content and pleased with the routine, leave it alone but occasionally offer a minor variation.

You or the trainer can introduce variations by manipulating the variables—the exercises, the combinations of weight, the reps, the sets, and the rest intervals. A few variations are useful not only to keep your SE's muscles from going stale but also to prevent boredom if that becomes a problem. But don't move too fast. See "Introducing the Exercises Gradually" on page 72.

With some thought, you can find enough variations to make each session interesting, even if you train your SE for years. Note that some older people want to be challenged, so you will need to communicate very well with your SE to find out.

Easy-to-Hard Progression

Many people forget an important part of the term *progressive*—it gets harder, but *it starts easy*. It should and must be easy at first. Psychologically, it needs to be so painless that your SE might become impatient or might say, "This is too easy. When does it become work?"

This question is a great sign. Nurture a little bit of impatience and mention that the exercises will get harder and the weights will get heavier.

Starts easy, gets harder—that's progressive resistance training in a nutshell.

Controlling the Variables

Exercises, reps, sets, weights—these are the basic variables. For each training session, plan which of these will stay the same as in the previous session and which of them you will change to suit the circumstances, such as adding more weight as your SE grows stronger.

Pay attention to other variables as well. For instance, try to schedule the strength training sessions at the same *time of day*. Find out when her energy level is at its highest, and schedule the sessions during that time, if possible. To convince yourself that time of day is an important variable, experiment with your own workout schedule. For example, if you have always worked out at 6:00 PM, just try one session at 9:00 AM. Chances are you won't feel as strong as you do at 6:00 PM. Your SE will have similar variations in strength unless her sessions are at the same time of day.

Keep an eye on the clock so that the rest intervals are consistent. You may find that your SE needs longer or shorter rest intervals after certain exercises. Certainly after heavy exercises like chair squats or dead lifts, your SE may require two minutes, maybe more, to recover, but try to keep the rest periods consistent. Generally, one to two minutes after a hard set is sufficient.

Finally, try to schedule a workout for two or three hours after a meal, and encourage your SE to eat something within an hour after each training session.

Keeping Good Records

A good scientific principle is to keep careful records. Strength training is a progressive activity. It will be necessary, especially for the first six months, to write down the specific exercises, the amount of weight lifted or resistance provided, the number of sets and reps, and any notes or observations you have made that you think are worthy of writing down. Example observations might include the relative difficulty of a particular exercise or your SE's attitude toward it. The Appendix includes a sample workout log to help you keep good records.

One of the important reasons for recording each session is to use the charts to inspire your SE later on. After six months of lifting weights, your SE is virtually guaranteed to lift between 30% and 300% more weight than at the beginning. If her interest or enthusiasm flags, you can point out the progress and encourage her to maintain or increase her strength.

Keeping good records is particularly important for the manual exercises in which you will be using your own strength as the resistance mechanism. Although it will take some practice to decide how hard to push against your SE's shoulders, for example, you will soon be able to feel the difference in her strength as she presses back. Before you begin training her, it's a good idea to practice a few times with someone else so you can gauge the degree of strength and balance you will need to use in providing resistance for the manual exercises.

Setting Goals

At the beginning, your SE may not know what goals to set because she will probably be unaware of what strength training can do for her. She may think she's on a persistent decline. You can prompt her for goals by mentioning some activity you know she can do right now, such as walking her dog, and ask whether she would like to stay strong enough to keep on doing that for the rest of her life.

The goal can be as simple as opening jars or as complex as intense gardening. If she has lost the capacity to do something she used to enjoy, you can ask if she would like to get strong enough to do it again.

People old and young seem to think that loss of function late in life is permanent and irreversible. Usually it's not, and making this discovery through strength training with your SE is almost like magic. It's a real Aha! moment for both of you.

> The important point about goal setting is to state a few goals, no matter what they are, to give you and your SE something to aim for.

If you can't draw out any specific goals, then you can take the scientific approach and tell her that your goal is to improve her strength in each muscle group by 30%. When you reach that goal, you can set higher goals if you both want to.

Frances

For example, Frances at age 84 couldn't state a goal when she first started training with John because she wasn't sure what strength training was all about. But after several months, she could see the improvements and readily stated her ongoing goals: "Well, I want to continue doing what I'm doing because I can tell that I have more strength and endurance. My blood pressure has improved so much. I attribute that to working out."

Medical Clearance and Diagnostics

Before you train your SE, you must first ask her doctor to consider her medical history and give his or her okay, if possible. Basically, you will ask your SE's family doctor, Can she work out or not? The answer is one of three: *Yes*, *Yes with restrictions*, or *No*. If you get a *No*, find out why the doctor said this.

If the doctor is against exercise in general, then get a second opinion from a more exercise-friendly doctor, especially if your SE scored above average on her Physical Inventory in Chapter 1. Most older people get a *Yes with restrictions*. It's your job or the personal trainer's job to find out more about those restrictions by conducting some diagnostic exercises.

Medical and Diagnostic Forms in the Appendix

The Appendix provides the following information for you to use in diagnosing and working with your SE:

- **Physician's Referral**. Everyone who hasn't exercised lately must obtain a physical exam and a doctor's consent.

- **Client's Medical History**. You or the personal trainer must know your SE's history and current state of health.

- **Shoulder Diagnostic Tests**. Diagnostic tests to discover shoulder problems, if any. Also see the introduction to "Testing the Shoulders" on page 63.

Testing the Joints

Before you start training anyone, especially your SE, take her through some very basic motions. Check the range of motion through the major joints: ankles, knees, hips, elbows, wrists, and neck. The shoulder joint is so important that you need to diagnose any shoulder problems separately. See the Appendix.

These diagnostic tests are more complete and rigorous than those in the Physical Inventory in Chapter 1. The main point is to take your SE through several movements to see what her range of motion is and whether any activity causes pain. If she never complains, look for a grimace, a wince, or a sharp intake of breath. These are often the visual equivalents of pain.

To test her joints, ask your SE to do the following:

- Stand and march in place several times for each leg. If she can raise her feet only an inch or two off the floor, emphasize the seated hip flexor exercise on page 129.

- Walk a more-or-less straight line. If she veers off course, emphasize all of the leg exercises, especially the abductor and adductor exercises on pages 159-161.

- Get up and down from a straight chair, and see how much effort that takes. If she has to use her arms to push off or has to rock back and forth, emphasize the chair squat exercise on page 124.

- Raise her arms to the side and, if possible, overhead. This is a very limited motion for many older people. If she can't reach the vertical, if she has pain, or both, emphasize the lateral raise exercise on page 130.

- Stand on tiptoes to see if there are any problems in her ankle joints. If she wobbles, can't raise her heels at least an inch, or has any pain, emphasize the heel raise exercise on page 127.

- Bend forward from the waist and hang in a forward bend. You are checking for spinal flexibility. Make sure you assist her in resuming the upright position, if needed, because this test may make her dizzy. If she doesn't get dizzy, emphasize the good morning exercise on page 132.

During these tests, take note, in particular, of the action of raising the arms overhead. She may tilt her head too far back and raise her hands too far back. If she has a pronounced curvature in her upper spine and neck (advanced kyphosis), this motion can block blood flow to the brain. Occasionally, a person with this condition may black out momentarily while raising her arms overhead, but not often. Be prepared to catch her if she loses her balance and then help her sit down and rest right away.

Testing the Shoulders

Older people tend to have more problems with their shoulders than with hips and knees as long as they are still able to walk. Many older people have almost quit using their arms, especially for reaching up. With patience and care, you can help her regain a great deal of the function she may have lost over the years.

In the Appendix on page 259, we adapt a set of rehabilitative exercises to test your SE's shoulder function. Take each step slowly and carefully as you ask your SE to attempt to perform the pictured actions. Caution her to stop at the first sign of pain or discomfort. See the accompanying text for advice on how to proceed if your SE has limited shoulder function.

Testing Stamina

If your SE has trouble breathing, her stamina may be low. Walk with her at her normal speed and listen to her breathing. If she huffs and puffs in less than a minute or two, you will know that she may have little endurance in a strength training session. The same is true if she can't walk and talk at the same time without experiencing shortness of breath.

In this case, reduce the number of reps in each set and give longer rest intervals. If your SE is overweight, her stamina is likely to be on the low side as well. She may find it difficult to breathe if she lies down to do the bench press, for example. Chapter 7 may give you some ideas on how to help her eat right to improve her stamina. For people with breathing or weight problems, emphasize exercises that she can perform in a seated position.

Starting the Training with Chapter 5

Even if your SE passes the preceding tests with full range of motion, without pain, and with good stamina, we still advise starting the training sessions with Chapter 5. Later on, you can gradually introduce the three advanced exercises in Chapter 6.

There's nothing to be gained by being macho with your SE. Start where she needs to start.

Communicating with Your SE

Maybe you have always had an easy time talking with your SE. If so, you probably got her involved in the decision process from the first moment you thought about being her Advocate and encouraging her to take up strength training. It will be equally easy to communicate with her throughout a training session if you take the role of Spotter or Strength Coach.

However, if communications tend to be somewhat strained or uncomfortable between you, then strength training can be a great way to improve your whole relationship. Whether you see yourself as practicing altruism or enlightened self-interest, you can establish an ease of communication that you may never have had before. Two communication tools will help you the most—banter and touch.

Using Banter Positively

All athletic endeavors seem to have a built-in banter factor. Ranging from private locker-room exchanges to the highest public award ceremonies, the language of banter goes along with the territory of sports. Light humor can provide a great basis for talking with your SE during your strength training sessions.

Good-natured joking about mistakes and missteps that you will *both* make will promote much more progress than criticism, sarcasm, anger, and the other negative feelings.

It's important to keep everything positive in a training session, including the talking. For example, if your SE can't seem to anchor her right foot during the Triangle pose in the warm-up on page 77, you can joke about looking around for some tape to hold the foot in place.

If she raises her left arm when you ask her to raise her right, you can nudge her shoulder in the appropriate direction and say, "Sorry. I meant *this* one." When she succeeds at an exercise that's especially difficult for her, you can joke about getting Mom a Wonder Woman outfit or Dad a Superman costume.

Gentle humor can do a great deal to improve the atmosphere of a training session, but be careful not to let the jokes slip into condescension or hurtful humor. Even if your SE is quite negative and sarcastic, make every attempt to keep things light, positive, and wholesome. When a formerly negative person starts joking back at you with positive banter, you will know that you have achieved great success as a promoter of good physical and mental health for your SE.

Since rest intervals of 30 to 120 seconds or more are built in to every training session, be prepared to carry the conversational ball, so to speak, during these times. Even if your SE is quite talkative, take a little time before each training session to look for jokes in such publications as the *Readers' Digest.* You can also recall amusing work and family incidents to tell her. Most of the time, she will make an excellent and appreciative audience.

Another good practice is to ask her some specific, non-threatening questions about her life. "Did you take physical education when you were in high school?" for example. In short, keep the conversation going whenever she isn't actually lifting weights. Don't banter during the lifts, of course, so she can focus completely on what she's trying to do.

Esther

Don't be surprised if your SE complains a great deal as long as her tone of voice is humorous or there's a glint in her eye.

"What are you trying to do—kill me?" complained Esther, 92, during a training session. Later the same day, as she was writing her check to John, she added, "I can't believe I actually pay you good money to hurt me like this." And yet, she's very proud of her accomplishments and doesn't miss a session.

Minnie Ree

Be prepared for your SE to banter right back at you. One day after a particularly successful session, John gave Minnie Ree a hug as he does with all his clients and said, "That was a great workout, Minnie Ree. I love you."

Attractive, thrice-married Minnie Ree, then 89, looked up at him with a twinkle in her eye and responded, "I love you too, John—but only as a friend."

Marie

Known far and wide as a complainer, someone we will call Marie, 85, sometimes realizes that she has made nothing but negative comments during an entire training session.

When she does, she invites John to what she calls a "whine and cheese" party. This comment gives John license to banter with something like this, "Okay, Marie, do you want a little cheese with that whine?" They both smile, and the mood is lighter.

Using Touch Positively

Some older people lead such lonely and isolated lives that they haven't felt the warmth of a friendly touch on the shoulder for years. They will be touched a lot in strength training, and touch, although they yearn for it, may be somewhat threatening to them.

If your SE flinches from touch, you can allay her fears by touching your own knees when you demonstrate the dead lift exercise, for example, and then it will seem more natural when you touch her knees to make sure they don't move too far forward.

When training young people, personal trainers usually don't need to use touch as much. They just demonstrate the exercises and the clients catch on. When training your SE, however, you will need to touch her with almost every exercise. You will clasp her hands to improve her balance, and you will touch her shoulder blades to remind her to keep them together. You will be right there to catch her if she falls.

Using touch is one of the best ways to keep your SE safe as she performs the exercises, especially those that require a pretty good sense of balance.

Another very good use of touch is to give your SE a gentle neck rub or shoulder massage after she finishes a particularly hard exercise. A 30-second massage of the trapezius muscles feels good and is a great reward for a heavy lift as well as a good way to increase the number of tactile experiences she has. It's well known that babies who aren't touched don't thrive. The same can be said about older people. They too need appropriate touching, especially from someone they love.

If you are an Advocate who will screen personal trainers on behalf of your SE, pay careful attention to the type and amount of contact he or she makes with older clients' bodies. Some touching is fine and even necessary, but make sure it's always appropriate and gentle.

Equipment

Maybe you have plenty of money and want to buy your SE a gym membership or a lot of equipment for home use. Maybe she lives in a retirement community that has an exercise room or a rehabilitation facility. However, if you need to supply the equipment for her strength training sessions, you will be happy to see that you won't have to spend much money at all. In fact, with a little ingenuity, you can fashion some homemade equipment for free.

Straight Chair

One item that you will definitely need is a firm, sturdy armchair, preferably one in which the seat is at about the level of your SE's knees. The wider the base, the better. This is the only truly essential piece of equipment.

You will use the chair for several abdominal exercises, the upper back exercise, the seated hip flexor exercise, the chair squat, the abductor and adductor exercises, and others. She can also use the chair for the rest intervals. For many of the exercises, you will also need to sit in a chair, but it doesn't need to be as sturdy as hers.

Benches, Barbells, and Dumbbells

It's unnecessary to buy very much equipment to use in strength training your SE. However, if you want to spend a little extra, you can usually get what you need at garage sales or from ads in the classified pages of your newspaper. Here are some items to look for:

- **A strength training bench**, which is a flat, narrow bench 3 1/2' to 5' long and hard but upholstered. It should be no more than 10" to a foot wide. It doesn't have to be costly, but it does have to be stable. Look for a wide base. Some are adjustable so that you can raise one end and lock it in place at various angles. Some have vertical supports for use with the bench press exercise. If you want to invest a little more, you can get a bench with a lat pull-down attachment. This will open the door to a number of good exercises. A new bench might cost anywhere from $50 to $150.

- **A set of weights** if you want to buy one instead of using homemade weights. You can pick up a reasonably useful set for between $50 and $75. Look for a steel bar or **barbell** about 5' long and weighing between 15 and 25 pounds. You will also want various iron plates to go on the bar. They come in 10-, 5-, 2 1/2-, and sometimes 1 1/4-pound increments. Make sure you get the spring clips, too, that hold the plates in place. You can also get a set of **dumbbells**, which you will buy in pairs weighing between 1 and 8 pounds. Weights generally cost between $0.50 and $1.00 per pound, so you could spend $30.00 or so.

- **An exercise band or tube.** A great upper back exercise—the band pull—uses rubber tubing with handles. Some have a door anchor. These are widely available, but John recommends JC Santana all-purpose exercise bands for under $20.00 available at www.performbetter.com. Order the travel band in fuchsia pink for lightest resistance.

Homemade Equipment

You can make weights out of anything that your SE can grasp firmly. For example, cans of soup make pretty good dumbbells. You can also make weights by adding sand to empty one-quart plastic cartons that have handles. These can substitute for dumbbells and for the plates that you would add to a barbell. The barbell can be a sawed-off and well sanded broom handle or something similar.

Using homemade equipment might appeal to the frugality of those who grew up during the Great Depression, but a small investment in equipment turns lifting into a different kind of activity, something special. Psychologically, it's probably a good idea to invest in a few pieces of equipment.

Shoes, Clothing, and Gloves

Ideally, your SE needs to wear a good pair of athletic shoes for strength training. Cross-trainers work well, and she can also use them for walking. At the very least, discourage her from working out in hose and pumps. If your SE is a woman who wouldn't be caught dead in a pair of pants, let alone shorts, then you can suggest that a pair of culottes would be appropriate. Take her shopping.

It may be difficult to get older people into T-shirts and sweat pants because they may prefer to wear out their old clothes. To many older people, it seems silly to have a special set of clothes for strength training. Just make sure that her blouse or his shirt is loose enough to permit a broad range of motion.

You might consider presenting her with a pair of strength training gloves for use with the dumbbell and barbell exercises because they will protect her palms from calluses.

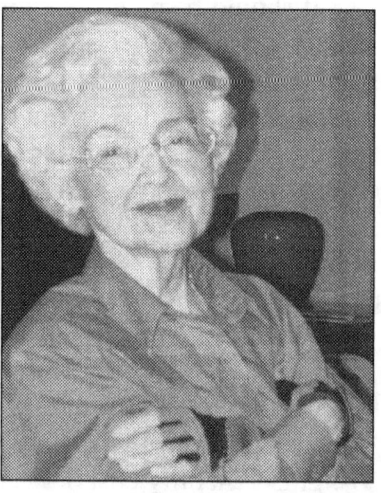

Some gloves are made of washable leather or similar material, which can be important in warm climates. A pair may cost between $5.00 and $20.00.

Figure 3-1 shows the cutaway fingers of a typical glove.

Figure 3-1. Frances proudly wears her gloves.

68

The First Things to Teach

Standing and sitting correctly and breathing properly—these are skills you will need to present gently because, of course, your SE has been standing, sitting, and breathing her own way for 65 to 95 years. However, there's a right way to do these for strength training.

Give these skills a fancy name, and she may take right to them—the Universal Stance, the Athletic Seated Posture, and Resistance Breathing. Don't feel that you have wasted your time if you have to spend a lot of time in the first several training sessions on these three skills. They are very important. Spend as much time on them as needed, both at the beginning and throughout the training sessions.

The Universal Stance

For nearly all of the standing exercises that your SE will perform, teach her to use the Universal Stance. Ask her to do the following:

- Stand and point her toes slightly outward.

- Place her feet shoulder width apart. If you dropped a plumb line from the outer edge of the left shoulder, the inside of the left foot should be even with the plumb line, and similarly for the right side. If you're training a man with very broad shoulders, however, ask him to place his foot at the center of the plumb line.

- Flex her knees slightly. Keep them soft and slightly flexed instead of locked into place.

- Keep her weight in the back half of her foot. Make sure she doesn't rock back on the heels. She needs to feel that most of her weight is coming down directly through her lower leg and ankle and then into the entire heel pad.

- Keep her spine in a neutral position with a slight concavity in the lower back and a slight convexity in the upper back. Most people, not just older folks, have a tendency to slump over, so you may need to remind her regularly at first.

- Keep her head up and her line of vision horizontal or slightly elevated.

- Keep her shoulder blades down and together in the retracted position. Keeping the shoulder blades together is such an important requirement for nearly every exercise that you need to check often to ensure that she's holding the correct posture. If her back has become too rounded over the years, you may have to work up to this skill.

- Lean very slightly forward at the waist so that she looks as if she's just about to sit down. If this position feels awkward to her, ask her not to lean forward quite so much. She needs a feeling of stability, not uneasiness.

The Athletic Seated Posture

If standing would be a problem, you can ask your SE to perform most of the exercises in a seated position. Even seated, however, she will need to sit up straight with her chest up, her shoulders back, her shoulder blades together, her spine straight, her head upright, and both feet firmly on the floor. Most seated exercises require her to sit at the front edge of the chair so that her back has no support. For a few seated exercises, she will sit all the way back in the chair with her hips and back against the back of the chair.

Resistance Breathing

The breath provides some of the fuel for strength training, so it's important that you teach your SE how to get the most from her breathing. She needs to breathe properly on each and every rep. Professional trainers apply specific, scientific terms to the correct way of breathing, but there are also translations into plain English:

- She inhales on the *eccentric* motion, the motion that returns the weight to its original position after the lift. For many exercises, she **inhales on the preparation**, that is, before she lifts (while she is getting ready) or while she is lowering the weight.

- She exhales on the *concentric* motion, the motion that does the work of the lift. For many exercises, she **exhales on the performance** of the exercise, that is, when she's pushing or pulling against resistance or against gravity.

Incorrect breathing isn't dangerous—*not* breathing is.
Encourage your SE to breathe deeply and well.

Breathing correctly takes time. Breathe along with her to provide a useful reminder. Encourage her to lift to the rhythm of her breathing, rather than vice versa. This habit, once cultivated, makes the entire weightlifting process feel smoother, more graceful, and more integrated with her body. It's a source of self-awareness. Chapter 9 contains more information on this topic.

Also, encourage her to breathe through her mouth and to make a noise when she exhales, such as expressing air with a "hooooo" or "sssssss" sound between slightly open lips. The sound will let you hear the pattern of her breathing. Many people of all ages start out with the reverse (incorrect) pattern in their breathing and then wonder why they get so tired or fail to make much progress. Give your SE the advantage of using her breath as fuel for the exercises.

In gyms around the world, you will hear a lot of grunting on the heavier lifts. There's no need to encourage your SE to grunt—she will do it when she needs to. If those last two or three chair squats cause a little "uhn" sound, you will know she's working hard and making progress.

The Warm-up and the Cool-down/Calm-down

When your SE is comfortable with standing, sitting, and breathing properly, then you can start teaching her the moves for the warm-up and the simple things to do during the cool-down. See "The Importance of the Warm-up" on page 72. For the cool-down, which is also a calm-down, see page 135.

The Elements of a Training Session

Some people like the inductive method of experiencing life, in which they come to an understanding of a new activity by jumping in and doing it or doing what the trainer tells them. They leave the explanations and interpretations for later.

If your SE prefers the deductive method, however, and wants to know in advance what to expect in a training session, you can mention that in addition to social time and rest periods, a training session contains three basic parts:

- The warm-up of at least 5 to 10 minutes covered below.

- The exercises of 35 to 45 minutes detailed in Chapters 5 and 6.

- The cool-down/calm-down of 5 to 10 minutes on page 135.

Demonstrate the exercises you will use, after practicing first on your own, and explain the purpose of each one. Since you are aiming for strength and mobility with your SE, you will want to emphasize that there's no substitute for muscular strength in conducting the activities of daily living. Strength will let her continue doing the things she enjoys.

Tweet

If your SE is like one of John's clients, Tweet, 84, she will think she should always be delicate and composed. Tweet never wants to feel that she's working, much less sweating and grunting. Tweet frequently complains, "I'm a lady. I don't think this is good for me."

"But you're a *strong* lady, aren't you?" John answers. She smiles. Sometimes she buys it, sometimes not. They laugh about it. The important point is that she keeps coming back to the workout room.

Slowly and gently, get your SE accustomed to the workouts. Be patient. Add one rep per week. Tell her what to expect and tell her about the changes you see—improved posture, deeper breathing, and more energy. You may even be able to tell her that she looks younger than she did before starting strength training. Who doesn't like to hear that?

Sequence of the Exercises

In addition to learning how to teach and supervise the exercises, you will also learn a good sequence in which to introduce the exercises during a training session. The basic principle is to perform multi-joint exercises first and then alternate upper body with lower body exercises. Each training session begins with less taxing exercises, builds up to more taxing exercises that require maximum effort, and tapers off with less taxing exercises. Many of the exercises focus on leg strength because mobility is one of the most important aspects of maintaining independence and self-confidence.

With your SE, you will want to cover the most difficult and beneficial exercises in the early and middle parts of a training session. Do this in case the rest periods take longer than you anticipate and the session seems to be taking more time than you both like. Even if she becomes too tired to finish the session, she will have completed some of the more challenging work before she tires. A short session is better than none at all.

Introducing the Exercises Gradually

To make the exercises as safe as possible, introduce them into the training sessions over time, taking two or three sessions or more for her to learn all of the exercises in Chapter 5. Provide light resistance at first so she can experience the happiness of a successful performance. Ask her to do only six to eight reps while you teach correct technique. Ask her to do only one or two sets of each exercise, especially if she has been living a largely sedentary lifestyle.

Increase the number of repetitions to 12-15 before increasing the resistance or weight of these exercises. Back off at the first sign of distress.

For any of the standing warm-ups and exercises, be prepared to stabilize her if there's any sign that she's losing her balance. If it takes weeks to complete a full training session, then that's what it takes. But *always* ask her to do the warm-up and the cool-down/calm-down, even if she gets through fewer than half of the exercises you have planned. Learning new things takes time at any age. Learning something new late in life has its challenges, but the rewards are so great that you can take comfort in knowing that you are doing the right thing.

Minnie Ree

When your SE is comfortable doing 15 reps, she may feel like Minnie Ree, who at age 90 remarked to another of John's clients, "If he ever learns to count past 15, we're *all* in trouble."

The Importance of the Warm-up

The descriptions that follow provide the words for you to use in teaching your SE the appropriate motions for each step of the warm-up, which should be five to ten minutes.

Make sure your SE warms up before she lifts weights.

If your SE becomes unwilling to warm up, remind her that if she doesn't stretch, she could easily hurt herself because her muscles will be cold and stiff. The muscles must be warm, relaxed, and pliant in order to move correctly and cut down on injuries. Many younger lifters use 20 minutes of running on the treadmill or a similar cardiovascular activity to warm up. For older lifters, however, there's a better way.

In general, ask her to do five to ten minutes of very gentle yoga-like movements and stretches. These movements build from the extremely easy and relaxing—moving the hips from side to side or rocking back and forth from toe to heel. Then they progress to reasonably difficult motions such as the modified Triangle pose in yoga.

The reason the yoga-based warm-up is so useful is that it's very efficient. The steps require your SE to do at least two and sometimes three or four movements and stretches at once. Each step encourages her to concentrate and to focus on her breath and on body awareness.

Another purpose of these warm-ups is to loosen the major joints and give you a way to assess the joint motions before you launch into the training session. If one day your SE's lower back seems tight and painful, for example, you will know that she needs to do more than her usual number of gentle stretches for the back during the warm-up.

You will also know to pay extra attention when she does the lower back exercise during the training session. The trainer or Strength Coach who minimizes the warm-up will miss one of the best diagnostic tools available for use at the start of each training session.

After you have moved on to the three advanced exercises in Chapter 6, you may need to revert to the gentler exercise in Chapter 5 for the muscle group that remains somewhat stiff or causes a slight twinge of pain during the warm-up. Nearly all of the warm-up motions ought to feel good. If they don't, then decrease the range of motion and the intensity of the stretch, but increase the number of times she performs the gentler motion.

The Start Position for the Warm-up

To start the warm-up, stand facing your SE about an arm's length away and make sure there's a chair about a foot behind her in case she needs to sit suddenly or loses her balance. The chair is the safety net behind her, and you are the safety net in front of her. If she has balance problems, you can either clasp her hands or place your hands lightly on the sides of her shoulders to provide stability. This warm-up routine stretches and loosens the muscles of the hips, the neck, the shoulders, the upper back and chest, and the lower back. It concludes with a whole-body stretch from yoga, the Triangle pose. Stretching the muscles helps her achieve the maximum range of motion for the joints.

Stretch and Loosen the Hips

Ask your SE to stand in a relaxed, upright posture with the toes pointed slightly inward and her weight distributed evenly on both feet. Her weight is on the front of the heel pads. Ask her to do the following motions four to eight times at each of the three steps:

1. Gently rock the hips from side to side. Encourage her to breathe deeply throughout each step.

2. Shift the weight from the front of the foot to the back of the foot and then to the front again. Come down softly on the heels. Over time, some older people can rise up on tiptoes during the front swing, but your SE probably shouldn't try to lift her toes during the back swing because this motion requires a high degree of balancing ability.

3. Rotate the hips in a circle, first in one direction and then in the other direction as if using a hula hoop from the 1950's. Some older people have trouble making this motion at first, so you can help by breaking it down into its parts: "Move your hips to the left. Move your hips to the front. Move your hips to the right. Move your hips to the back." Then repeat for the other direction.

Stretch and Loosen the Neck

Ask your SE to stand as she did in the preceding stretch and do the following:

1. Inhale. Stand tall and lengthen the spine.

2. Exhale and let the chin sink to the chest.

3. Pull the head to the chest and feel a light stretch along the back of the neck.

4. Take another deep breath, relax during the exhale, and slowly roll the head and neck in a big circle, first in one direction and then in the other direction. Make sure your SE takes at least 30 seconds for one complete rotation.

5. Ask her to do these neck rolls only once or twice in each direction, but tell her that she needs to do these every day on her own. When she discovers that this motion is easy to do, feels good, and relaxes the neck and upper shoulder (trapezius) muscles where many people carry a great deal of tension, she will probably be convinced that she should incorporate neck rolls into her daily life.

If your SE feels discomfort with the neck roll, use an alternative stretch. After she has pulled her chin to her chest as in the neck roll, ask her to raise her head and make a circle in the air with her nose. Start with a circle the size of a golf ball in both directions. Don't be surprised if the motion isn't smooth and circular. If the motion is jerky or square but free from pain, move on to a larger circle the size of an apple and then one the size of a large Texas grapefruit. If she has no discomfort, then ask her to roll her head and neck in the largest circle she can manage while remaining free of pain.

Stretch and Loosen the Shoulders

Ask your SE to take the Universal Stance and do the following:

1. Lean forward a couple of inches and swing the arms loosely back and forth in front of the body. Let the trunk rotate with the arm swings.

2. If your SE moves her arms in a stiff, robotic fashion, that is, she moves only her shoulders and does not rotate her trunk, you can use a slightly different motion. Ask her to rotate her body back and forth, letting her arms relax and flop. Ask her to turn her head in the same direction as she rotates her body. This motion will also relax the shoulders, which is the point of this step.

3. Remind her to breathe deeply whenever she needs to.

Stretch and Loosen the Upper Back and Chest

Ask your SE to imagine that she's a child standing at the edge of a swimming pool just about to dive in. Ask her to do the following:

1. Bend the knees slightly and push the hips back slightly.

2. Take a deep breath and extend the arms straight out in front with the palms facing down. Cross one hand over the other in a diving posture.

3. During the exhale, round the back as much as possible, drop the head, and separate the shoulder blades. Feel the stretch across the muscles of the upper back.

4. Inhale, straighten up, and open the arms out to each side as wide as possible while looking up, lifting the chest, and pulling the shoulder blades together. Feel the stretch across the muscles of the chest.

5. As a transition to the next stretch in the warm-up, ask her to swing her arms loosely across the body a few times as in the step for loosening the shoulders.

6. Roll the shoulders forward a few times and then to the back. Many older people love the shoulder roll because it feels so good.

Stretch and Loosen the Lower Back

A good stretch for the lower back resembles the yoga pose called the Sun Salutation. You will ask her to do it only a couple of times. Ask her to stand as she has done for the preceding stretches and do the following:

1. Place her palms together in front of the body at about the level of the chest.

2. Inhale and, during the exhale, lower the hands to the sides.

3. Inhale and lift the arms forward and upward with the palms facing the ceiling.

4. Continue to bring the arms upward and over the head while keeping the arms nearly straight.

5. Near the top of the arc, rotate the palms inward as far as possible without causing pain. This motion provides a good but gentle stretch of the rotator cuff muscles.

6. Turn the head and eyes upward and feel the stretch along the lower back, rib cage, and shoulders.

7. Now exhale and lower the arms to the sides.

8. At the same time, roll the back slowly forward and down so that the head and arms hang toward the floor in a kind of rag doll posture with the head down, the neck relaxed, and the knees slightly bent. See Figure 3-2 below.

9. Slowly return to the upright position. Roll up with the back and spine as rounded as possible. Imagine stacking the vertebrae one by one, beginning with the tailbone.

10. Keep the knees bent throughout the roll upwards. When about halfway up, bend the knees a little more and tuck the hips underneath the torso. This technique removes stress from the lower back and hamstrings. Then continue to roll up.

11. Lift the neck and head only when the back is upright and long. Roll the neck and head up slowly.

12. Repeat steps 1-11 smoothly a second time, depending on the condition of her lower back. When she has become adept at the Sun Salutation, ask her to rise up on tiptoes a bit at the top of the arc where the palms almost touch. This additional feature provides a very pleasant feeling of almost letting the whole body rise upwards. It also provides an additional stretch for the back.

Notes: Since this lower back warm-up is a complex motion, you will need to check on a number of things:

1. Make sure she bends her knees as she rolls forward so that the motion feels relaxed. Bending the knees takes the stress off the lower back and hamstrings and helps her feel good in this position.

2. If she always feels faint or dizzy when her head goes below the level of her heart, take it slowly and help her build up to this stretch. Make sure you are right there to stabilize her, especially on the upward roll. Until she is able to perform this stretch, you can substitute the part-way stretch pictured in Figure 3-3, which also improves shoulder flexibility.

3. If your SE feels discomfort in the neck or shoulders, modify this stretch so that she raises her arms and head only as far as she can without pain.

To perform a good stretch called the trust pose, pictured in Figure 3-3, face each other at least one foot apart with her feet shoulder width apart. Place one of your feet forward and the other back for balance. Grasp each others' wrists with yours on the bottom. Ask her to bend her knees and sit down and back. Counterbalance her weight by leaning back slightly. Carefully assist her in rising after the stretch.

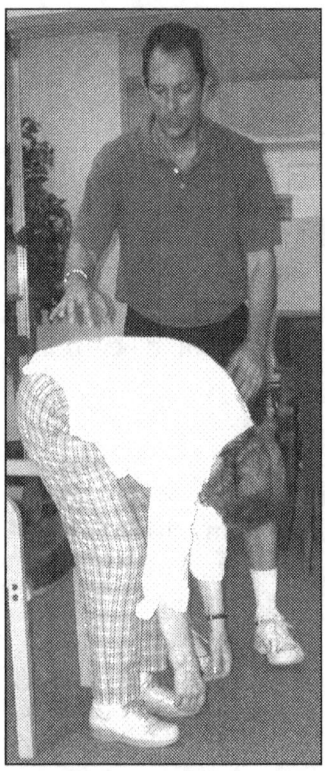

Figure 3-2. Ann does the rag doll.

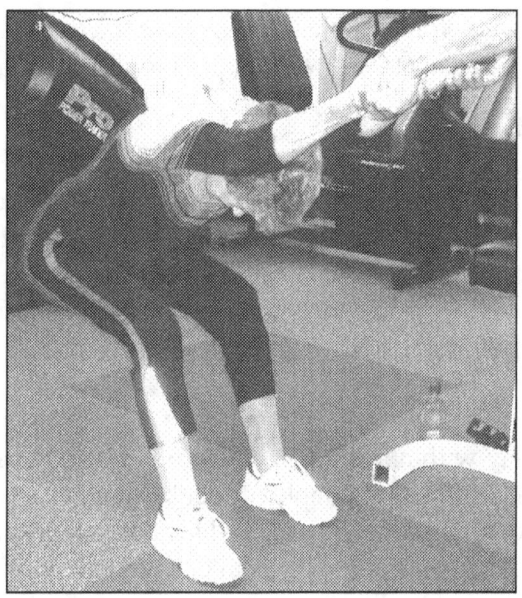

Figure 3-3. Virginia stretches deeply.

Stretch and Loosen the Whole Body with the Triangle

The preceding stretches should be so gentle that your SE feels good throughout and has little or no sensation of working hard. The final step of the warm-up provides a transition into the harder work she will do in the training session. Over time, watch for that fine line between boredom and discomfort. If this whole-body stretch becomes too easy, her attention may wander; if it's too hard, she will feel stressed.

This final part of the warm-up is intense because it stretches half a dozen muscle groups at the same time. It also requires presence of mind and some degree of balance. It resembles the Triangle pose in yoga, but you may have to modify some of it to match your SE's abilities, especially at first. If she has any difficulty at any point, you can show her how to ease off. You can gradually help her work up to the pose in Figure 3-4 on page 80.

Unless you have practiced yoga for some time, you will need to master this full-body stretch on your own before you attempt to teach it to your SE. Because of its intensity and complexity, this final stretch is divided into sections on preparation and performance. The performance section is divided into subsections for each body part as it comes into play. Teach the Triangle pose bit by bit, and don't be in a rush to complete the whole stretch.

Some older people won't be able to complete all of the subsections. Take your SE only as far as she can go without pain or discomfort.

Preparation

Talk her through the mental image of an ancient Egyptian hieroglyphic in which the human figures are two-dimensional. Tell her that she needs to strive for that same kind of flat appearance. Any part of the body that sticks out to the front or the rear isn't very Egyptian. Later on, you can talk about errors of technique. Take many training sessions to help her develop the ability to place all parts of her body in a single plane. Gently remind her of the goal from time to time.

Stay within arm's length in front of her in case her balance or concentration falters. Also, place a chair a couple of feet behind her to be the rear safety net in case she needs to sit down suddenly. It's a good idea to perform this stretch along with her but in mirror image so that she can take visual cues from your body position, but always be prepared to stabilize her if necessary. To prepare for this stretch, ask her to do the following:

1. Stand with very good upright posture.

2. Place her feet about hip width apart with her toes very slightly turned inward.

3. Leaving the left foot in place, step out to the right about 12 inches or a little less if she's short or frail.

4. Shift the weight on the right foot toward the heel and turn her toes to the right so that her right foot is perpendicular to her left foot.

5. Shift the weight on her left foot toward the ball of the foot and slide the heel of the left foot outward so that the left foot is at a 45-degree angle from its starting position.

6. Look down at the feet and make sure that a line drawn through the right foot to the left foot would go through the instep of the left foot.

Performance

When she is reasonably comfortable in the ready position, ask her to start the first phase of the Triangle pose.

Keep the Hips Flat

1. Rotate her hips back to the starting position facing you if her hips have turned toward the right foot. This turn is almost inevitable.

2. Feel the twisting or rotational stretch on her lower back, pelvis, and upper thighs.

3. Take a deep breath and relax from the waist up so that the stress doesn't go up into the neck and shoulders.

Cock the Hips

1. With a straight spine, cock the hips to the left so that the torso is at an angle to the lower body.

2. Lean to the right without curving the spine until she feels a stretch in the hamstring and inner thigh of the left leg. The more she cocks her hips and leans, the more she will feel the stretch.

Extend the Right Arm

1. Keeping the spine straight and the hips facing toward you, ask her to extend the right arm straight out over the right foot and as high as possible.

2. Then make the right arm an extra inch longer by extending the shoulder to the right.

3. Without curving the spine, lower the right arm until it contacts the right leg, usually at the thigh but sometimes at the knee if she's pretty flexible; over time, she may be able to reach her shin.

4. Grasp the right leg and lean slightly on the right arm.

5. Keep the right leg straight with no bending of the knee.

Rotate the Shoulders

1. Raise the left arm up, out, and to the left side as high as possible, with the palm up, if possible. If she has shoulder pain, ask her to rotate the palm forward toward you, not toward the ceiling. If she still has pain, ask her to move her left shoulder slightly forward toward you until the pain subsides. If there's still pain, ask her to just let the left arm hang down by her side. Later on, she may be able to raise her arm.

2. Relax the trapezius muscles between the upper part of the shoulder and the neck.

3. Pull the shoulder blades back to the retracted position.

Turn the Head and Neck

1. Turn the head to the left, cock the chin up a little, and look up and over the left shoulder.

2. If the hips have shifted toward the right, pull the left hip back and push the right hip forward.

Breathe and Stretch

1. Breathe and focus on the breathing.

2. When she inhales, she should feel the stretches.

3. When she exhales, she should feel relaxed.

4. Try to stay in the Triangle pose for two complete breaths. Later on, she will probably be able to increase the number of breaths to five or more.

5. Return to the starting position—lower the left arm, straighten the torso to the erect position, and move the feet closer together.

After a few moments of rest, ask her to repeat the entire stretch in reverse by stepping out to the left—all of the steps of the preparation and all of the steps of the performance.

Then ask her to sit and rest for a minute or two before going into the exercises of the training session presented in Chapters 5 and 6.

In Figure 3-4, Faye mirrors John in the Triangle.

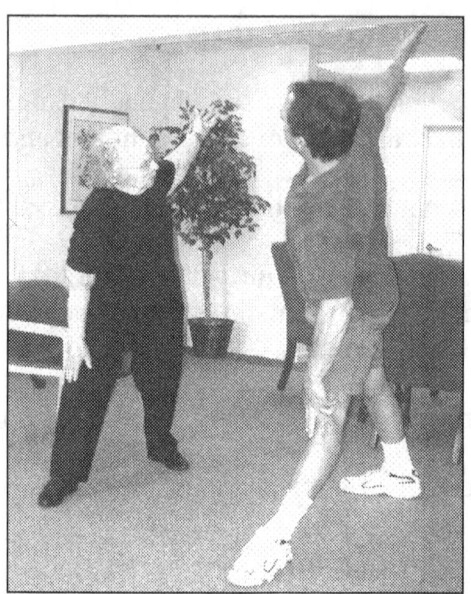

Figure 3-4. Faye performs the Triangle

A Note to Certified Personal Trainers

The main topic in this chapter that may not be familiar to you is the idea of incorporating yoga stretches into the warm-up. Feel free to use your own methods for the warm-up, of course, but for your oldest clients, over age 85, consider adopting any of these steps that make sense to you. They are very gentle but effective.

The idea of using your sense of touch as a means of communication may seem foreign or excessive to you. However, if an older client seems unable to respond to what you say and demonstrate, then a gentle touch on the shoulder blades or lower spine may be just the right technique to use in order to get through to her about posture. All of the manual exercises require you to touch her and to use your body weight as the resistance. If you prefer, use free weights or resistance machines instead. Remember:

*   Always have your older clients do a warm-up that includes stretching.

*   Use appropriate banter and touch as important communication tools.

- Pay particular attention to your older clients' shoulder joints. Use the diagnostic form in the Appendix to uncover any functional problems.

Summary of the Main Points

- The basic principles and terminology of strength training are easy to grasp. There is no reason to be apprehensive about the lingo or about strength training in general.

- Before you begin, get a medical clearance from your SE's doctor.

- Teach her the Universal Stance, the Athletic Seated Posture, and the correct Resistance Breathing technique. Gently remind her about these elements as often as needed.

- Communicate with your SE at every step of the way on her journey to health and strength. Banter and touch can be helpful tools.

- Consider buying a small amount of equipment:

  - A sturdy chair with arms   Free. Use one that you have.
  - A set of dumbbells up through eight pounds   About $30.00 new.
  - A set of plates and a barbell   About $60.00 new.
  - Weightlifting bench   About $100.00 new.
  - Total $190.00, less if second-hand.
  - **Your SE's physical wellbeing**   **Beyond any price**

- A strength training session contains three parts: The warm-up, the exercises, and the cool-down/calm-down.

- Never neglect the warm-up. If your SE doesn't want to warm up, find a way to help her see the necessity of getting her muscles warm, pliant, and flexible before working them.

What's Next?

The next chapter on safety is of supreme importance. Do *not* skip it. If you haven't taken a basic first aid course in some time or ever, then you must equip yourself with the necessary safety skills before you start training with your SE. Certified trainers must take first aid, and you should too. You will also need to assemble a first-aid kit to keep in the strength training area. Finally, become intimately familiar with her medical history and current physical limitations, if any.

Chapter 4. Keeping Your Significant Elder Safe

How to Cope with Safety, Injuries, and Recovery

"One hundred percent of the injuries I've had since I became a trainer, when I'm supposed to be older and wiser, have come from being impatient and stupid. Either I didn't warm up sufficiently, or I didn't listen to my own body."
  John, 54, Certified Personal Trainer, Advocate, and Strength Coach

Important Points for Advocates: The main idea to absorb from this chapter is to realize that your SE will be safe with a certified personal trainer. If an injury or illness occurs, you may have an important role to play in encouraging your SE to resume strength training when it is safe for him to do so. For some useful techniques on overcoming reluctance and staying positive, see page 100.

Safety First—Really

Safety is crucial for all activities and all athletes. Recreational strength training is one of the safer sports,[15] but the image of older folks pumping iron seems alarming to some caregivers who might otherwise be interested in strength training with their Significant Elders. You can overcome this reluctance by emphasizing safety at all times.

Strength training prevents *far* more injuries than it causes.
Strong people are *much* less likely to fall and hurt themselves.

Spotters and Strength Coaches must learn safety techniques, and Advocates need to know something about them as well. After all, overseeing your SE's program from thousands of miles away will be easier if you can talk with his doctors, physical therapists, occupational therapists, trainers, and others while using the appropriate vocabulary.

In training your SE, you do need to learn or review safety practices (see page 83), take precautions, and be consistent. But your worst fears are highly unlikely—there's very little chance that your SE will suddenly have a heart attack or stroke during strength training. Basically, safety means expecting the best and being prepared for the worst.

---

[15] "Injuries in Recreational Adult Fitness Activities," *American Journal of Sports Medicine*, V. 32 (3), pp. 461-467 (1993). The number of injuries per 1000 hours of strength training is 4. Walking has a rate of 2.

If an injury occurs, it's much more probable that it will happen in your SE's daily life and not in the strength training room, where knowing how to prevent injuries is the key to safety (see page 92). You will learn which joints and muscle groups are the most susceptible to injuries and which exercises are the most likely to result in injuries. You will learn which injuries you can treat yourself and which ones you can't. But you will also learn the steps to take, such as warm-up, technique, and focus, to protect your SE.

If your SE does sustain an injury, you will learn how to assist in the recovery on page 97. If the injury is serious enough to require extensive medical help, you will see how to approach the situation positively. You will also learn how and when to use strength training as an extension of the medical treatment. Best of all, you will feel good about knowing how to help. You will definitely be prepared.

Preparing for Safety

If you are at all worried, and even if you aren't, you will be and feel safer as the Advocate and the Spotter or Strength Coach for your SE if you do what professional trainers do—take safety courses.

Just in case, you will also feel better if you know how to recognize the warning signs of a heart attack and stroke, even if your SE is healthy, and if you learn what to do in case you see these signs, page 90 and following. Further, you will feel more comfortable if you know what to watch out for in a training session and how to protect your SE against the most common training injuries.

Using a Heart Monitor

For about $50.00, you can purchase a heart monitor for your SE. It consists of a strap to be worn around his chest and a display that straps onto his wrist or yours. The monitor gives you an easy way to keep track of his pulse. Subtract his age from 220 to find his maximum rate of exertion. However, his working rate should be about 60% of the maximum rate. Keep an eye on the display while he is performing the most taxing exercises. Ask him to rest for a few moments if his heart rate exceeds the working rate before he finishes the set. These numbers don't apply if your SE is taking blood pressure medication. Instead, use the Borg Scale on page 101 to monitor his level of exertion.

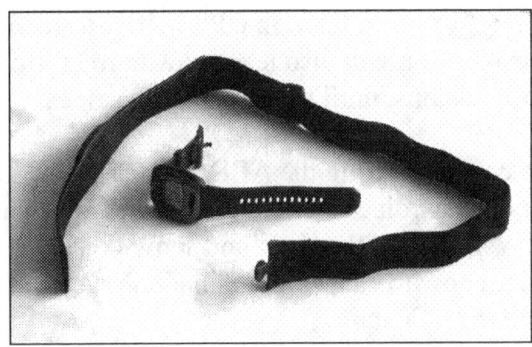

Figure 4-1. A typical heart monitor and display

Taking Courses

Taking safety courses is a little like buying home and car insurance. You may never need it, but if you do, you will be very glad you have it. Check with your local Red Cross on costs—quite reasonable—and schedules—usually quite convenient—for the mandatory courses:

- Cardiopulmonary resuscitation (CPR) and using the automated external defibrillator (AED).

- Basic first aid, including the Heimlich maneuver for choking victims.

These courses are often taught together. You won't need to know how to handle snakebites and drowning, but it will feel good to master the latest practices for first aid and to learn about the latest products. Keep your certifications up to date by periodically taking refresher courses because CPR techniques in particular change from time to time.

If your SE lives in a retirement community that's big on safety, there may be an AED at some location in the facility. If so, the nurses or other staff members may be trained to use this device. If an AED is available in the strength training room, consider learning how to use it. It's always better to be over-prepared than under-prepared, and you may be able to help other people besides your SE in an emergency. Since AEDs are being installed in many public places, you could save your SE's life or a stranger's life.

CPR and AED

The chance that you will ever need to use CPR or an AED on your SE is quite small, but, again, do what the professional trainers do and take the course. One of the most important things you will learn in CPR is how to recognize the warning signs of heart attack and stroke. You will also learn how to treat life-threatening emergencies, such as choking and convulsions, until the ambulance arrives.

A course in using the AED will teach you how to administer early defibrillation in case of sudden cardiac arrest. Most courses also teach you a little about the anatomy and physiology of the heart and show you when to use the AED and when not to. You may also learn how to clean and maintain the AED. Ensure that the AED has not been recalled by the manufacturer.

There is an approved version of the AED for home use. Although these devices are somewhat pricey for many budgets, ranging from about $2,000 to $3,500, you might consider buying one if you are seriously worried about your SE's heart. However, heart attacks frequently give enough warning that you can call EMS and get your SE to a hospital in time for effective treatment.

Don't delay in calling EMS.

Basic First Aid

Injuries of various types are inevitable. They happen to everyone even though strength training and its equipment are quite safe. Dumbbells and barbells don't have sharp edges, and weight benches are padded. However, in addition to the expected muscle strains, it's possible to bang a finger between two dumbbells, to fall and bump the forehead on a chair, to drop a weight on the toes, and so on.

It's much better to have the training and a first aid kit that you never use than not to have them when you need them.

The first aid rules you may have learned as a Boy or Girl Scout, or that you have used with your own children, are still useful for minor cuts or scrapes. But there have been some significant changes in other areas that a good first aid course will teach you.

After you take the course, you will want to assemble a first aid kit to keep handy wherever your SE works out. Focus on two types of products—those for treating cuts and scrapes and those for treating bruises, muscle pains, and joint sprains. Also have water available for your SE throughout the strength training session.

Products for Treating Cuts and Scrapes

Most commercial first aid kits that you can buy already assembled anticipate that you will want to take elaborate precautions against coming into contact with the injured person's blood. However, if you know for sure that your SE doesn't have HIV, Hepatitis C, or another blood-borne infectious disease, you won't need protective gowns, gloves, and masks.

The basic first aid course will show you how to sterilize the wound, how to apply pressure to stop the bleeding, how to dress the wound, and whether or when to seek medical help. The supplies you will need include the following:

- Antiseptics.

- Bandaging materials.

- Adhesive and elastic tape.

Products for Treating Bruises, Muscle Pains, and Joint Sprains

Products to treat bruises, muscle pains, and joint sprains have improved a lot over the last several decades. For example, the instant cold pack is an essential element of any first aid kit because it can treat all three types of injuries. A cold pack is useful because it reduces the swelling and inflammation that can cause much of the pain.

The kit should also contain a roll of athletic bandaging material in case you need to stabilize a joint, such as an ankle, that suddenly feels painful. If a doctor says that your SE can take ibuprofen or acetaminophen, keep those products in the kit to treat pains and sprains. For more information on preventing these types of injuries, see page 97. To sum up, the first aid kit should contain the following:

- Instant cold packs.

- Elastic bandaging material.

- A pain reliever that your SE's doctor has approved for his use.

Water

If you exercise at all, you know the importance of drinking enough, but not too much, water. However, you may need to remind your SE to drink water, not only during strength training sessions but also during the rest of his day. Dehydration poses a significant problem for some older people, especially those with heart disease or diabetes.

Without enough water, even healthy people can experience mental confusion, headaches, fatigue, lethargy, muscle weakness, muscle cramps, dizziness, nausea, forgetfulness, deep rapid breathing, or an increased heart rate. Dehydration is a serious condition, and older people sometimes have a reduced sense of thirst. It's one of the more frequent causes of hospitalization for people age 65 and older.[16]

Ideally, the strength training area will provide a water fountain so you won't need to bring bottled water. If it doesn't, then consider giving your SE an aluminum or stainless steel reusable water bottle. It could be a reward for achieving an early milestone such as completing two sessions. These bottles, costing about $15-$25, are easy to wash with soap, hot water, and a bottle brush after each use. Some can also go in the dishwasher.

Everyone has reused plastic water bottles with no ill effect, but bacteria can accumulate in them. Reusing the same water bottle after you recover from a head cold or similar infectious illness can cause a recurrence. In the interests of your SE's safety and health, discourage him from reusing plastic water bottles unless he washes them with soap, hot water, and a bottle brush.

Staying Current

A basic problem with learning emergency medical procedures is that crises seldom happen. What we don't use, we forget. The American Red Cross (ARC) certifications are good for two years, but that's far too long for everyone except emergency medical technicians and fire fighters who use the information almost daily.

---

[16] See http://www.aging-parents-and-elder-care.com/Pages/Signs_of_Dehydration.html and many other sources.

After taking the courses, review the basics periodically for 10 minutes once a month, for example, to keep the information fresh in your mind. ARC courses come with excellent word-and-picture outlines, which make ideal review materials. A good time to review is just before a training session or during the first several minutes of a session. Include your SE in the process because his knowledge and focus can also be helpful.

Handling Health Issues Safely

Along with taking safety courses, learn your SE's limitations and be thoroughly familiar with his medical history and current physical status. Apply common sense to his specific condition. Following are several conditions or diseases and suggestions on how to handle them in strength training:

- **A heart condition.** Learn the distress signs to look for and keep the phone number for EMS handy. Call EMS before you call his primary care physician. As medical professionals say, "Time lost is myocardium (heart muscle) lost." Your safety courses will train you to spot the symptoms of a heart attack. The American Heart Association recommends exercise for heart patients and has added physical *inactivity* to its list of risk factors for heart disease. Since heart disease is the number one killer of both men and women, strongly encourage your SE to exercise.

- **Cancer.** Design very gentle workouts, and be prepared to go even lighter when the medical treatments cause weakness and fatigue.

- **Diabetes.** Diabetics who exercise have a low risk of diabetic coma caused by ketoacidosis unless they are already ill or have not complied with their medications and diet program. Diabetics are also at low risk of hyperosmolar coma unless their glucose is very high, which is usually caused by non-compliance with their medications and diet program. However, diabetics are at much higher risk of hypoglycemia or low blood glucose, so keep some real fruit juice handy, not the kind containing a sugar substitute. If your SE becomes shaky, anxious, or very tired, he will probably recognize these symptoms of low sugar. Encourage him to use a home glucose monitoring set and to check his serum glucose before, during, and after exercising. Stop exercising if his glucose is unusually low.

- **Peripheral neuropathy in diabetics.** If your SE has decreased sensation in his hands and especially his feet, he won't be able to tell when he has injured or even fractured a bone. Nor will he be able to determine whether his shoes fit correctly. He will need supportive shoes that don't rub or compress his feet anywhere. A podiatrist can assist with purchasing these shoes. After each strength training session, check his feet for redness, blistering, deformity, or any signs of infection. If you see any of these, take him immediately to his physician or podiatrist.

- **High blood pressure.** Know whether he's taking medications and, if so, what side effects they may cause. For example, if you want to take his pulse at the beginning and the end of the cool-down/calm-down, these readings may not be valid indicators of his state of recovery because many blood pressure medications tend to slow the pulse rate.

- **Epilepsy.** Watch for an impending episode and know what to do if one occurs. Read up on the disease and talk with your SE and his doctor. The Epilepsy Foundation provides helpful information on what to do if an episode occurs. See http://www.epilepsyfoundation.org/answerplace/Medical/firstaid/firstaidkeys.cfm.

- **Balance problems.** Stay close to your SE and know how to stabilize him if he stumbles, seems about to fall, suddenly loses mental focus, or has had previous falls.

- **Advanced kyphosis.** The upper spine and back are severely rounded, the shoulders hunch forward, and the neck juts forward before curving back upwards. Pay careful attention to the safety issues discussed on page 92.

- **Osteoporosis.** Protect those fragile, brittle bones, but encourage your SE to do strength training because it's one of the most effective osteogenic exercises. It can increase bone mineral density and bone strength. You will need to start slowly and proceed carefully. Read up on it and talk with your SE and his doctor.

- **Osteoarthritis.** Incorporate gentle stretching into the warm-up and pay particular attention to strengthening the muscles surrounding the affected joints. Encourage cold therapy or heat therapy after each workout, whichever feels better on your SE's joints.

- **Short-term memory loss or dementia.** Introduce each exercise as if it were the first time you have taught it. Give only one instruction at the time. Be prepared to repeat the purpose and the instructions for every step. Patience is the key.

- **Stoicism about pain or a strong urge to please you**. Be alert for signs of fatigue. Every few minutes, ask, "How do you feel? How ya' doing?" Don't take "I'm fine," especially with gritted teeth, as the true indicator. Watch for the wince. Listen to the breathing. Observe the posture, observe the effort, such as muscles that are trembling with exertion, and try to spot the glazed, glassy look that shows fatigue. Have him take a longer rest period before the next set of exercises.

- **Lack of body awareness** such as raising the right arm when you ask for the left. Think, watch, and concentrate during a session, at least at the beginning. Use your SE's rest periods to take your own mental and emotional breaks. The same is true for older people who are so **trusting** and confident of your abilities that they either fail to pay close attention or are unable to tell you when fatigue or trouble sets in.

- **Hypochondria or being fearful or negative**. Emphasize the positive results of strength training as well as the safety precautions you have taken. Try to josh him into a more positive frame of mind with bits of humor. If he complains, "This will kill me!" you can respond, "But you will look great." For more information on motivation, see Chapters 8, 9, and 10.

Review "Is There Anyone Who Can't Work Out?" on page 8 for a few diseases or conditions that make exercise inadvisable or that require placing limits on the amount of weight to lift.

Agnes

It's very likely that you will worry more about safety than your SE will. Many older people are quite calm and accepting about their limitations and may even make light of them if the opportunity presents itself.

For example, an octogenarian we will call Agnes had an interesting experience. After a routine office visit to her doctor, she was trying to phone for her ride home but couldn't see well enough in the dim waiting room to punch the correct numbers.

Two other people were sitting in the room, a fellow octogenarian and her middle-aged daughter. When the daughter offered to make the phone call, Agnes said, "Thank you. I'm half deaf and mostly blind. If I were a horse, they'd shoot me."

The other older lady piped up: "For God's sake, don't break your leg or you'll be a goner for sure."

Virginia

Although hospitalized in the spring of 2005, Virginia, 93, doesn't seem worried. Like many people her age, she has made peace with life and death, and is ready for whatever happens. See her in action in the next two chapters.

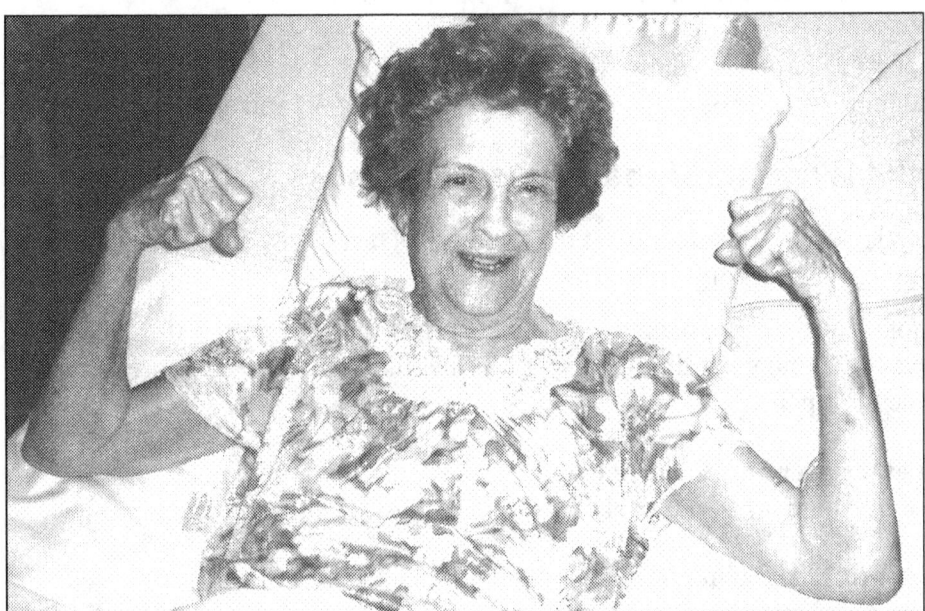

Figure 4-2. Virginia shows her biceps.

The Worst Thing about Inactivity—It Kills

The only way to avoid all risk of pain and injury is for your SE to sit on the sofa all day, but this practice has even worse risks. The results of inactivity kill far more people over age 65 than exercise ever could.

Keep in mind that strength training will actually help your SE prevent, avoid, or alleviate injuries. Fortified with good information, you can take the necessary precautions to keep your SE safe.

> Sofas ought to come with warning labels. A couch can kill you.

Arming Yourself with Knowledge

In Chapters 5 and 6, the finer points for each exercise include specific tips that are geared toward safety. "Rules for the Workout Area" on page 94 will also minimize the minor injuries that are inevitable at all ages and in all sports. Shoulders and knees are especially susceptible to injuries in older people, whether they do strength training exercises or not. Recovering from these and other types of injuries can take more time and care than for younger people. However, strength training is *safe* for people over age 65.

Regardless, it's important to recognize the warning signs of heart attack and stroke. You will learn these and more in courses at the Red Cross or a similar organization.

Recognizing the Warning Signs of a Heart Attack

For a quick introduction or review, read what the American Heart Association provides on its web site, www.americanheart.org:

- **Chest discomfort.** Most heart attacks involve discomfort in the center of the chest that lasts more than a few minutes or that recurs. It can feel like uncomfortable pressure, squeezing, fullness, or pain.

- **Discomfort in other areas of the upper body.** Symptoms can include pain or discomfort in one or both arms, the back, the neck, the jaw, or the stomach.

- **Shortness of breath.** The feeling of being unable to breathe well often precedes or accompanies chest discomfort.

- **Other signs:** These may include breaking out in a cold sweat and feeling nauseated or lightheaded.

Women's Symptoms: According to the American Heart Association, women suffering a heart attack are more likely to experience the following symptoms:

Sweating, nausea, fatigue, and pain in the jaw.

> Call EMS immediately if you think your SE could be having a heart attack or a stroke. Time lost is heart muscle lost, and time lost is brain tissue lost.

Recognizing the Warning Signs of a Stroke

The warning signs of a stroke, also called a brain attack or a cerebrovascular accident, and a transient ischemic attack (TIA) are similar, but the TIA is temporary and causes little or no brain damage while the stroke lasts longer and causes damage or death. One or more TIAs may be a warning sign that a more disabling event may happen in the future.

For a quick introduction or review, read what the American Stroke Association provides on its web site, www.strokeassociation.org:

- Sudden **numbness** or **weakness** of the face, arm, or leg, especially on one side of the body.

- Sudden **confusion** or trouble speaking or understanding.

- Sudden **trouble seeing** with one or both eyes.

- Sudden **dizziness**, trouble with walking, or loss of balance or coordination.

- Sudden, severe **headache** with no known cause.

Taking Care of Yourself

In addition to taking care of your SE, you will also need to monitor yourself. You may feel frightened or panicky if you notice heart attack or stroke symptoms, but fear and panic won't help you or your SE in a crisis. Do whatever it takes to stay calm—take a deep breath and relax for a moment. Then make the call for help, get your SE into a comfortable position, and do what is necessary until the professionals arrive.

The after-effects of any emergency may trouble your SE and you as well. You may feel as if your entire body has been pulled through a ten-inch pipe. Acknowledge the stress and pamper yourself over the next several days and week.

Do whatever works for you—massage, talk therapy, ice cream, vigorous workouts, support from people who love you, and so on. Even if you feel hesitant, don't be afraid to resume your role as Strength Coach or Spotter as soon as your SE receives medical clearance. Continuing the strength training will help both of you.

Understanding the Legal Issues

Red Cross safety courses cover the legal concerns to be aware of when you treat injuries. The main point to remember is that there is a difference between treating someone who is blood kin and someone who is not, such as your mother- or father-in-law, an aunt or uncle by marriage, or your stepfather or stepmother. Carefully note the legal implications and be prepared to act in the best interests of the person you are treating for an injury.

See the Appendix on page 257 for a typical consent form that all professional trainers ask their clients to sign in order to protect themselves against frivolous or malicious lawsuits. You may or may not want your SE to sign such a form, but consider discussing the possibilities with him and perhaps his attorney.

Protecting Your Significant Elder

Protecting your SE from injuries is the primary job of the Spotter. Some of the most beneficial strength training exercises, such as dead lifts, chair squats, bench presses, and the big pulls, are also the exercises that require the most vigilance on your part. In these exercises, your SE will be working several body parts at once, so you may feel as if you are scoring several tennis matches simultaneously.

You will be coaching, watching, listening to the breathing, troubleshooting the potential mistakes, correcting technique errors, and encouraging progress all at once. Keep focused and vigilant and you will be successful with safety.

Chances are good that your SE will never get hurt while doing strength training exercises, but watch him closely so that you can spot the signs of trouble and jump in to assist if necessary. Be especially vigilant when your SE attempts two types of motions:

- Exercises that require raising the arms above the head.

- Exercises that may cause dizziness.

Raising the Arms above the Head

For anyone with advanced kyphosis, lifting the arms overhead will be difficult or impossible. Those with this condition may never attain the flexibility needed for complete overhead lifts, and you shouldn't push it. Encourage partial completion of the exercise because this will still provide a good workout. Shoulder and chest exercises are the most common lifts that require the arms to go higher than head level.

If you are working with an obese person or someone with breathing problems, be aware that lying almost flat on the back can sometimes appear to compress the breathing mechanism. To prevent gasping, shortness of breath, or other problems, start with the bench back inclined at 35 or 40 degrees, and carefully check that his breathing is normal. If you hear even the smallest difficulty, raise the bench back until your SE can breathe comfortably.

Also, instead of keeping your SE in the semi-reclined position between sets, assist him to sit upright for the rest period. You can gradually experiment with moving the bench back closer and closer to flat, but there's no need to push it. Your SE will get a good chest workout even if you never reach the almost-flat position. Remember that the bench shouldn't be completely flat because you want his head above the level of his heart.

Frances

After Frances, 84, attained the almost-flat position on the bench, she continued to bring a small satin pillow to her strength training sessions. Sometimes she matched her outfit to its peachy pink color. When John told her that she didn't really need to use the pillow any longer, she said, "I'm not giving it up. It keeps my hair neat."

Watching Out for Dizziness

The dizziness caused by a sudden drop in blood pressure that anyone may feel when standing up too fast is called *orthostatic hypotension*. In strength training, it is most commonly induced when the head is lowered below the level of the heart and then raised too suddenly.

The exercises in Chapters 5 and 6 that are most likely to result in this phenomenon are the bench press and the good morning exercise. Also, the Sun Salutation and any of the seated exercises are likely candidates for causing dizziness if your SE stands up too quickly. Encourage a brief rest in the same seated position used for performing the exercise and then assist him to stand up slowly and carefully. Have him wait a few moments before walking.

Other exercises that might cause dizziness are those that require a down-and-up motion, such as dead lifts and good mornings. Also, any exercise that your SE may try to perform too quickly for his current fitness level may cause dizziness.

If your SE is competitive and impatient, you may have to watch that he doesn't overdo it. Don't let anyone get the better of your good judgment. As the Spotter or Strength Coach, you are the boss in the strength training room and it's your responsibility to keep your SE from overdoing it. If he continues to press too hard, consider ending the session early. See what happened to J. C.

J. C.

Some inexperienced older people will try to perform all of the exercises as fast as they can with no rest periods in between. They will wind up dizzy, exhausted, and unable to continue. Early in his training, J. C., 88, became impatient with what he perceived as slow progress. "I'm ready. Let's go. Why aren't we doing anything? This is a waste of time," he complained.

Over and over, John tried to convince J. C. that he needed rest intervals and that he needed to build up slowly to the faster workout routine that he wanted. Nothing worked to stop J. C.'s demands. "Fine," John said one day. "Let's just work continuously and see what happens."

John had to stop the session in 20 minutes because J. C. became dizzy and tired. He was simply out of gas. Never again has John let a client, even a client in good shape, goad him into such a potentially dangerous situation.

A Note on Falling Safely

Aging, loss of strength, falls, and broken hips—a recipe for disaster. Virtually everyone over age 70 or 75 is concerned, at least a little, about falling; people in their 80s and 90s may be so worried that they stop doing some of their favorite activities. Performing the leg exercises in Chapters 5 and 6 and doing Tai Chi regularly are among the best ways to prevent falls.

However, while your SE is on the road to becoming stronger, you can coach him in how to fall as safely as possible and how to get up safely from the floor after a fall or after exercising. Falling is an accident that gives very little warning, but you can teach your SE to fall safely with just a few simple principles:

1. When he feels unsteady and senses that a fall is imminent, just let it happen.

2. Relax his muscles and go with the momentum of the fall.

3. If he is falling forward, try to make himself into a ball—tuck his chin to his chest, bring his arms up to cradle and protect his head, collapse his body by sinking to his knees, and try to roll onto one hip and shoulder. Even if he lands on his knees and elbows, he can still protect his head with his hands. Rolling over onto his side after impact can also minimize the damage to his knees, elbows, and hands.

4. If he is falling backward, try to place his arms behind him so the elbows or palms will be in position to stabilize him. This action may keep his torso upright. Sitting down hard can be painful, but not as painful as falling all the way backwards and bumping his head. However, caution him not to keep his arms so straight and stiff that they absorb most of the impact. Let the buttocks do that, and use the arms or elbows only to keep his head up off the floor.

Ensure that you show him how to get up safely after a fall by practicing the techniques detailed on page 95.

Practicing Deliberate Falls

Consider asking your SE to practice falling on purpose. It's not as scary as it sounds, especially if you ask him to practice on a bed while you help him at every step.

The Forward Fall-and-Roll

Practice the forward fall-and-roll technique first. It's less frightening because he will be better able to see what's happening. In as few as half a dozen tries, spaced over two or three sessions, he may master the technique. However, consider asking him to do a refresher session every few weeks or months, depending on his strength and state of health.

Break the forward fall into two sections, assisted and unassisted. In the assisted portion, stand in front of him and hold his hands while he lowers himself to his knees. After he has performed this motion a few times, let go of his hands and ask him to tuck his chin, cradle his head, go to his knees, and roll onto one side. Stay close enough to keep one hand lightly on his shoulder or back to let him know you are right there for him.

The Backward Fall-and-Sit

The backward fall is more difficult to practice because he will feel out of control. It's best to begin by holding his hands in front while he lowers his seat to the bed and bends his knees. Ask another person to help if he's large and you're small, each of you taking one of his hands. After a few assisted downward motions, move behind him and ask him to fall-and-sit. You will be right there to prevent his head from hitting hard in case he goes over backwards. Then show him how to place his palms or elbows into position to keep himself upright.

Getting Up from the Floor Safely

The exercises in Chapters 5 and 6 don't require your SE to get down on the floor. The reason is that getting back up is difficult for many older people. However, there is a safe method of getting up, whether your SE went down deliberately or as the result of a fall, provided he experienced no major injuries.

Despite the fallen-and-can't-get-up television commercials a few years ago, many people who fall can use this safe method of getting up. The first is for those who have been exercising on the floor, such as doing crunches on a mat. The other is for those who have fallen accidentally.

Getting Up after Exercising

It's a good idea to demonstrate the motions and then take your SE through the correct steps. The instructions begin with him in the supine position lying flat on his back. Ask him to:

1. Roll over onto his side, bend his knees and bring them up to hip or waist level, and bring his elbows in front of his torso.

2. Roll and push himself onto his hands and knees and reach for or crawl over to a sturdy piece of furniture for support.

3. Lean his torso on the furniture and push against it to raise his torso and place his weight on his knees.

4. Bring one knee up, and place that foot flat on the floor. Continuing to push against the support, bring the other knee up, and place that foot flat on the floor.

5. Extend the legs and push the hips up, still leaning over on the support. Slowly extend the back and raise the upper body.

6. Remain still in the standing position for a few moments, especially if he feels dizzy or shaky. When he is steady on his feet, take a few steps while remaining near the piece of furniture for support.

Getting Up after a Fall

If he falls onto his back, which is common after slipping on ice or water and losing his balance, the steps are the same as those above. The only additional note is for him to lie still for a minute or two to assess his possible injuries. If he hit harder on his left side, for example, he needs to roll onto his right side in Step 1 above because his right arm will be stronger. Caution him to take his time so he can assess his physical and mental condition.

If he falls forward, which is common after tripping over something on the floor, he may find himself spread-eagled on his stomach, possibly with his arms underneath his body. Or he may have landed on one side. In both situations, he needs to assess his condition first. If he is able, he then rolls onto his stronger (uninjured) side and continues with Step 2 above. Again, caution him to move slowly and carefully as he makes his way to a standing position.

Setting Rules for the Workout Area

It's a good idea to make posters for the workout room that list common safety rules. If you look around your own gym, you will probably see several courtesy rules, such as Replace Your Weights on This Rack, Wipe Up Your Sweat, and the like. For your SE, consider some of the following statements.

Eat Before You Work Out—Don't Skip Breakfast
Warm Up Before You Work Out—Don't Start Cold
Keep Your Eyes Open—It Helps Your Balance
Breathe—Don't Hold Your Breath while Exercising
Inhale on Preparation—Exhale out on Performance
Take the Universal Stance—Flex Your Knees
Take Your Time—Rest when You Need To

See page 106 for a large-font version of these safety rules. Photocopy them and place them strategically around the strength training room if you like. Reminders are good for everyone but especially for older people who may be exercising for the first time in a long while and who may also be a little forgetful.

Further, seeing the posters will reinforce what you have been saying all along. Putting up posters is just one more thing you can do to keep your SE safe. It's up to you to enforce these rules and to encourage your SE to follow them.

Helping Your Significant Elder Recover from Injuries

An injury is anything that causes physical damage to the body, usually with accompanying pain. Injuries require that the injured person discontinue or limit the activity that caused the injury. In older people, many injuries are due to a lack of strength caused by a sedentary life style. Falls, sprains, and strains are much more likely to occur in the weak and frail. Thus, a strong, active person is less prone to a variety of injuries.

In the early stages of strength training, your SE may be at some risk of injury because of muscular weakness and unfamiliarity with the exercises. Even then, however, it's much more likely that the activities of daily living, not the exercise, will cause discomfort or pain. John estimates that 95 to 98% of the injuries sustained by his older clients occur *outside* the training setting. But you still need to be prepared.

Coping with Immediate, Short-term Treatment

If an injury occurs in the exercise room, you will be the right person to treat it, and you want to be well prepared. As you will learn in your basic first aid course, the best way to treat muscle and joint injuries on the scene is with PRICE—Protection, Rest, Ice, Compression, and Elevation:

- **Protection** means that immediately after an injury occurs, protect the site of the injury from further damage. Don't let your SE use the injured muscles or joints. Help him avoid putting weight on the injury. Support the injured area.

- **Rest** means not only avoiding any activities that cause pain to the injured area but also resting the entire body to allow the injury to heal optimally. Before the pain kicks in on an ankle injury, it's probably okay for your SE to hop a couple of steps to a chair with your assistance, but no farther. Thereafter, make sure the injury site is free of stress and does not bear his weight.

- **Ice** means to apply an instant cold pack to the site of the injury as soon as possible. The cold pack will reduce swelling and inflammation. Apply additional ice packs for 15-20 minutes of each hour for the first several hours. Afterwards, your SE may need to use an ice pack several times a day until the pain and swelling clear up.

- **Compression** means applying pressure to the site, usually right after the first treatment with a cold pack. Either use hand pressure or bind the painful area with an elastic bandage to cut down on swelling. You shouldn't wrap an injury so tightly that the area goes numb, tingles, or turns purple. Your SE should always remove the bandage at night for sleeping. As the injury heals, wrap the area with athletic tape to provide some support. The basic first aid course will show you how to wrap an injury correctly.

- **Elevation** means raising the injured area to a level above the heart to reduce the pain and swelling. If you can't get the injured area above heart level, then raise it as high as you can without causing discomfort.

Practicing PRICE is an excellent way to help your SE recover from a minor injury with a minimum of discomfort and a maximum of healing. If you feel that the injury requires more care than you can provide, or if your SE wants medical help, then get it. After most minor injuries, though, your SE can resume exercise sessions as soon as the pain and swelling have gone away or decreased significantly, usually in only a few days. If the swelling remains, take him to his physician for an X-ray as there could be a broken bone.

Depending upon the seriousness of the injury, your SE may need to skip some sessions. When you resume, allow for several lighter-than-usual workouts. The important thing is to have a plan for returning your SE to strength training as soon as it's safely possible. If you can't be the Spotter or Strength Coach for a while, then be the Advocate by talking with his doctor and developing a recovery plan for resuming exercise.

Be aware that there's a large gray area between injuries that you can treat on the basis of your first aid training and those that you can't treat. Always err on the side of caution. You may have done a commendable job with icing and bandaging an ankle injury, for example, but you may be completely unaware that the training accident also fractured a small bone in the foot. If you are in doubt, get your SE to a medical professional.

Coping with Ongoing, Long-term Treatment

Whether injured in the exercise room or somewhere else, your SE may have to undergo surgery, wear a cast or splint for some time, go through a period of physical or occupational therapy, or all of the above. During the treatment period, you will have access to the medical professionals when you accompany your SE to the hospital or to subsequent check-ups. Ask questions, understand the nature of the injury, and discuss when and how to resume exercise. Long-distance Advocates can keep abreast of the situation by phone.

Particularly in cases of physical and occupational therapy, it's important to develop a plan with the therapist so that after therapy ends, usually when the insurance runs out, you can incorporate the essential home therapy exercises into your SE's strength training program. Explain to the therapist the exercises your SE has been doing, and get a good idea of the treatment the therapist is using. If possible, watch the therapist work with your SE. Together, develop a plan to make a smooth transition from therapy to strength training.

As injured muscles or the muscles supporting injured joints become stronger, there will be less likelihood of subsequent injuries to that area. If you and your SE have any questions or concerns after returning home, call the therapist to make sure you are doing the home exercises properly.

Returning to Training during and after Recovery

After a minor injury, your SE may want to resume strength training exercises before you think he's ready. Overcome your aversion and foster his desire as soon as the medical professionals agree that it's time for him to exercise.

After an injury, *plan* for your Significant Elder to
return to strength training. Don't leave it to chance.

If your SE has been largely inactive for a period of time during recovery, however, then plan on lighter workouts for a while. Ask your SE to do three sets of ten repetitions according to the scale below. If the discomfort becomes obvious at any point before rep 6 or 7 of the third set, then stop the exercise and lower the weights at the next session:

- For one or two weeks of inactivity, reduce the amount of weight on each exercise by 10% to 20%. For the manual exercises, reduce your level of resistance.

- For three to four weeks of inactivity, reduce the amount of weight on each exercise by 20% to 30%. Adjust your resistance on the manual exercises.

- For two to three months of inactivity, reduce the amount of weight on each exercise by 35% to 40% or more if necessary. You may need to provide no resistance on the manual exercises, only using your strength to support him.

For longer periods of inactivity, you may need to return to the weights and exercises that you used at the beginning of your SE's strength training. This time, however, you will definitely see more rapid progress than you did at first because he is now experienced at strength training and has some muscle memory of the exercises. Always take things slow and easy, and reduce the weights and the number of repetitions at the first sign of discomfort.

The most important points to impress upon your SE are these:

- Strength training will continue.

- The time spent on home exercises prescribed by his physician or therapist are more important in his recovery than the time spent in strength training sessions.

- The recovery exercises that the therapist prescribes will probably need to continue daily, sometimes several times a day, over several weeks or months.

- Your SE needs to do the prescribed recovery exercises faithfully.

- A home health therapist may be available after your SE leaves the hospital or doctor's office, especially if there was significant loss of function or strength.

You need to check up on these medically prescribed exercises. Make sure that your SE does them with the correct technique and at the appropriate times during the day. Devote part of the training sessions to these recovery exercises, if necessary. If you are the Advocate, phone your SE right after he is supposed to have done the exercises and ask, for example, "How's that knee feeling? Do you have less pain?" Give him all due praise for continuing his exercises. In short, make every effort to ensure a successful recovery.

It's hard to tell how often physical or occupational therapy fails due to clients' neglecting to comply with the prescribed post-clinical routine. But the number is probably high. Don't let this happen to your SE.

Dave

It's a good thing Dave Brady, 69, is in such great shape. In his early 60s, he suffered a heart attack complicated by blood filling his chest cavity. He had only 20% of his normal lung capacity before undergoing surgery to correct the problem.

Two weeks after his heart attack, he entered cardio rehab where he walked on the treadmill and rode a stationary bicycle for 5-, 10-, and 15- minute intervals, pausing for the physical therapist to monitor his heart. All went well. Three weeks after his heart attack, he was back in the gym. He took it slow, used very light weights, and listened to his body. It was several weeks before he resumed his heavy lifts, but resume he did.

On another occasion, he tore his rotator cuff and went through 28 weeks of rehab. It worked because he got back to his same strength level. By the way, Dave is a state, national, and world record holder in his age group in power lifting. Here are his best lifts:

- Squat—363 pounds.

- Bench press—275 pounds.

- Dead lift—342 pounds.

- Meet total—957 pounds.

In power sport competitions, his best total for the combined bench press and dead lift is 617 pounds. The world record is 622 pounds, and Dave expects to beat it at his next competition. Dave looks forward to turning 70 so he will be in a different age group and can go after a new set of world records. Dave inspires everyone who knows him. He is the first to state that strength training won't prevent medical crises altogether, but he insists that it shortens his recovery time.

Helping the Reluctant to Resume Exercise

If your SE is unwilling to return to strength training after a major injury, you can certainly sympathize with the fears behind the reluctance or the lingering pain. However, at some point, the doctor or the therapist will write a prescription for home exercises. As the healing progresses, you can then help to implement this prescription by returning to your duties as Spotter or Strength Coach.

Always encourage your SE to return to strength training as soon as the doctor approves.

One useful tool for diagnosing how much pain your SE is really feeling is to use a scale of perceived pain, such as *Borg's Perceived Exertion and Pain Scales*, by Gunnar Borg.[17] Or you could simply ask your SE to rate the pain between zero and ten, with ten being the most painful. If the number stays at nine for three weeks, for example, you can instigate another trip to the doctor to determine why the healing isn't going as well as expected. You may suspect as much malingering as you like, but never voice any of it. Always stay positive.

You can also ask your SE for an assessment of how hard he thinks he's working if he seems to be taking an unusually long time in returning to the level of exertion he achieved before the injury occurred. Using the Borg Scale can help. Instructions for the Borg Rating of Perceived Exertion (RPE) Scale are widely available.[18]

> While doing physical activity, we want you to rate your perception of exertion. This feeling should reflect how heavy and strenuous the exercise feels to you, combining all sensations and feelings of physical stress, effort, and fatigue. Do not concern yourself with any one factor such as leg pain or shortness of breath, but try to focus on your total feeling of exertion.
>
> Look at the rating scale below while you are engaging in an activity; it ranges from 6 to 20, where 6 means "no exertion at all" and 20 means "maximal exertion." Choose the number from below that best describes your level of exertion. This will give you a good idea of the intensity level of your activity, and you can use this information to speed up or slow down your movements to reach your desired range.
>
> Try to appraise your feeling of exertion as honestly as possible, without thinking about what the actual physical load is. Your own feeling of effort and exertion is important, not how it compares to other people's. Look at the scales and the expressions and then give a number.

---

6 No exertion at all
7
Extremely light (7.5)
8
9 Very light
10

---

[17] Chicago: Human Kinetics, 1998.
[18] See the Web site of the Centers for Disease Control and Prevention at http://www.cdc.gov/nccdphp/dnpa/physical/measuring/perceived_exertion.htm:

11	Light
12	
13	Somewhat hard
14	
15	Hard (heavy)
16	
17	Very hard
18	
19	Extremely hard
20	Maximal exertion

Notes:

9 corresponds to "very light" exercise. For a healthy person, it is like walking slowly at his or her own pace for some minutes.

13 on the scale is "somewhat hard" exercise, but it still feels OK to continue.

17 "very hard" is very strenuous. A healthy person can still go on, but he or she really has to push him- or herself. It feels very heavy, and the person is very tired.

19 on the scale is an extremely strenuous exercise level. For most people this is the most strenuous exercise they have ever experienced.

The Borg scale was designed to correspond to the typical heart rate at rest and during progressively harder exercise. It is most accurate for young, healthy people, but it's also useful for older people as a rough indication of effort.

Staying Positive

On an upbeat note, consider an injury to one part of the body as a golden opportunity to work other parts of the body until the injury heals. A wrist injury, for example, is a great time to work the legs and the abdominal muscles. Similarly, an ankle injury gives you the perfect chance to work the upper body. In short, no minor injury is an excuse to skip more than a few workouts, and very few major injuries should cause a permanent halt to your SE's exercise program.

You can also stay positive by encouraging and participating in activities that put little or no stress on the body, such as easy yoga, water aerobics, swimming, walking, or Tai Chi. See Chapter 9 for some additional benefits of these activities. The important thing is to help your SE avoid sitting on the couch or lying in bed for extended periods. As long as the medical professionals have cleared your SE to resume activities, then these are what he shall have.

An Inspiring Footrace—Kirk and Wang

Safety information has its somber side, and you may be wondering by now whether to even try to get your SE off the sofa and into the strength training room. You may be thinking that older people have far too many issues with health and safety for you to feel comfortable working with them. Take heart. For an uplifting tale, consider the story of two elite athletes in their 90s. At the World Veteran Games in 1989, Wang Chingchang, then age 94, and Herbert S. Kirk, then age 90, competed fiercely in the men's 200-meter dash:

> Wang bolted to a 5-m lead off the turn. But Kirk charged with 80 meters to go and passed Wang with 40 left, as the crowd stood roaring. Wang, amazingly, dug down and re-passed Kirk, winning by a foot, 52.21 to 52.33 sec. But this race wasn't over. Kirk, who had given up tennis at 86 because he could no longer see the ball, didn't see the finish line either. He kept right on sprinting. Wang, fiercely competitive, went with him, and they dueled for another 70 meters before they were stopped. As they trotted back, it was in front of a delirious, tearful throng.[19]

More Inspiration—Track and Field after Age 75

Les Amey competes in senior sports at age 101. Rosari Iglesias began running competitively at 79. She still does so at 90. Wally Dashiell throws the javelin at age 78. Melvin Larsen and Hugo Delgado, both 77, tied in a 100-meter race at 14.43 seconds. Many men in their 40s can run 100 meters in 11 seconds. The record is 9.79 seconds, set by Maurice Greene at age 28.[20]

Not all of these older athletes are life-long competitors, and not all are genetically endowed, but they show something important about the human potential. They also show that your SE probably can exercise and become much stronger than either of you realizes.

A Note to Certified Personal Trainers

If you have always worked with younger clients, this chapter shows you how to support older clients who have undergone extensive physical or occupational therapy. It is vitally important that you work closely with health care providers, if possible, when or if older clients sustain injuries. You will also need to be prepared for considerable interaction with your clients' grown children and may need to assure and reassure them that you will do everything in your power to keep Mom or Dad safe.

John always makes a point of trying to meet with the physical and occupational therapists to go over treatment plans so he can continue the good work in the training sessions. A few therapists have been known to show little regard for the benefits of strength training, but if you approach them respectfully and on behalf of the client you have in common, most will work with you to achieve what's best for the client.

For example, when Esther, 92, had severe neck pain, her physical therapist used ultrasound, massage, and deep muscle exercises to solve the problem. The physical therapist compared

---

[19] Moore, K "The Times of Their Lives." *Runner's World* (1992), vol. 20, pp. 44-47. Cited in Spirduso, Waneen W. *Physical Dimensions of Aging*. Chicago: Human Kinetics, 1995, pp. 390-391.

[20] Dowling, Tim. "Older and Better," SAGA Magazine, October 2002, pp. 58-62. On the cover, don't miss the 80-year-old pole vaulter.

notes with John, who immediately saw how to provide exercises that continued strengthening her neck and shoulder muscles.

John also takes responsibility for checking up on whether his older clients faithfully perform the motions prescribed by doctors or physical therapists on days when he doesn't train them. Sometimes he has to kid them along to motivate them. Remember:

- Use extra precautions for safety with older clients.

- Work with medical personnel and physical and occupational therapists after an injury.

Summary of the Main Points

Safety, injuries, and recovery are important but not necessarily frightening aspects of strength training with your SE. To be as well prepared as possible, keep these main points in mind:

- Practice safety by knowing your SE extremely well and by taking safety courses at the Red Cross or a similar organization.

- Protect your SE by knowing how to guard against injuries on the most difficult exercises and by establishing good safety rules in the strength training room.

- Know how to help your SE recover from injuries by practicing PRICE and by knowing how to return safely to strength training during the recovery period.

- Cultivate a safe frame of mind. Be knowledgeable, alert, and relaxed just like the professional trainers.

What's Next?

Part II, "Getting Going," starts with the actual training sessions for your SE. It's a good idea to begin the training sessions with Chapter 5. Even if you believe he is strong enough to start with Chapter 6, it will do no harm to spend a few weeks or months on the beginning exercises.

There are two reasons to start gradually. One is to make sure you aren't overestimating his strength and abilities. The other is to gain thorough knowledge of the exercises you may need to revert to in case an injury, an illness, or a long vacation causes an extended layoff from strength training.

In Chapter 5, you will learn how to provide the safest starting point for your SE. These exercises will enhance his life, help him feel good, improve his health, and restore a significant amount of his former strength.

Each exercise contains sections on the *preparation*, the *performance*, and the *finer points*. An *additional note on safety* is included for some of the exercises so that you can assure yourself and your SE that the exercises are as safe as humanly possible.

Move on to Chapter 6 only when your SE is ready and able to perform these slightly more difficult exercises.

Then Chapter 7 helps you see how to improve the eating and sleeping habits of your SE so that he will receive the maximum benefit from the exercises.

Safety Rules for Significant Elders

Eat Before You Work Out—Don't Skip Breakfast

Warm Up Before You Lift—Don't Start Cold

Keep Your Eyes Open—It Helps Your Balance

Breathe—Don't Hold Your Breath while Lifting

Inhale on Preparation—Exhale on Performance

Take the Universal Stance—Flex Your Knees

Take Your Time—Rest when You Need To

PART II. GETTING GOING

"If anyone had told me that when I reached my sixth decade I would begin lifting free weights and working out on weight-training machinery, I would have called them crazy... The thought of lifting weights was ridiculous to me ...I think in some ways Debra [Richards' personal trainer] saved my life."
    Ann Richards, former Governor of Texas[21]

Now that you have gotten ready, Part II presents what you need to know to get going in strength training with your Significant Elder or how to be truly supportive if you take the role of Advocate. You will learn:

- The top 10 exercises to teach first. These will help your Significant Elder regain strength and health.

- The next 12 exercises to add as soon as your SE is able. These exercises will help maintain her strength and health throughout life. Three of the exercises are considered advanced, but the other nine are available for variety as soon as your SE has mastered Chapter 5.

- The best practices for nutrition and rest. This knowledge will keep your SE well fueled for strength training.

When you finish Part II, you will be ready to get ahead by seeing some inspiring information in the case studies, enhancing your SE's performance with mind-body awareness, and empowering your Significant Elder.

---

[21] Ann Richards with Richard U. Levine, *I'm Not Slowing Down: Winning My Battle with Osteoporosis* (New York: Dutton, 2003), p. 131, 136, 137.

Chapter 5. Top 10 Exercises for Reclaiming Strength

Helping your Significant Elder Regain Strength for the Activities of Daily Living

"I tried to go to those group sessions, but I couldn't keep up with them. I thought if I couldn't do it, they were more advanced than I was. And I just felt like I wanted somebody who could work with me with the ability that I have."
   Frances, "84 years young"

Note: A physician's examination is recommended for all exercise participants with any restrictions and for those persons over forty (40) years of age. Fitness evaluation participants in these categories who have not had a physical examination in the past year must acknowledge that they have been informed of its importance and, therefore, accept full responsibility for their health and wellbeing. Participants understand that no responsibility is assumed by a personal trainer or the authors of this book. If you intend to train your SE, take four to six lessons with a certified personal trainer so that you can teach the correct techniques.

Important Points for Advocates: To help you follow up in your weekly phone calls, learn the name of each exercise and the muscle group or groups that it engages. Consider buying your SE the exercise band pictured in Figure 5-6 on page 116. If you want to expand your knowledge about the muscles, we recommend two books.[22]

Introduction

These beginning exercises are designed for regaining physical function so that your Significant Elder can continue or resume doing the activities of daily living. Before teaching an exercise, however, review the section on the universal stance, page 69, and the athletic seated posture and resistance breathing, both on page 70. You may need to devote much of the first several strength training sessions to these principles.

Note: Do not ask your SE to perform these exercises until she has warmed up thoroughly. See page 72.

---

[22] Biel, Andrew. *Trail Guide to the Body: How to Locate Muscles, Bones, and More.* (Boulder, CO: Books of Discovery, 2001) and Frederic Delavier. *Strength Training Anatomy.* (Chicago: Human Kinetics, 2001).

Each exercise in this chapter contains a section on:

- **Preparation**—getting ready to do the exercise.

- **Performance**—exactly what to do to complete the exercise.

- **Finer points**—the expert knowledge that will increase your SE's strength and health *safely*.

The last exercise in the chapter provides **an additional note on safety** on page 134 so that you can be on the lookout for the things that sometimes lead to injuries in doing that exercise. You want to prevent mishaps to the best of your ability.

These exercises are presented in the order in which you need to use them in a training session. Be prepared to demonstrate each exercise repeatedly until your SE can do it correctly with a minimum of instruction. Even then, refreshers at each training session may be necessary.

There are three good reasons why it's a good idea to start with these top 10 exercises unless your SE is extraordinarily strong *and* you have a history of showing the ropes to inexperienced lifters in the gym. These reasons relate to age or frailty, safety and recovery, and inexperience or fear.

Before you teach these exercises to your SE, master them yourself under the supervision of a certified personal trainer. Demonstrate each exercise several times. You may need to remind your SE at each training session.

Age or Frailty

You will want to start with these exercises if your SE is over age 75 or 80 just to be on the safe side. If it turns out that she's stronger than you thought, you can move on to the exercises in Chapter 6 after only a few sessions or a few weeks with these beginning exercises. In this case, listen carefully for her first complaints that the exercises are too easy or that she doesn't feel that she's getting anywhere with the training sessions. However, recall that J. C. on page 93 pushed too hard and couldn't complete his workout.

Some older people, who have been sedentary for so long that they are already frail or close to it may need to do these exercises for many months before they will be strong enough to move on to Chapter 6. In fact, they may never master all of those exercises, but over time, you can probably introduce several of the Chapter 6 exercises if your SE is willing and able. See the discussion of frailty on page 21.

You certainly need to start with these beginning exercises if your SE has lost some of her former abilities, such as:

- Crouching to pick up something and then standing up straight with good posture.

- Walking with a confident, non-shuffling stride while carrying bags of groceries.

- Reaching straight overhead to place something fairly heavy on a high shelf.

- Standing up from a chair without rocking back and forth first or pushing up with her hands and arms.

These and other activities of daily living are usually recoverable if she can regain enough muscular strength and flexibility through strength training.

Safety and Recovery

The exercises in Chapter 6 are certainly not *un*safe, but those in this chapter are safer because your SE can perform many of them in a seated position or with your assistance. Even if her balance is unsteady, she won't fall and hurt herself before you can steady her. Also, these exercises use little or no equipment. Instead, use your body weight[23] in several of them and will place your hands on her shoulders or clasp her hands in yours to provide stability. These exercises are very, very safe.

Another point is that later on after you have moved on to the exercises in Chapter 6, you can always revert to one or more of the beginning exercises if your SE experiences sore muscles or a minor injury or illness. You won't want your SE to stop training altogether during the recovery period.

Finally, if you teach the beginning exercises first before moving on to those in Chapter 6, you will find it easier to go back to them as needed. When she has a minor injury or illness, her motivation and interest in learning new exercises can decrease or disappear. However, if she already knows the beginning exercises in this chapter, she's more likely to embrace them as old friends during the challenging times when she may need lighter workouts.

Inexperience or Fear

If you want to be the Spotter or Strength Coach but have little experience in training other people, you need to begin with the exercises in this chapter even if your SE seems strong enough for those in Chapter 6. You will feel more secure as a newcomer if you can conduct much of the training session with her in a seated position instead of standing.

Prevail over any objections that your sturdy, under-70, athletic father, for example, might state about these exercises by explaining that they are the training wheels for both of you. He will need them for a few weeks if he's never done strength training before or hasn't

---

[23] Alan Hedrick, strength coach at the U. S. Air Force Academy in Colorado Springs, CO, developed dozens of manual exercises that use body weight instead of machines to provide resistance. Some of them are adapted for use with Significant Elders.

exercised in a long time, and you will need them for a while because you haven't trained anyone before.

Finally, your SE may be somewhat fearful or nervous about strength training, indeed, about taking up anything new late in life. If so, you can ease her apprehensions by demonstrating each exercise a couple of times—prove to her that it's non-threatening. Let her watch the training session of someone in her age group and at her approximate level of physical ability. She will probably take heart and realize that she can do it, too.

> Age, frailty, inexperience, and fear are *great* reasons to work out safely.

The Abdominal Muscles—Two Exercises

Starting a training session by exercising the abdominal muscles is a good idea because everyone claims to hate abdominal or ab exercises. Doing them first is a good way to get them over early in the training session when your resolution—and your SE's—is high. In addition, contracting the abs is a relatively short, simple motion, which makes the chances of muscle strain very small. In many respects, exercising the abs provides a transition between the warm-up and the exercises for the other major muscle groups.

The primary function of the abdominal muscles is to support the spine, that is, to keep the spine upright. Many older people who fall do so because they lose their balance and stick out an arm or a foot to brace themselves. But if they lack the lower back and abdominal strength, their body can't support them and they will fall. A bad fall can result in major injuries or even death.

> 300,000 people are admitted to U. S. emergency rooms each year with a broken hip, many due to a fall. Often, osteoporosis makes a fracture even worse.[24]

---

[24] *Exercise: A Guide from the National Institute on Aging* at http://weboflife.ksc.nasa.gov/exerciseandaging/chapter4_balance.html.

The Seated Push

The seated push is a good ab exercise for your SE because there's no chance of her getting hurt. This exercise requires one sturdy straight chair with arms for your SE. Sit in a second chair while you provide resistance during the exercise.

Preparation

Ask your SE to do the following:

- Sit at the front edge of the chair with both feet on the floor, knees about a foot apart. If her feet don't touch the floor firmly, place something—a small bench, books, or possibly your own feet—under hers.

- Sit as upright as possible with the shoulder blades pushed down or depressed and pulled together or retracted.

- Inhale and prepare to push forward as you provide gentle resistance with your hands.

Sit in front of her, as John does in Figure 5-1 with Mary, 91. Make sure you are close enough to reach across and place the heels of your hands on the front of her shoulders.

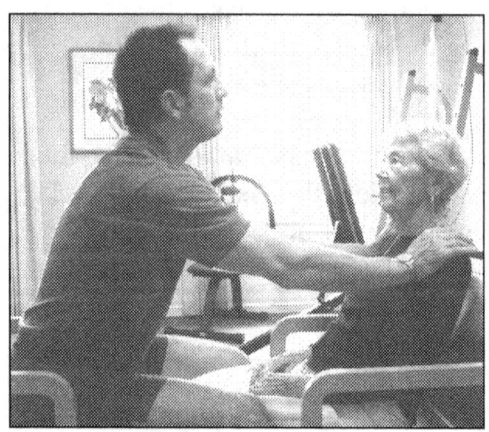

Figure 5-1. Mary prepares for the seated push.

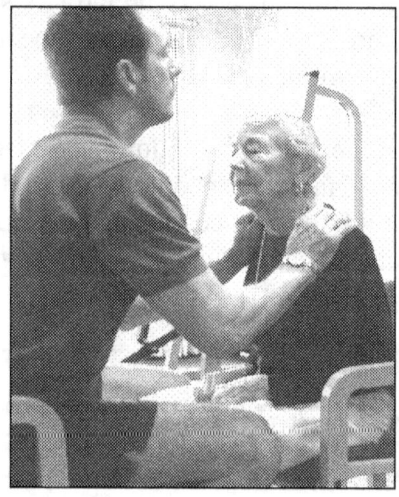

Figure 5-2. Mary performs the seated push.

Performance

Ask your SE to do the following while keeping her back strong and flat:

- Exhale and push as far forward as possible while still keeping the back flat and straight, as Mary does in Figure 5-2. Return to the original position while inhaling.

- Repeat up to 10-15 reps.

- Rest for 30 seconds to one minute.

You will apply enough resistance to make the push somewhat difficult but easy enough for her to do it at least 10 times. A little practice will help you understand how much resistance to apply. Increase the resistance over time. As with all exercises in which you provide the resistance for your SE, develop a scale for estimating how hard you push. Or use the scale suggested on page 57:

1 = Very Light, 2 = Light, 3 = Medium, 4 = Heavy, 5 = Very Heavy

Finer Points

At first, your SE may not understand the purpose of this exercise for strengthening the abs. Here are some common mistakes:

- Extending her neck too far forward.

- Pushing only her shoulders forward, an action that doesn't actively engage the abs.

- Rounding her back so that she can thus use all of her strength.

None of these mistakes will prevent her abs from contracting. However, for the safest and most efficient technique, your SE should try to be a single moving unit that is hinged at the hips and flat all along the back. Play it by ear. Give yourself some time—three or four sessions—for her to perform the exercise correctly. Eventually, her body will remember the correct motion. This is a very good, safe, and interactive exercise for the abdominal muscles.

As she becomes proficient, you can increase the difficulty of the exercise by employing an important but often under-taught skill: ask her to *yield with strength* as she returns to the upright position. She will keep her abs tight and will continue to push against your hands on the return motion.

Chair Crunches

The main difference between crunches for your SE and crunches for people of your own age is that she will do them seated in a chair while you generally lie on the floor or on a bench. The reason for using a chair is that getting down on the floor may be hard or impossible, and getting back up may take too much effort. Also, chair crunches are safer because this exercise recruits additional muscle groups for assistance.

Note that the hip flexors are the muscles that actually cause the upward motion of her feet in this exercise. The abdominal muscles are recruited as stabilizers, so she will still get quite a bit of ab work. As long as you ensure that she keeps her knees bent, not straightening her legs out in front, she will keep the hip flexor involvement to a minimum.

Preparation

Ask your SE to do the following:

- Sit in the chair with her hips and the small of her back firmly against the back of the chair.

- Place her feet about a foot apart on the floor.

- Place her elbows and forearms on the arms of the chair and grasp the arms firmly.

- Use her hands and arms to brace herself and to keep her lower back and hips pushed against the back of the chair.

Sit in another chair at a right angle with her knees. Place the palm and heel of your hand on the front of her shoulder that's nearer to you. For example, if you are seated perpendicular to her on her right, then place your left hand on her right shoulder.

The purpose of your touch is to remind her not to lean forward when she performs this exercise. The purpose is not to restrain her or to provide resistance. Figures 5-3 and 5-4 show Frances, 84, preparing for and performing the chair crunch.

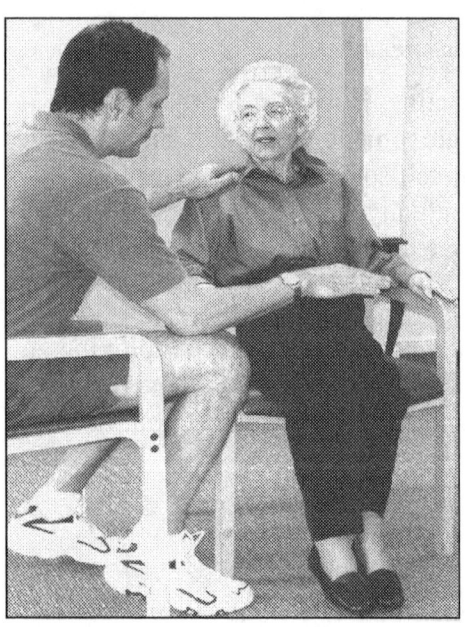

Figure 5-3. Frances prepares for the chair crunch.

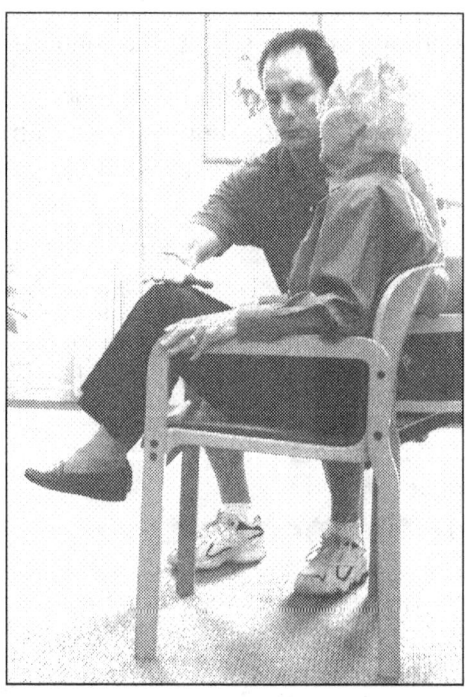

Figure 5-4. Frances performs the chair crunch.

Performance

Ask your SE to do the following:

- Inhale.

- While exhaling, slowly and steadily lift both knees as high as she can, usually only an inch or two at first, but see how high Frances can lift her feet!

- While inhaling, slowly and steadily lower her feet to touch the floor.

- Repeat for 8-12 reps.

- Relax and rest for 30-60 seconds.

Finer Points

It's okay if you feel her shoulder coming forward during the set because her body is attempting to actively contract the abs. However, remind her with gentle pressure on her shoulder, and a few words if necessary, to keep her lower back against the back of the chair. Ask her to press the small of her back against the chair.

A potential technique problem to watch for is scooting her seat a few inches forward in the chair. If she moves her back and seat forward, she will usually be able to raise her knees higher, which she might mistake for the purpose of the exercise. However, the point is to fatigue her stomach muscles.

Another point is to ask her to relax her shoulders or to pull her shoulder blades back and together to help her focus her energies on her abs. As she tires, she may yank or jerk violently to recruit the lower back muscles. Warn her not to do this because she can place harmful stress on her lower back.

As she gets the hang of this exercise, you can hold your free hand—your right if you have your left hand on her shoulder—a few inches above her knees to give her a target to aim for. When she consistently hits your hand each time during a set, then raise it an inch or so next time. Continue gradually raising your hand over time to provide just a little more challenge.

Eventually, you can also ask her not to touch the floor but to keep her abs tight and raise her feet without touching down until the end of the set.

The Upper Back Muscles—The Seated Band Pull

Pulling is the essential exercise for the latissimus dorsi, lower trapezius, and rhomboid muscles. The upper back pull is the best action to improve the posture. The older person who pulls regularly is no slouch and won't slump over. Pulling is the hardest exercise to do in a home setting because in a gym, it takes special equipment. Recall the seated row on page iii. Using a band, pictured in Figure 5-5, is an excellent substitute.

The seated band pull is the first and simplest of all the band exercises. When your SE is sitting, she will need little sense of balance in order to complete the exercise. In addition to a sturdy chair or bench, you will need two items:

- A door that closes securely or a sturdy weight-bearing pole or column. If you are extremely strong, you can consider holding one end of the band in place, but be extra careful. The backlash from a band is enormously painful and could cause serious injury.

- A 4- or 5-foot length of rubber tubing with a hand grip on each end.

A therapeutic rubber band, such as a Theraband™, works reasonably well, but it doesn't feel as comfortable in the hands as a tube with handles such as the band pictured in Figure 5-5. The band also has an extension piece to fit through the space between a door and its jamb when the door is securely closed. The advantage of this product is that you can raise or lower the level of the tube to match your SE's seated height.[25]

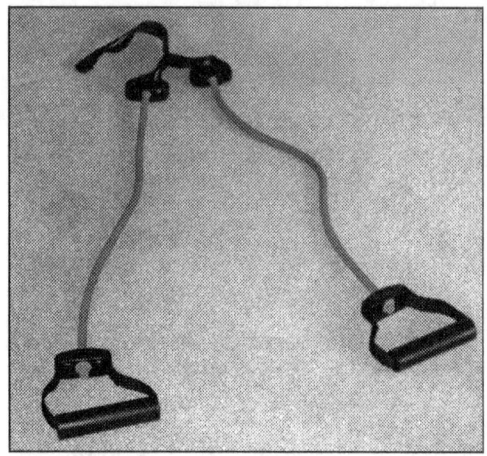

Figure 5-5. The handles provide a good grip.

Preparation

Ask your SE to:

- Use the athletic seated posture and sit on the front edge of the chair facing the doorjamb with the knees apart and the feet on the floor.

- Grasp the handles of the bands.

As the Strength Coach or Spotter, you will do the following:

- Insert the band in the space between the door and the jamb and close the door securely.

---

[25] John recommends the J. C. Santana travel band in fuchsia pink available at www.performbetter.com.

- Help your SE move the chair far enough away from the jamb so that, when she grasps the bands with her arms outstretched, there is no slack in the bands.

Performance

Ask your SE to do the following:

- Inhale. Then exhale and simultaneously pull both bands toward her as far as she can, pulling her shoulder blades together or retracting them as she does so. Retain the upright posture. Do not lean back. See Figures 5-6 and 5-7.

- Inhale as she returns her hands to the original position.

- Repeat 8-12 times.

- Rest for 30 seconds to a minute.

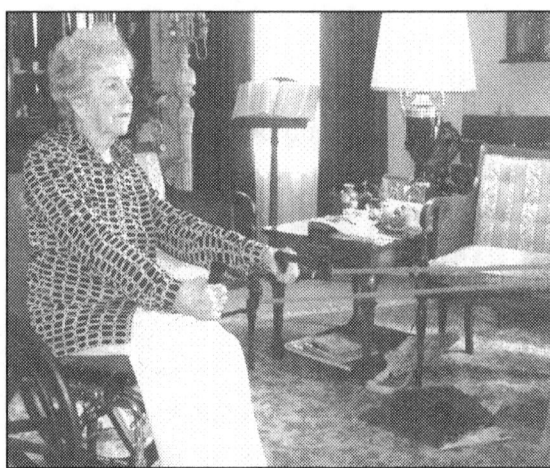

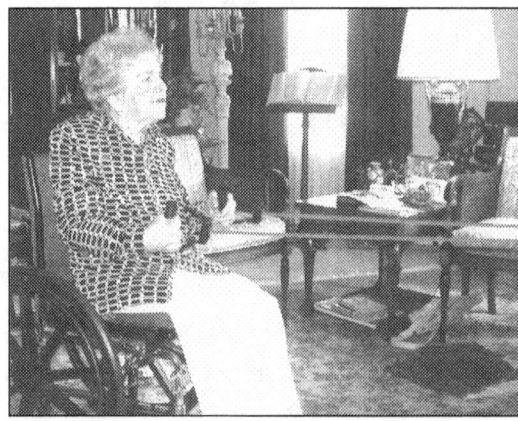

Figure 5-7. Lyn pulls both hands toward her.

Figure 5-6. Lyn prepares for the seated band pull.

Finer Points

The seated band pull is an extremely important exercise. It is easy to perform but there are several requirements that your SE will use again and again:

- She must maintain good, upright posture. If she has trouble with full shoulder blade retraction when pulling the hands close to the body, ask her to thrust her chest forward.

- She needs to focus, physically and mentally, on the position of her shoulder blades. Throughout the exercise the shoulder blades need to be depressed or down and retracted or together.

- During the return motion, she should make an effort not to protract or separate the shoulder blades.

- When she has mastered the two-handed pull, you can ask her to pull one arm at the time, as Lyn does in Figures 5-8 and 5-9. This action requires better control, so always start with two hands.

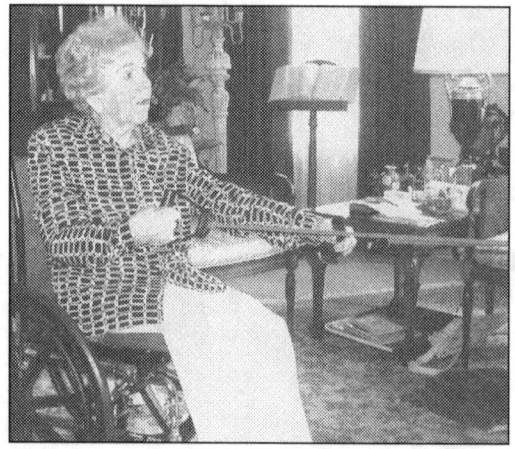

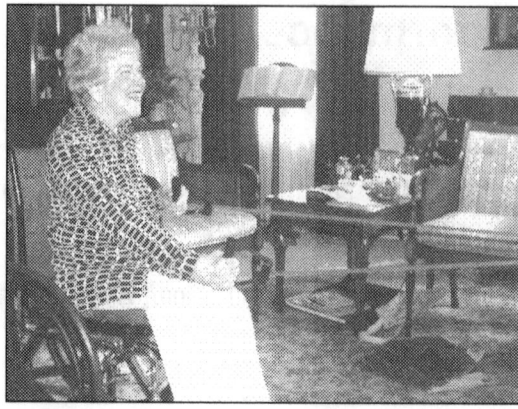

Figure 5-9. One more pull and Lyn has finished.

Figure 5-8. Lyn pulls one hand at the time.

Your SE's posture must be at its very best. When she is in the pulling phase of this exercise, have her stop and become aware of her posture when she's in full pull position. Tell her that this is how she needs to sit all the time, even on the sofa.

The Chest Muscles—Two Exercises

The main chest muscles, pectoralis major, are used primarily for hugging and pushing motions. When your SE pushes open a door or embraces someone, she's using her chest muscles. The main reasons for exercising these muscles are not only to retain the functions of hugging and pushing but also to achieve good muscle balance with the muscles of the upper back.

Pushing is a multi-joint motion involving the shoulder and elbow joints. This motion recruits the chest, shoulder, and triceps muscles in the back of the upper arm. For this reason, a separate triceps exercise is not included in this chapter.

For the hugging motion, teach your SE the butterfly exercise. For the pushing motion, teach her the wall press exercise.

The Butterfly

The butterfly works the hugging motions of the chest muscles. An advantage of this exercise is that your SE can perform it in a seated position so that balance won't be a problem. Another advantage is that it's less likely to cause pain to the shoulder joints than other chest exercises.

The butterfly is easier on the shoulder joints than the bench press on page 143 or the wall press on page 121. It's not a multi-joint exercise and requires motion only in the shoulder joint. While the pectoral muscles are exercised, adjoining muscles such as parts of the shoulder and the triceps are not used. This exercise requires two sturdy straight chairs.

Preparation

Ask your SE to do the following:

- Sit in a chair with her back and hips firmly against the chair back.

- Place her feet on the floor with her knees spread apart a little bit.

- Raise her arms straight out in front of her so that they are horizontal to the floor.

Sit in another chair close to and facing your SE. Extend your arms out in front of you parallel to the floor and just to the inside of her arms. Have her grab the backs of your hands or your thumbs with both her palms. Your palms are facing inward. Then ask her to do the following:

- Push her shoulders down.

- Push down and pull her shoulder blades together in the retracted position.

- Rotate her elbows outwards and flex them about 10 to 20 degrees and keep her elbows up. She needs to keep her elbows in this slightly angled position throughout the exercise.

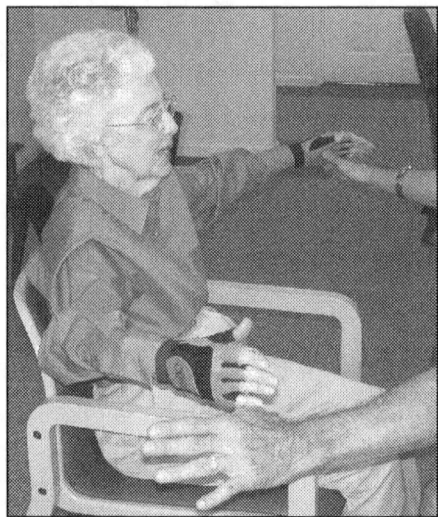

Figure 5-10. Frances gets ready.

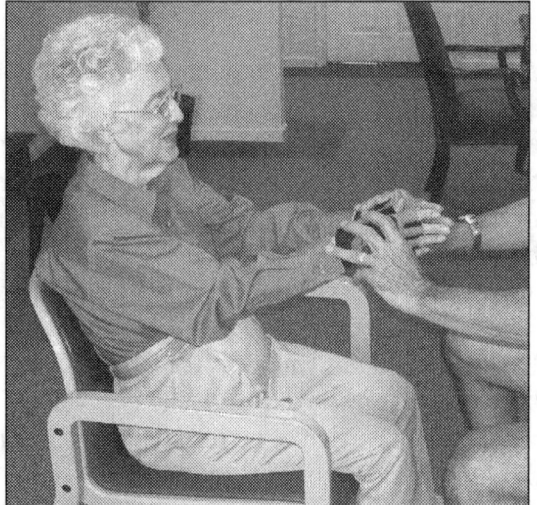

Figure 5-11. Frances performs the butterfly.

Performance

Ask your SE to do the following:

- Inhale and open her arms wide while she's holding on to your hands.

- Exhale and bring her hands together in a hugging or pincer-like motion without bending or straightening the elbows.

- Repeat for 8-12 reps.

- Rest for one minute.

Apply resistance to her hands while she performs the hugging motion. John is the strength machine for Frances in Figures 5-10 and 5-11 above.

Finer Points

Use these suggestions for safety:

- When she has brought her arms out to her sides in a straight line, be sure she comes to a complete stop before pressing her hands together in the hugging motion. Tell her, "Make sure the first things you squeeze are your chest muscles."

- Ensure that she keeps her elbows raised and her arms relatively parallel to the floor. The tendency is to let the elbows fall far below the level of the hands.

- Make sure she doesn't yank or make sudden movements because these will put a strain on the shoulder joints.

- Make sure she remains seated with excellent posture and with both feet firmly on the floor.

As she gets tired, she may begin to hunch her shoulders forward, raise her hands, bend her elbows, move her shoulder blades apart, or do a combination of any or all of these technical errors. Watch to see that she is using the right technique and always encourage her to feel the chest muscles working. The amount of resistance you use as she makes the hugging motion needs to be such that she can perform 8 to 12 repetitions. More important, she will be tired during the last two or three repetitions. Determining how much resistance to use as an art, and you will find your way as you go along.

Err on the side of caution. It's better to be too easy than too hard, but you will quickly get to know how strong your SE is. This is one of the nicer parts of interactive training, using your body to provide the resistance for her body. You will actually be able to feel her strength increase over time.

As her strength and technique improve, provide resistance during the yielding or eccentric motion. She will keep her chest muscles engaged as she spreads her arms wide, and you will provide a little resistance for her to press against.

The Wall Press

Ask your SE to stand at arm's length away from a bare, open wall. When she's standing with her shoulder blades pulled back, well retracted, she should be barely able to touch the wall with her fingertips. You will stand to the side and slightly behind her.

Preparation

Ask your SE to do the following:

- Place her palms against the wall about shoulder width apart. She will now be standing straight but leaning forward slightly.

- Move her palms down the wall until they are level with the middle of her chest unless she has already placed her palms at the correct height.

- Keep her feet parallel or her toes turned slightly out. Her feet should be approximately hip or shoulder width apart. She should keep her knees and hips straight. Before the exercise begins, she will be at a leaning attention position.

- Rotate her palms inward about 45 degrees, as Ann does in Figure 5-12.

The line joining her wrists is horizontal. The line from the base to the top of the triangle is vertical. Note that this hand position accomplishes two things:

1. With the hands lowered and the fingertips turned inward, she will place her arms and shoulders in the correct position to exercise the chest muscles and remove the stress from the shoulder joints.

2. With the fingertips turned inward, she won't put excessive stress on the wrist joints.

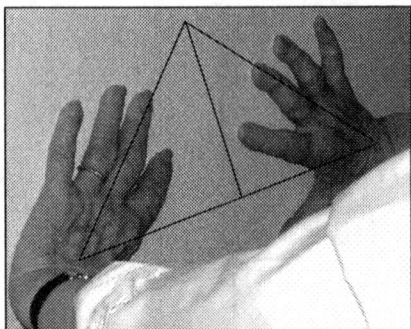

Figure 5-12. Ann places her hands correctly.

Remind her to push her shoulders down and not to let them ride up. Remind her to pull her shoulder blades together and to keep her elbows straight.

When she's in the ready position as in Figure 5-13, place the palm of your hand lightly between her shoulder blades. Leave your palm there, suspended in space, during her performance.

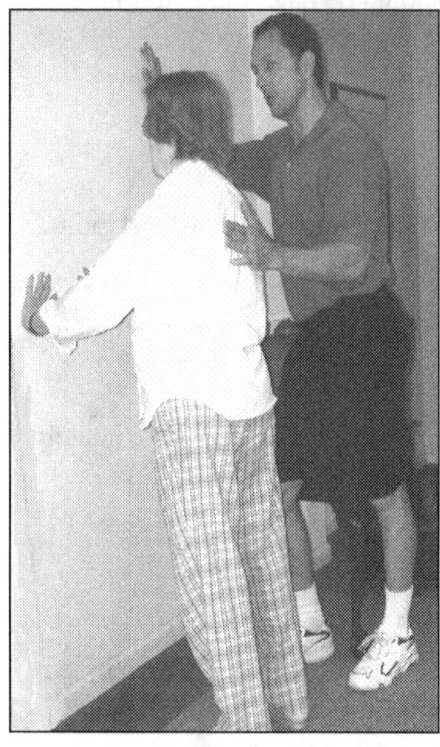

Figure 5-13. Ann prepares for the wall press.

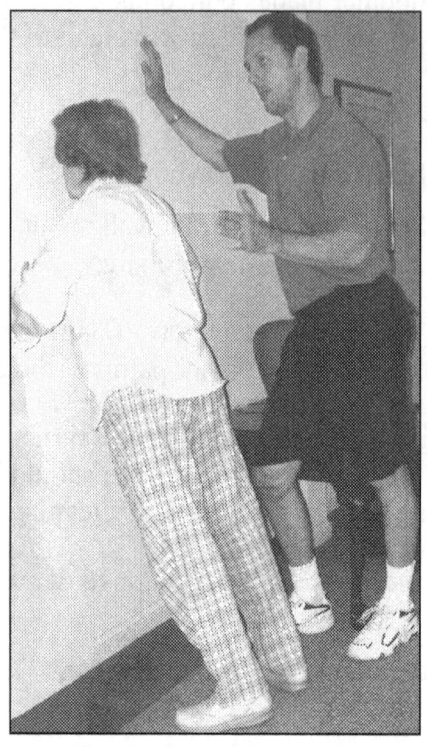

Figure 5-14. Ann performs the wall press.

Performance

Ask your SE to do the following:

- Inhale and move her upper body toward the wall by bending her elbows outward so that her forehead or nose touches the wall, if possible; if not, ensure that she comes as close to the wall as she can without pain.

- As she lowers herself toward the wall, her heels will leave the floor. That's quite all right.

- Exhale and push away from the wall, straightening or extending her elbows so that she returns to the original leaning attention position.

When her elbows are almost straight, make sure she doesn't extend her shoulders. Ask her not to separate her shoulder blades, but try to keep them retracted.

- When her back touches your suspended palm, the repetition is complete.

- Repeat for a set of 8-12 reps.

- Rest for one to two minutes.

Finer Points

Ensure that she keeps a straight line from her ankles through her knees and hips to her shoulders.

Note that you will use your sense of touch during this exercise. The most common and most hazardous error in technique is for her to spread the shoulder blades apart as she straightens her elbows.

Spreading the shoulder blades puts the rotator cuff muscles of the shoulder joint in jeopardy. The touch of your suspended palm is her tactile cue to stop before the shoulder blades can separate or protract.

Continue to encourage her to keep her shoulder blades together or retracted and down or depressed every time she performs this exercise.

As the reps get higher and the exercise gets harder, the other common technique flaws are likely to be the following.

- Separating the shoulder blades on the pushing motion.

- Extending the shoulder joints at the end of each repetition. This puts the shoulder joints in jeopardy of injury.

- Failing to keep the elbows pointing outward and downward at about a 45-degree angle. If the elbows point too far toward the floor, the exercise works the triceps muscles. If the elbows point too high toward the horizontal, the exercise is hard on the shoulder joints.

- Bending forward or backward at the waist. Your touch on her lower back and verbal instruction will remind her to remain as straight and stiff as a two-by-four.

The Leg Muscles—Three Exercises

Since mobility is so important for your SE's feeling of power and independence, this chapter provides three exercises for the leg muscles.

The chair squat, heel raise, and seated hip flexor exercises will help your SE regain good walking ability. It's hard to live independently if you can't walk, and it's even harder to feel independent if you can't get around by yourself.

You may see a harmful progression in your SE's life: she has a near miss with a fall, begins fearing for her safety, starts hanging onto walls and railings, shuffles her feet, and loses leg strength. Then she really does fall.

Break the vicious cycle of growing weak, falling, and growing even weaker by focusing on exercises that strengthen your SE's leg muscles. Ask her to do chair squats during nearly every training session.

Use the heel raise and seated hip flexor exercises as alternate or additional leg exercises, but place them later in the session. Let her leg muscles recover from chair squats. A good time for heel raise and seated hip flexor exercises is after the shoulder exercises. Make sure your SE has enough time and energy for them as well. If you have to select just one leg exercise, make it chair squats.

The Chair Squat

If there's a magic exercise, it's the squat. A person could remain reasonably fit her whole life just by doing squats. The squat is the core exercise for *any* strength training program for *anyone*, from the adolescent to the nonagenarian to the professional football player. Without the squat, your program will ever be fully realized. With it, you can be assured that your SE is getting the most universally beneficial strength training exercise she can get.

The squatting motion, which everyone does daily, is basically raising and lowering one's center of gravity. However, squats have to be done properly and safely, and learning the technique takes a little time.

Anyone over 65 needs to start with a version called the chair squat: starting to take a sitting position until the buttocks just touch the chair and standing back up again. The utility of this exercise is apparent. It's basically getting up and down from a seated position without using the arms for leverage.

Most of the muscles of the trunk, hips, legs, and feet are used to do this exercise. It is *the* major exercise for thighs and hips and one of the major exercises for the lower back. That's what makes it so special. This exercise involves so much muscle mass and requires so much energy every time she performs it that it places very high oxygen and energy demands on her body. Expect to see your SE huffing and puffing in order to get through this exercise. This is actually a good thing.

Minnie Ree

The always colorful Minnie Ree, 89, used to call chair squats *temptations*: "When you get up and down a few times, it's such a temptation to just sit there."

Preparation

Ask your SE to do the following:

- Assume the universal stance with the feet approximately shoulder width apart and the toes pointing slightly outward.

- Keep the head up and the line of vision slightly elevated and focused on a stationary point on the wall.

- Keep the shoulder blades down and together and the spine long and flat.

- Keep the lower back very, very rigid. In fact, keep the whole back as rigid as possible.

Start with no weights and then add dumbbells as her strength improves, as John does in Figure 5-15. Sit next to your SE, facing her profile so you can watch her touch down and keep an eye on the position of her knees.

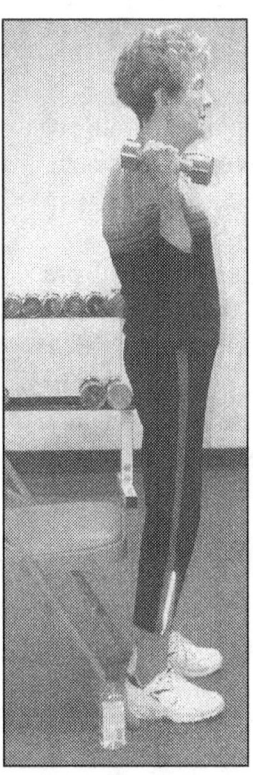

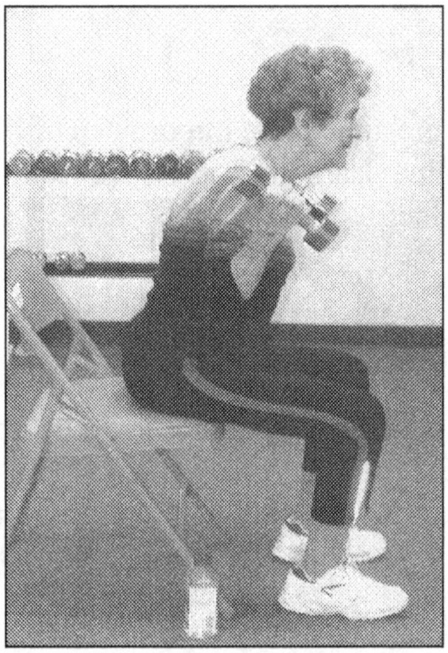

Figure 5-16. Virginia touches down.

Figure 5-15. Virginia gets ready.

Performance

Ask your SE to do the following:

- Push the hips backward and slightly bend the knees. Extend the arms forward only if needed, for balance.

- Lower the body until the buttocks touch, but don't rest on, the chair.

- With her weight firmly on the back half of her feet and without letting her weight shift forward to her toes, return to the standing position.

- Repeat for a total of ten reps.

- Sit and rest for one or two minutes.

Hold one hand near the small of your SE's back to provide a reminder for her to keep a *tight* back that is flat or extended and to support her if necessary. Watch *carefully* for correct posture: back flat, head up, and knees over the toes, not forward of the toes. Give verbal feedback as necessary.

If she can't touch down in the chair at first, place a firm cushion or pad in the seat to raise its level. Ideally, in the lowest position of the squat, the hip joint is level with or slightly below the knee joint. She may have to work for some time to achieve this position.

Finer Points

You can't overestimate the importance of this exercise. If you don't do squats in your own workout routine, learn how and learn well. They will cause major improvement in your physical wellbeing and in your SE's.

Note that the squat feels awkward at first to many people. The awkwardness comes from long practice of depending on the front thigh muscles (quadriceps) to do the work of sitting down and then standing up. The thighs are major movers in this exercise, but what we are trying to do is involve the gluteus and hamstring muscles of the hips and posterior thighs. These muscles come into play when Mom sticks her rear end backwards and sits down. When she stands up again, the gluteal and hamstring muscles extend the hip joint. In a nutshell, the keys to good squatting are for your SE to do the following:

- Keep her knees directly above her feet. Don't let them move inward as she squats or stands.

- As she squats, don't let her knees extend forward past her toes.

- Don't plop down on the chair and don't relax—just barely touch it and then stand back up.

- The shorter your SE is, the easier this exercise will be. As she improves, have her squat with a lower chair or place a one- or two-inch board in front of the chair for her to stand on. Even an inch or two will make a big difference. Naturally, a taller SE may need to start with a higher chair.

Big chest, tight back. She will need to hear it over and over and over again. As her performance improves, draw her hands closer to shoulder level.

When she masters this position, begin adding weight by having her hold a dumbbell in each hand, as Virginia does in Figures 5-15 and 5-16.

When her strength increases, encourage her to use a small stool, as Kathleen, 77, does in Figure 5-17. The lower the chair or stool, the more difficult the exercise—and the greater the benefit.

Help your SE avoid the "point and shoot" method of eyeing the chair over her shoulder and then just plopping down on it. She basically falls the last 8 or 10 inches.

This method uses none of the gluteal and hamstring muscles that we are trying to engage in the chair squat. Be patient with your SE. Changing a lifetime of habit takes time. It's definitely worth the effort to learn and practice the chair squat.

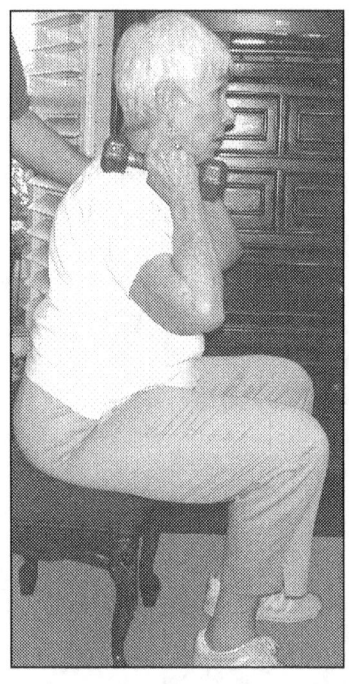

Figure 5-17. Kathleen goes low.

The Heel Raise

The calves are important muscles for maintaining balance and support while standing still and for providing the push-off in order to walk. They help lift the feet from the floor, an action that lessens or prevents the dragging, shuffling walk seen in many older people. The easiest calf-strengthening exercise is to raise the body up on tiptoes in the heel raise exercise.

Preparation

Ask your SE to do the following:

• Stand with the feet 6 to 10 inches apart and the toes pointing forward.

• Keep the body tall and erect.

• Focus the eyes on something in the background at eye level.

You will stand in front of her and grasp her hands with yours, as John does in Figure 5-18 below. During the performance of this exercise, you won't be providing any of the muscle, but you will help stabilize her and give her the confidence that she can do this motion without toppling over.

Performance

Ask your SE to do the following:

- Take a deep breath.

- While exhaling, rise up onto her tiptoes.

- Hold the position for a count of one-one thousand.

- Inhale and slowly lower back down to the standing position.

- Repeat up to a total of 8-12 reps.

- Rest for 30 seconds.

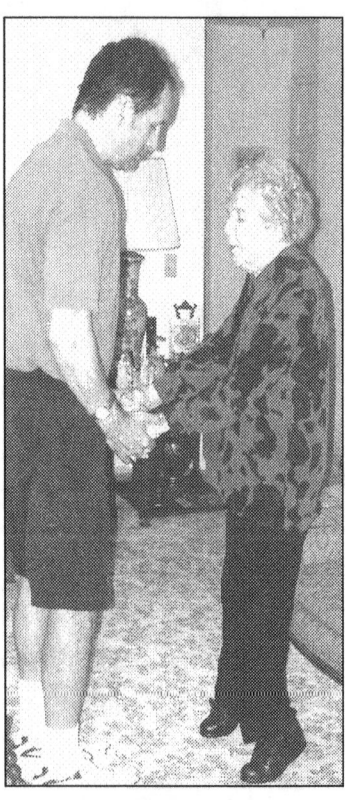

Figure 5-18. Lyn performs the heel raise.

Finer Points

When she's ready to stop holding onto your hands, you can still assist or spot her in order to prevent a fall. Provide support for the skill of balancing by doing the following:

- Stand to one side and place your hands gently on the front and back of one of her shoulders.

- Watch her ankles and caution her to place her weight on her big toes. Ensure that her ankles don't wobble out to the sides or in toward each other.

- As she goes up on tiptoes, provide balance as needed, but ensure that she doesn't lean her weight on you.

The purpose of your assistance is to give your SE confidence about not falling and to be right there in case she loses her balance. In the beginning, provide a lot of support so that your SE has to think of nothing but going up on tiptoes. As her balance improves, gradually discontinue the support. For as long as you train your SE, however, stand very close by and watch vigilantly for any signs of fatigue, wobbling, or distress. Be right there to catch and support her.

Seated Hip Flexor March

The hip flexors enable your SE to lift her knees, which is an important part of walking and going up stairs. Lifting the knees, like pushing off with the toes, keeps her from shuffling. If the hip flexor muscles get too weak, she will tend to drag her feet. The basic exercise is very simple and is good even for someone who lacks good balance. This exercise requires only a sturdy armchair.

Preparation

Ask your SE to do the following:

- Sit in the chair, with the hips and back touching the back of the chair.

- Hold onto the arms of the chair and push her back against the back of the chair.

Your position is right beside her, seated if you like. Place one hand on her shoulder and the other hand an inch or two above her knees to give her a target. See Figure 5-19 below.

Performance

Ask your SE to raise one foot and then the other:

- Lift one knee and touch your hand.

- While lowering it, lift the other knee and touch your hand.

- Keep marching in a seated position for 10-15 lifts on each side. Ensure that she breathes throughout the exercise.

- Rest for 30 seconds to one minute.

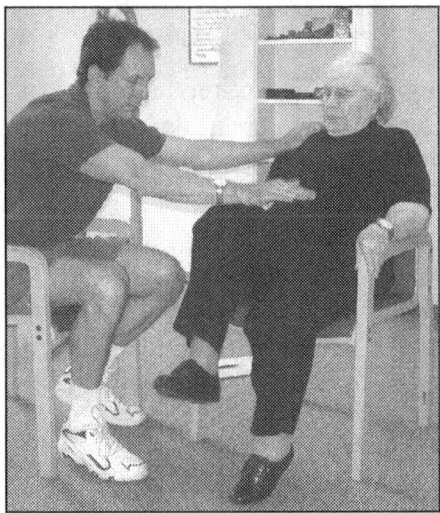

Figure 5-19. Faye does the seated hip flexor march.

Finer Points

After a few sessions, begin raising the height of your hand to ensure progressive strengthening of the hip flexor muscles.

Later on, add resistance by placing your hands or fingers on her knees and pressing down gently as she lifts. As her strength improves over the weeks and months, increase the resistance.

When she begins to tire, she may start arching her back, shifting her hips forward, or jerking her knees upward. Discourage these motions because they place unnecessary strain on the lower back.

Later on, your SE may move to the standing hip flexor march, as Ann demonstrates in Figure 5-20.

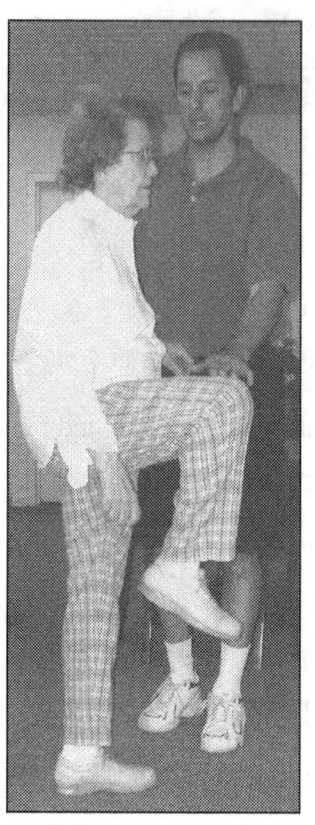

Figure 5-20. Ann does the standing version.

The Shoulder Muscles—The Lateral Raise

The next area to work is the shoulder muscles. The standard shoulder motion that incorporates the largest number of muscles is the overhead or military press, done with dumbbells or barbells. However, note that putting a bar overhead with both arms is difficult to impossible for many older people.

If your SE can't get her arms overhead within 30 degrees of vertical, use the lateral raise. The lat raise means you are laterally—out to your sides—raising the dumbbells. It requires only two small dumbbells of equal weight. After you teach the motion with no weights at all, then start with one-pound dumbbells. If balance is a problem, you can modify this exercise so that your SE can perform it in a seated position.

Preparation

Ask your SE to do the following:

- Take the universal stance.

- Pick up two small dumbbells. At first, you will hand the dumbbells to her.

- Hold the dumbbells in front of her thighs, as Kathleen does in Figure 5-21 below.

- Bring the thumbs together in front of her body below the waist.

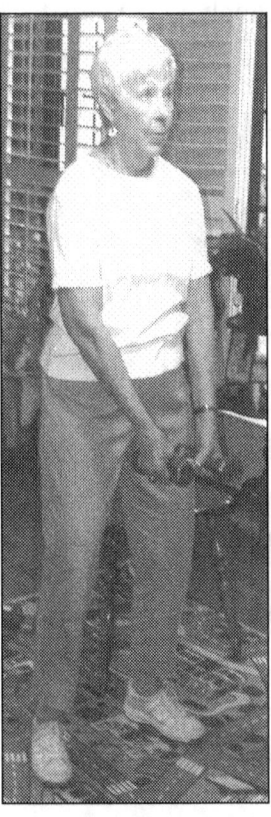

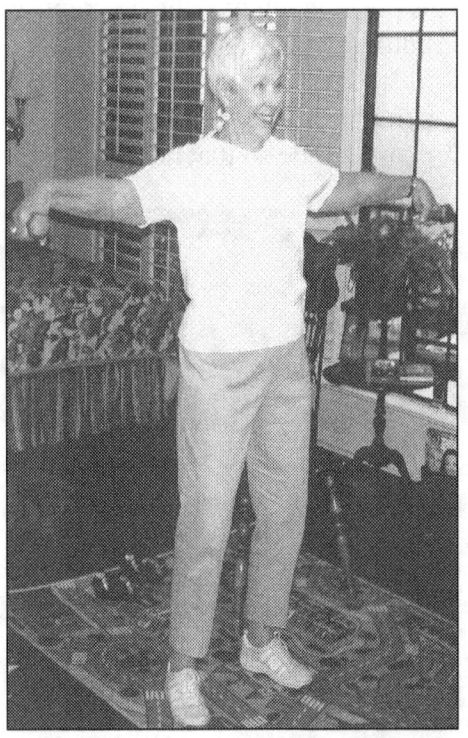

Figure 5-22. Kathleen performs the lat raise.

Figure 5-21. Kathleen gets ready.

Performance

The easiest and safest way to do this exercise is as follows:

- Inhale.

- While exhaling, lift the weights up and out to the sides until the arms are parallel to the floor but no higher. At first she may not be able to reach the parallel position, so ask her just to raise the weights as high as she can manage.

- Inhale and lower the dumbbells to the starting position in front of the body.

- Repeat for 8-12 reps.

- Rest for one minute.

Finer Points

Don't expect your SE to keep her wrists locked in a straight line with her arms. Instead, have her relax her wrists so that her hands and fingers point downward at the top of the lift, as Kathleen does in Figure 5-22. Thus, the dumbbells will be an inch or so lower than the arms. This position relieves the wrist muscles, leaving more energy to apply to the target shoulder muscles.

If she has trouble raising the dumbbells out to her sides, you can suggest that she bring her hands forward a little so that her arms come forward about 30 degrees.

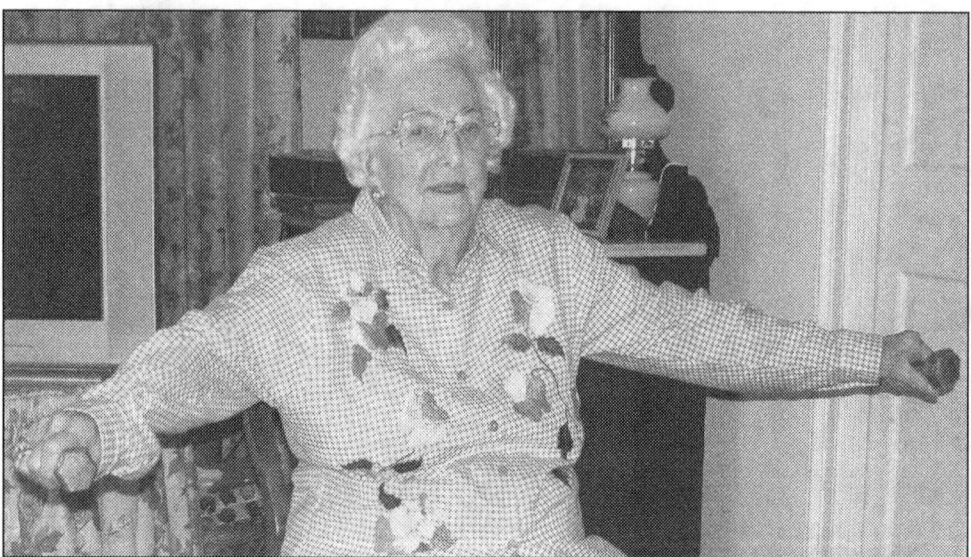

Figure 5-23. Anna Fay performs the seated lat raise.

If your SE has balance problems, she can perform this exercise by sitting on the front edge of a chair without arms, as Anna Fay does in Figure 5-23. She will move her hands underneath her thighs on the lowest portion of the arc. Ensure that there is enough space between the chair legs and her calves for the dumbbells to complete the swing without bumping her body or the chair. Anna Fay holds a one-pound weight in her right hand and a two-pound weight in her left hand because of a problem with her right shoulder.

The Lower Back Muscles—The Good Morning Exercise

These days you hear this a lot: The key to a healthy, pain-free lower back is strong abs. After all, the primary function of the abs is to support the spine and help keep it erect from the anterior or front side of the body. An out-of-shape abdomen—big belly, beer gut,

Dunlap disease, or whatever—pulls the lower back forward, causing lordosis or swayback as well as lower back strain and pain. Swayback can lead to herniated or ruptured lumbar discs.

All of the above is true and makes good sense except for one thing. Strong abs are only the second-best way to protect the lower back. The key to a healthy lower back is to develop a strong lower back. The good morning exercise will provide the means of ensuring strong lower back muscles.

Preparation

Ask your SE to do the following:

- Take the universal stance.

- Spread the feet approximately shoulder width apart and keep them parallel to each other or slightly turned out at the toes.

You will stand slightly to her side and watch her technique in profile to make sure she maintains good posture throughout the exercise.

Performance

Ask your SE to do the following:

- While inhaling, bow at the waist, bending the knees as much as necessary to maintain balance and relieve the over-stretching of the hamstrings.

- Keep her weight in the center and back part of her feet.

- Keep the spinal column long and flat.

- Keep the upper shoulders (trapezius muscles) relaxed.

- Keep the head and neck extended and the eyes slightly elevated.

- Bow as deeply as possible or until she can no longer maintain good posture with a flat back.

- Try to keep the line of vision elevated.

- While exhaling, return to the upright position by extending her hips and knees.

- Repeat for 8-12 reps.

- Rest for one minute.

You will sit or stand to the side and continue to observe both the posture and the performance in profile, as John does in Figure 5-25.

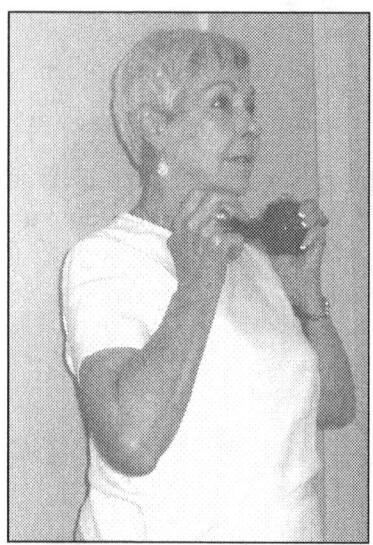

Figure 5-24. Kathleen gets ready.

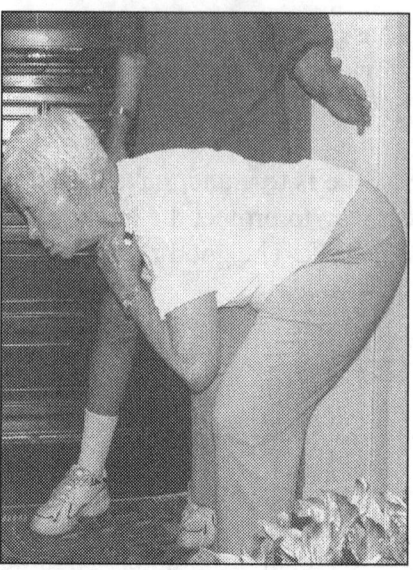

Figure 5-25. Kathleen bows low with a flat back.

Finer Points

If your SE lacks balance or leg strength at first, she may perform this exercise by sitting at the front edge of a chair. Ask her to do the same performance steps as for the standing good morning exercise.

You may want to put one hand an inch or two in front of her upper chest and the other hand an inch or two behind her middle back. In this way you will be ready to use the touch method to gently remind her to keep the lower back flat or slightly concave, keep the shoulder blades together, and keep her chest out.

As she improves and becomes more adept at performing the exercise, you can add some weight. Start with a two- or three-pound dumbbell that she holds at both ends as Kathleen does in Figures 5-24 and 5-25. Ensure that she holds the weight close to the upper part of her chest. Over time, she will increase her strength and will be able to "bow" holding quite a bit of weight.

An Additional Note on Safety

John finds that a common technique error in doing the standing good morning is bending the knees too much, thus requiring less work for the targeted lower back muscles. Older and younger people as well are hesitant to use the lower back at all for fear of hurting it, hence, the widespread use of industrial back belts in the workplace despite little scientific evidence that they protect the back—and these belts certainly don't *strengthen* the back.[26]

---

[26] "Back Belts: Do They Prevent Injury?" National Institute for Occupational Safety and Health, available at http://www.cdc.gov/niosh/backbelt.html.

Remind your SE of the purpose of this exercise. Ask her to flex forward at the hips (bow) only as far as she feels comfortable. Progress will come over time. Before the exercise ever starts, remind your SE:

- Not to lean too far forward.

- To keep the head and eyes up. If she has some kyphosis or over-rounding of the upper back, the eyes-up posture may not be possible for her. In this case, ask her to keep her head down but to keep her back straight and flat from the lower back on upward.

- To keep the knees and thighs in the same flexed position throughout the exercise.

- To focus on keeping the back straight.

After she has practiced for some time holding a small dumbbell to her chest, you can increase the intensity by giving her two heavier dumbbells to hold on her shoulders. Always place the dumbbells on your SE's shoulders instead of expecting her to get them into the correct position. Later on, her strength may improve so much that you can place a barbell across the back of her shoulders. However, be quite cautious with the bar.

After placing the bar across your SE's shoulders, make sure that her hands are positioned in a firm, wide grip. Then move to the front so that you are facing each other. Keep your hands lightly encircling the bar as your SE performs the downward and upward motions. You will want to be able to assist with lifting the weights if there's any trouble in raising herself back to the upright position.

The Cool-Down/Calm-Down

Often overlooked in the workouts of younger people, the cool-down/calm-down is very important for your SE, especially if she's worked out strenuously. The cool-down/calm-down doesn't need to take more than a few minutes and is as much a psychological evaluation—a calm-down—as a physical evaluation. Following are several suggestions for the cool-down/calm-down:

- Sit with your SE for a few moments at the end of a session. Your personal attention to her welfare will make her feel secure and cared for.

- Make sure that she seems to have no dizziness or mental confusion while seated.

- If your SE isn't taking blood pressure medication and you are familiar with reading a pulse, you can take hers, preferably the carotid pulse, at the beginning of the cool-down/calm-down period and at the end to determine whether she's returned to a pulse rate that's normal for her. However, if she's taking blood pressure medication, the readings won't be valid indicators because these medications tend to slow the pulse rate.

- Offer some water, or remind her to drink from her water bottle.

- Engage in a little positive conversation to ensure her that she is making progress. Go over her best lifts and congratulate her on a job well done.

- Stand up and see if she can also get up without assistance. Offer a pull up if necessary.

- Observe whether she seems steady on her feet. If not, encourage her to sit for a while longer.

- As soon as she's ready, walk around the exercise area with her to ensure that she can walk steadily.

- Ask her to do a few stretches and give her a brief neck and shoulder massage.

- If it takes her more than two or three minutes to stand, to walk a little, and to stretch lightly, she may have worked too strenuously. Ease up a little in the next training session.

- Sometimes, John feels that he needs to walk a client back to her apartment in the retirement center, and you may need to provide similar support after a particularly strenuous training session.

- Don't say goodbye until you are sure she feels fine and not just because she says so. Make sure she's really good to go.

- Remind her to rest and have a snack after she gets home.

A Note to Certified Personal Trainers

Nothing in this chapter ought to come as a surprise to you except, perhaps, the opportunity to do hands-on training with little or no equipment. If you prefer to teach the exercises you are more familiar with, you should feel free to do so, of course. However, you might keep the exercises in this chapter in mind in case one of your older clients needs to use them for a period of time, either at the beginning of training or during recovery from an illness or injury.

If the idea of supervising a client's cool-down/calm-down period is new to you, then it may seem unnecessary until you think about the need to calm down after a hard workout. Older people are adults, of course, who have lived long lives, but many of them need to be reminded about nearly all aspects of a training session, including the cool-down/calm-down. During each training session, John is on the lookout for some tiny improvement to discuss with the client. He really believes in giving as much positive reinforcement as possible. Remember:

- Use equipment if you prefer, or use the hands-on techniques in this chapter.

- Use the cool-down/calm-down to assess how your older clients feel after the workout so that you can make sure they are okay.

- If a client has a little trouble recovering from a workout, then lower the weights and reps or make other adjustments at the next training session.

Summary of the Main Points

This chapter shows you how to conduct a training session using the safest exercises for someone who is somewhat frail or seems to have lost some physical ability:

- Good technique is an absolute must for safety and health. Technique must be your main concern.

- Multi-joint exercises (the band pull, the wall press, and the chair squat) require more muscle, more energy, and better technique. They closely resemble everyday functions and provide the greatest benefit for your SE.

- Work the abdominal muscles first because they are a safe continuation of the warm-up discussed in Chapter 3.

- Work the upper back muscles next because upper back pulls are strenuous yet relatively safe and they are easy on the shoulders.

- Work the chest muscles next for upper body strength and for muscle balance with the upper back.

- Work all of the leg exercises because the leg muscles contribute the most to mobility. Take extra safety precautions. The chair squat is the most difficult and the most beneficial of the leg exercises.

- Work the shoulder muscles next and be careful to avoid injuries.

- Work the lower back muscles to prevent back pain and take extra safety precautions.

- The biceps and triceps are worked during the upper back and chest exercises. The next chapter presents specific exercises for these muscle groups.

- Always have your SE do a cool-down/calm-down.

- Be ready to repeat instructions a lot. Be patient with her and with yourself.

What's Next?

When your SE becomes stronger or gets bored or impatient with the exercises in this chapter, go to the next chapter. In the meantime, see the information on how to help your SE improve her eating and sleeping habits in Chapter 7.

Chapter 6. Top 12 Advanced, Add-on, and Supplemental Exercises

Helping Your Significant Elder Stay Fit and Interested

Question: "If someone had told you on your 65th birthday that when you reached your present age, you would be regularly and strenuously lifting weights, what would you have said?"
Answer: "I probably would have laughed. But it's really helped me stay mobile."
  Ann, age 91

Note: A physician's examination is recommended for all exercise participants with any restrictions and for those persons over forty (40) years of age. Fitness evaluation participants in these categories who have not had a physical examination in the past year must acknowledge that they have been informed of its importance and, therefore, accept full responsibility for their health and wellbeing. Participants understand that no responsibility is assumed by a personal trainer or the authors of this book.

Important Points for Advocates: As you did in the previous chapter, learn the names of the exercises and the muscle group or groups they engage. In particular, be prepared to congratulate your SE when he tells you he has moved on to an exercise in this chapter. Your interest and good wishes can be a powerful motivator for him to stick with his exercise program.

Introduction

The exercises in this chapter are intended for older people who are reasonably strong, mobile, and healthy. These exercises are also for the formerly frail who have increased their strength, stamina, balance, power, and flexibility enough to perform some or all of them. However, take particular care with the three advanced exercises and observe excellent safety precautions.

If you have been using the exercises in the previous chapter, as recommended, don't abandon them. Instead, continue using them while you introduce the exercises in this chapter one at the time over a period of weeks or months. Select an exercise you think your SE can perform and will enjoy. Then replace or supplement the beginning exercise with the exercise in this chapter for the corresponding muscle group. For example, if your SE needs to work on abdominal strength, then add the two in this chapter on pages 156 and 157.

In general, when your SE can perform the beginning exercises well—two sets of 8-12 reps with good technique—he's probably ready to move to the advanced exercises. The variety will help your SE increase his functional strength even more than sticking to the same exercises for every training session.

However, if your SE suffers an injury or has some other extended period away from strength training, it would be a good idea to go back to the exercises in the previous chapter until he has regained his former state of health.

The exercises in this chapter will increase even a strong, healthy older person's strength and help him to remain active for the rest of his life, barring major illnesses or injuries. You can readily see the benefit for older people of these standard gym exercises.

Before you begin teaching the exercises in this chapter to your SE, make sure that you have read Chapter 4.

Keep your Significant Elder safe at all times.

You also need to learn the exercises yourself, especially any that you don't use in your own workout routine, so that you can demonstrate them for your SE by using correct technique. You will then be able to describe how the muscle group that you are focusing on will feel to your SE as he performs the exercises. You will also know the risks of each exercise so that you can take the necessary precautions, and you will be better able to sympathize in case your SE experiences sore muscles or an injury.

These exercises are designed for functional strength so that your SE can keep on doing the activities of daily living—sitting up straight, reaching, standing, walking, picking up and carrying items, climbing the stairs, and so on. Along the way, your SE will improve his posture and gain a more compact appearance, improved aerobic capacity, and increased self-confidence, but the main focus is always on strength.

As in Chapter 5, each exercise contains a section on **preparation** or getting ready to do the exercise, a section on **performance** or exactly what to do to complete the exercise, and a section on the **finer points** or the expert knowledge that will help keep your SE strong and safe. Two exercises also include **an additional note on safety** because they require careful attention to technique so as to prevent injuries.

An important addition to this chapter is the **readiness indicators** for the advanced exercises so that you will know when to start introducing these exercises into your SE's training sessions. From time to time, you can test him to see whether his physical abilities have improved enough to ensure success with the advanced, add-on, and supplemental exercises.

You will also need to get a feel for whether his attitude and determination are equal to the challenge of becoming even stronger or whether he will need your encouragement to move him along. Most of John's clients are thrilled or at least willing to move up to a tougher challenge, but he never tries to force a client to do something he or she just doesn't want to do. Coaxing, cajoling, light pestering, arguing, and a little trickery, however, might be okay to use.

Before you teach these exercises to your SE, master them yourself under the supervision of a certified personal trainer. Demonstrate each exercise several times. You may need to remind your SE at each training session.

The Warm-up

Use the same warm-up presented on page 72. If you have access to a treadmill or an elliptical trainer, you can add 5-6 minutes to the warm-up by introducing these or similar machines. Taking a walk of equal duration is also good. In addition to warming and loosening the muscles, these activities can significantly improve your SE's cardiovascular system, especially if you increase the time by 30 seconds or a minute each week.

These aerobic exercises may also help him lose weight if he needs to shed a few pounds. However, make sure that he first has enough strength and stamina so that the additional effort won't wear him out and make the training session too difficult to complete. In short, add new things gradually.

Three Advanced Exercises

The three exercises described in this section are termed *advanced* because they require not only that your SE is reasonably strong and has a good sense of balance but also that you are experienced at training him and vigilant in keeping him safe.

Make sure you SE is ready for these exercises, both psychologically and physically, before you introduce them.

Upper Back Exercise—The Standing Band Pull

This exercise is similar to the seated band pull in the previous chapter except that your SE stands while performing it. Any fear that he may have had about losing his balance or falling while exercising must be long gone before you replace the seated exercise with this one.

Readiness Indicators

As soon as your SE can perform the seated band pull for two sets of 12-15 reps with confidence and good technique, you can suggest moving on to the standing version. Ensure that he has a good sense of balance and little or no fear of leaning backwards.

Preparation

Use the same band with handles as you did for the seated band pull on page 115. Test the security of the equipment by performing the exercise yourself a few times. Then ask your SE to do the following:

- Face the band and grip the hand pieces securely with his thumbs on top.

- With his arms fully extended, step far enough back that there is no slack in the band.

- Take the universal stance with shoulder blades down and together.

Stand behind and to one side of your SE in case you need to assist with his balance or his pull. Figure 6-1 shows the ready position. The performance is the same as for the seated band pull on page 117.

Performance

Ask your SE to do the following:

- Inhale on the pulling motion and exhale on the return motion.

- Pull the handles toward his body, sliding his elbows snug against his ribcage and pulling his hands to his waist. If he can't pull to his waist, ask him to take a step forward.

- Hold the pull for a second with his hands at waist level and squeeze his shoulder blades together.

- Return to the starting position smoothly without leaning forward and without letting the band pull him forward.

- Repeat for a total of 12-15 repetitions.

- Rest for 30-60 seconds.

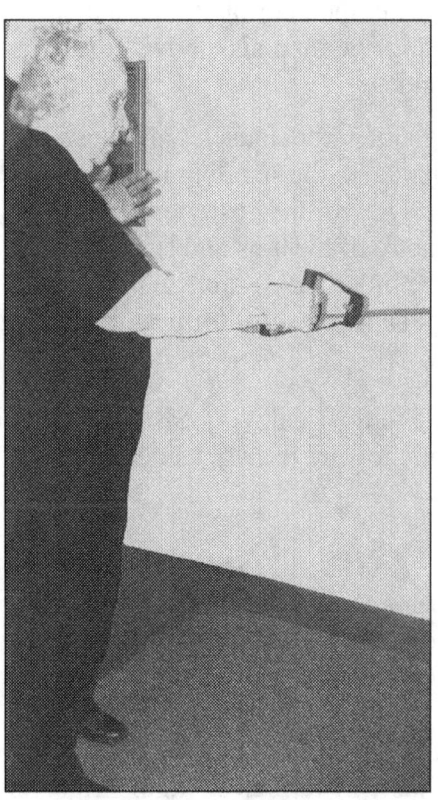

Figure 6-1. Faye starts the standing band pull.

Finer Points

Since this exercise will feel less secure than the seated band pull for both you and your SE, place your hands lightly on the back of his shoulders. You will then be in a position to catch him if needed. The return motion takes the most practice because he may lose his balance when the band is not tight.

To do the exercise well, ensure that he is doing the same things as with the seated band pull:

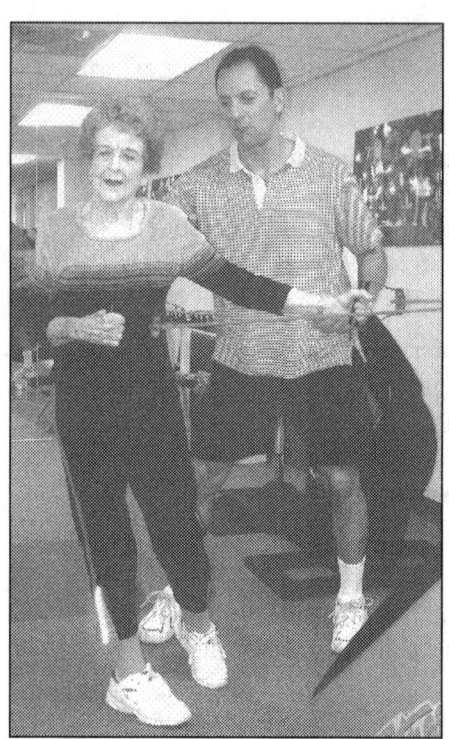

- Do not depend on the band to keep him from falling backward. His leg and core muscles need to keep him upright.

- Lean back as little as possible so he will work his upper back muscles.

- Keep his back long and straight from tailbone to head.

- Keep his shoulder blades pulled back and together and his elbows close to his sides.

Although the target muscles are those of the upper back, the standing band pull uses nearly all of the posterior musculature of the hips and legs as well as the feet in order to stabilize the body. It is a valuable exercise for posture and balance.

Figure 6-2. Virginia rotates to her right.

To rotate to the right, your SE will lift his left heel, turn his left toe inward, and pull his right hand toward the right side of his waist. He will also rotate his hips and torso to the right.

Ask him to do 10-12 to the right and then 10-12 to the left. In addition to exercising his upper back, he will feel a good stretch along his sides and lower back. Place your hands on his shoulders to reassure him that he won't lose his balance while performing this advanced exercise.

A Further Word on Bands: Bands are quite useful, especially in a home setting. They are available in various strengths from very easy, which we recommend for your SE, to very hard. Hundreds of band exercises have been developed[27] that imitate exercises usually done in gyms with expensive equipment. For a very low cost, your SE can perform many excellent exercises, such as the band rotation exercise in Figure 6-2.

The Chest Muscles—The Bench Press

The basic pushing exercise for the chest is the bench press, which requires your SE to lie supine on a flat or almost flat bench while lowering and raising a barbell over his chest. It's a demanding multi-joint exercise that simultaneously works the chest, triceps, and front shoulder muscles. For a description of the importance of the chest muscles, see page 118.

If performed improperly, it's the exercise that is most likely to result in an injury to the shoulder joints. If performed correctly, the bench press gives an enjoyable sensation of upper body strength and power that non-exercisers never experience.

The bench press exercise for your SE closely resembles the same exercise that you can see in any gym in the world, and his chest muscles will get just as strenuous a workout. But you will need to make a few adjustments so that the exercise will be both safe and beneficial. See "An Additional Note on Safety" on page 147.

Readiness Indicators

Note that there are two contraindications for the bench press:

- No one with severe kyphosis will ever be fully ready for this exercise because he won't be able to lie flat on his back, so continue with the butterfly and the wall press instead.

- If your SE can't breathe properly in the almost-supine position, which is sometimes associated with obesity, then always use an adjustable bench to ensure that he never lies completely flat on his back. He will do the modification known as the inclined bench press. You will raise the head of the bench 20 to 35 degrees toward the upright position. Then ask him to sit on the bench and lean back. Hand him the barbell to perform the exercise. Between sets, assist him in sitting up.

If neither of these contraindications applies to your SE, you can introduce the bench press as soon as his strength and confidence show that he is ready. If his strength and stamina are no longer challenged after three sets of 15 reps for the wall press, the time is ripe. However, you both need to take the preparations and the safety issues quite seriously.

Preparation

Ask your SE to do the following:

- Sit astride one end of the bench.

---

[27] See *Band Training* by J. C. Santana, available at www.performbetter.com.

- Lie back until he is almost supine. Assist him if necessary. Then stay at the head of the bench, looking down his body, as John does in Figure 6-3.

- If lying flat makes him dizzy, make sure that his head stays above the level of his heart by placing a small pillow under his head or by slightly raising the head of an adjustable bench.

- Make sure both of his feet are flat on the floor, legs bent at the knees. If his feet don't reach the floor, help him raise his feet onto the end of the bench.

- If there is a rack at the head of the bench, ask him to lie down on the bench so that his face is under the bar. He will reach up and grasp the barbell with his hands palm up and his thumbs facing each other. Ask him to grip the barbell with his hands a little farther apart than shoulder width. As soon as he takes his grip, you will grasp the barbell with your hands in between his hands. One of your hands takes an overhand grip and the other hand takes an underhand grip. As he lifts the barbell into position by extending his elbows, assist him with the placement of the barbell above his upper chest, making sure that it is right above his clavicle, shoulders, neck, or chin.

- If there is no rack, hand him the barbell with your hands already in the overhand-underhand position.

- Ask him to lock out his elbows so that his arms are perfectly straight.

- Remind him to keep his eyes open.

- Very importantly, remind him to keep his shoulder blades pulled back or retracted, not spread apart so that his shoulders raise up off the bench.

- It's a good idea to have him practice spreading and retracting his shoulder blades so that he gets the feel of retracted shoulder blades while he is lying on the bench. He needs to do this before he ever lowers the barbell for the exercise. In the supine position, help him practice balancing the barbell and moving his shoulder blades several times until the retracted position feels comfortable. Patience is a must with this exercise.

- Always keep your hands near the barbell so that you can help stabilize it if necessary.

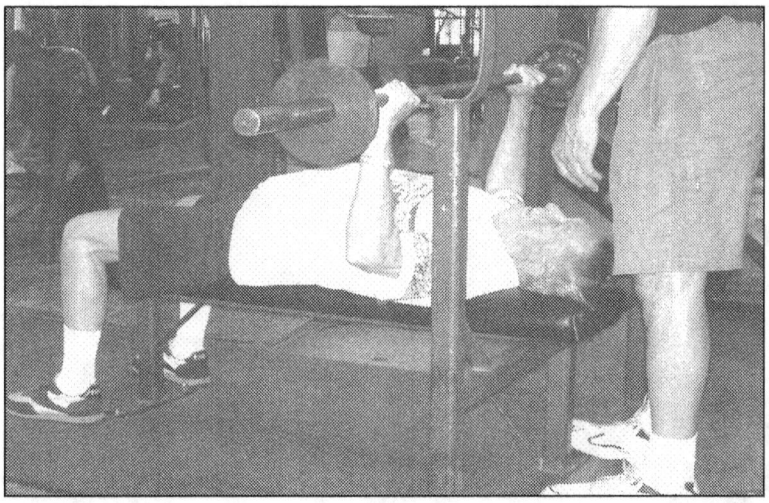

Figure 6-3. Jack lowers the barbell.

Performance

Ask your SE to do the following:

- Inhale and lower the barbell to a position 4" above his chest. The barbell will, of course, be perpendicular to the body and will approach the chest at the nipple line. The elbows will move out to the sides of the body under the bar and slightly toward his feet. He will feel a good stretch horizontally across the chest. Have him take two seconds for the downward motion.

- When the barbell comes near his chest, he will pause and exhale as he pushes it back to the starting position. His elbows will be extended completely, and the bar will be directly over his face.

- The shoulder joints do not extend upward because the shoulder blades are always retracted. Keep your hands very close to the bar, in fact, encircling it with your fingers. Make sure that the barbell stays in line, that is, parallel to the floor.

- One repetition of the exercise is from the highest to lowest and then back to the highest position. Ask your SE to do 8-12 reps.

- At the end of the last rep, take the barbell from his hands. Then step back and either place the barbell on the rack or put the barbell on the floor.

- Then ask him to rest for one to two minutes. Help him sit up for the rest period if he has trouble breathing in the supine position.

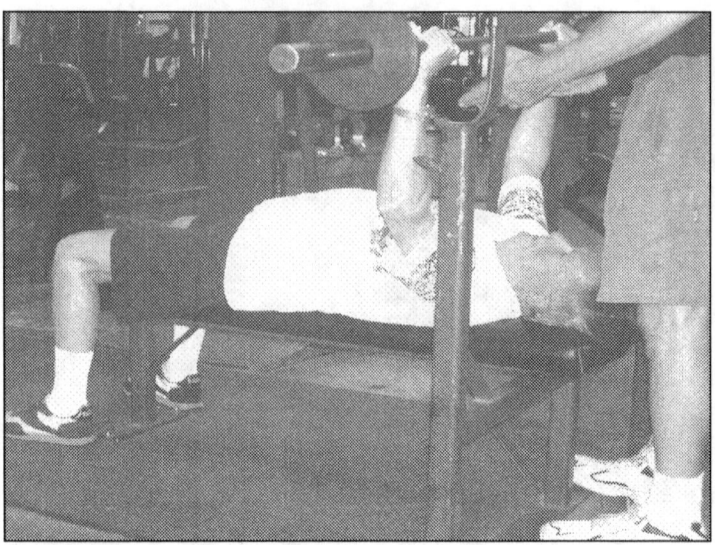

Figure 6-4. Jack nears the top of the bench press.

Finer Points

Remember that the barbell weighs 10 to 15 pounds by itself and may, over time, have additional plates on it to make it heavier. Your SE is in a vulnerable position when the barbell is overhead. So pay utmost care and attention to safety.

A key point for both you and your SE is that as he pushes the barbell upward by extending his elbows and horizontally adducting or flexing his shoulders, he still keeps his shoulder blades retracted. Always keep your hands under the bar as in Figure 6-4.

Resistance breathing is especially important. Ask your SE to inhale as he lowers the barbell and exhale vigorously as he lifts the bar.

> You can't overstress the importance of good technique for the bench press.

It's a good idea to spend quite some time doing partial bench presses, that is, lowering the barbell only about a quarter or half of the way down to his chest a few times. Then ask him to lower the barbell halfway down a few times. It's also a good idea to spend quite a lot of time practicing for this exercise before performing it—hold the barbell with elbows extended and shoulder blades retracted while balancing the barbell overhead.

When people are standing, it's a natural motion, when pushing both arms horizontally, to both extend the elbows and protract or spread the shoulder blades. For the bench press, however, your SE must to learn how to extend the elbows without abducting or spreading the shoulder blades. This technique is the key to safe performance on the bench press.

If your SE lowers the barbell to a point too high up on his chest, that is, near the clavicle, he will place less stress on the chest and more on the shoulder joints. This is what you are trying to prevent. Remember that the bench press is not primarily a shoulder exercise— it's a chest exercise. For many people, it feels very natural to lower the barbell too far up the chest. However, if your SE adheres strictly to good form, he will not only be safe but will also get maximum performance from the chest muscles.

Encourage him not to wriggle around on the bench during the exercise. A firm, non-moving spine (*tight back*) stabilizes the entire torso, providing a steady base from which to raise the barbell.

Failure to retract the shoulder blades is the major technique flaw of the bench press. This can result in injuries to the shoulder muscles, specifically to the rotator cuff muscles.

An Additional Note on Safety

The bench press requires the most vigilance on your part of any exercise in this chapter. Never lower the bench to the fully flat position because you will need to make sure that your SE's head is always a little above the level of the heart. If you are using a standard bench with upright supports for a weighted barbell, you might need to start by asking him to practice with a broom handle or with nothing at all but just going through the motions.

Make sure your SE feels comfortable with the motions of lowering and raising the arms before you apply any weight. Then you will want to make the weights as light as possible at first and to assist with both lowering and raising the arms with shoulder blades retracted.

After your SE gets comfortable with the motion, you will still want to follow the barbell down and up with your hands to provide a safety net in case of trouble. To ensure safety, use the following summary of techniques:

- Stand at the head of the bench.

- Lean forward over the barbell but keep your body well balanced.

- Grasp the barbell with your hands in between your SE's hands.

- Use an overhand grip with one hand and an underhand grip with the other.

- Provide a little guidance on the downward motion so that the barbell is placed in the proper position at the bottom portion of the motion until he is good at doing it by himself.

- On the upward motion, keep your hands close and help guide the bar if needed.

If your SE complains that you are helping too much, show your loose grip on the upward push and say, "It's all you. Good lift! I knew you could do it." Everyone likes praise and encouragement, especially on the more difficult exercises.

Be extra vigilant on that last two or three inches of the upward motion or the last few reps. This is the time when he's most likely to protract or spread his shoulder blades. If he does, take the weight in your hands and remind him, "Shoulder blades together." Make sure that your feet are planted but your knees are flexed.

Make sure that you are not leaning over your SE at more than about a 30-degree angle and that you are well balanced. If you suddenly have to support a 25- to 50-pound bar, you certainly don't want the weight to pull you forward and down on top of your SE.

The Lower Back Muscles—The Dead Lift

Despite the unpleasant name, the dead lift is a life-affirming exercise. Maybe it should be called "picking up and putting down heavy stuff." It's certainly one of the most challenging and athletic exercises you will introduce to your SE, but over time, it may become one of his favorites. The dead lift is the best exercise for strengthening the lower back and is a great producer of endorphins because it taxes the thighs, hips, and lower back muscles. It's also a nice exercise to photograph or tape so you can show him how cool he looks while doing it.

The dead lift can challenge people of any age, so make sure you see "An Additional Note on Safety" on page 150. This exercise works best if you use a barbell rather than dumbbells. It also works best if you demonstrate how to perform it correctly because good technique is essential. For a description of the importance of the lower back muscles, see page 132.

Readiness Indicators

The most important indicators that your SE is physically ready for the dead lift are these:

- He has reasonably good posture, especially in the upper back.

- He performs the good morning described on page 132 with good technique

- He performs the chair squat described on page 124, with good technique.

- His sense of balance is excellent.

- He has no problems with dizziness when lowering and raising his center of gravity.

Preparation

Ask your SE to do the following:

- Take the universal stance.

- Grasp the barbell that you hand him in an overhand grip with the palms facing back. His hands need to be a little farther apart than his knees.

- Keep the shoulders back and the shoulder blades pulled together (retracted).

- Stick the chest out and keep the head up.

- Focus the eyes on something stationary in front of him that's a little higher than eye level.

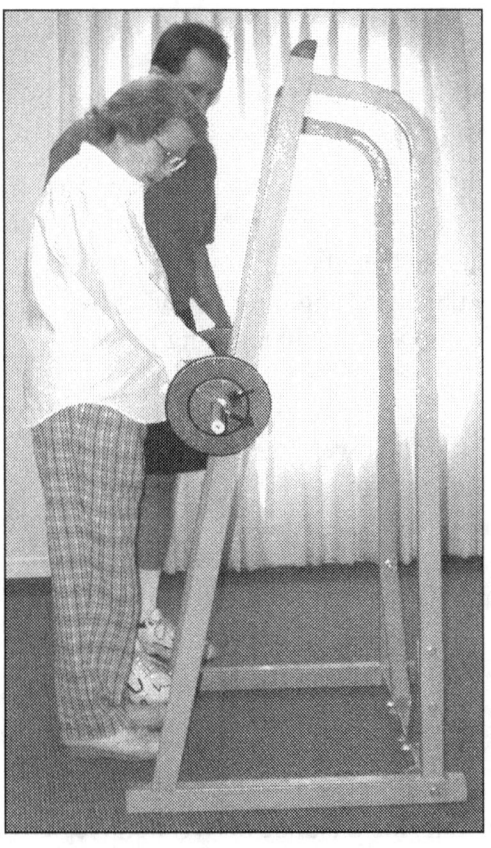

Figure 6-5. Ann takes the barbell from the rack.

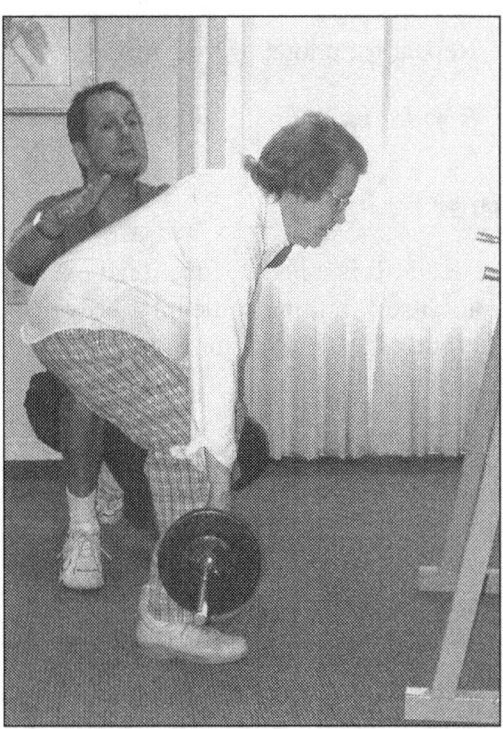

Figure 6-6. Ann dead lifts 40 pounds.

Performance

Ask your SE to do the following:

- Inhale and slowly lower the barbell by moving his hips back, bending his knees, and leaning forward.

- Keep the barbell within an inch of his legs at all times.

- Let his knees move no farther forward than the tips of his toes.

- Take two or three seconds to lower the barbell to mid-shin.

- Exhale and slowly extend (straighten) the hips and knees.

- When the barbell moves above the knees, extend the back.

- Raise himself up to the starting position with his chest out, his shoulder blades back, his hips and back fully extended, and his knees extended but not locked out. He will take two or three seconds to complete the raise.

- Repeat for a total of 8-12 reps.

- Rest for two minutes or more.

Finer Points

The dead lift is a highly functional exercise and a highly technical one. However, the motion itself, putting something heavy on the floor and then picking it up, is something everybody has done. Your SE already knows the basics, so your main teaching job is to refine his technique.

A good starting point is to ask him to hold a broomstick or a dowel, lower it to mid-shin, and straighten back up. Watching him closely will give you a good idea of what areas to focus on.

As the Spotter or Strength Coach for your SE, you can take several actions to ensure that he performs the dead lift correctly and safely:

- After handing him the barbell, move about a foot to one side and lower one knee to the floor.

- From this half-crouched position, you can observe the dead lift in profile and can watch his knee, back, shoulder, and hand positions, as well as the distance between his legs and the barbell.

- As he performs the exercise, keep one hand near the small of his back and get ready to remind him with a gentle tap on his lower back if it begins to round or flex.

- When he completes the exercise, move quickly to his front so that you can easily take the barbell from his hands.

- This exercise is demanding, so make sure he takes a long rest (two minutes or more).

An Additional Note on Safety

Although the potential for injury is relatively high with the dead lift, the exercise provides enormous benefits if done safely. To make the exercise as safe as possible, note the following:

- Be prepared for your SE to shift his weight onto the front half of the foot. Remind him to keep his weight on the back half of his foot. Ask him to "push through his heels."

- Watch to see that he doesn't round his shoulders. If he does, remind him to keep a big chest, that is, to keep his shoulder blades together and to stick his chest out.

- Anticipate that he may have trouble lowering the barbell below his knees. If he does, ask him to bend farther forward with his lower back and move his hips farther to the rear. Many people are reluctant to move in this way because they are fearful of using their lower backs at all.

- Be ready to rise suddenly from your half-crouch if he tires, loses his balance, or relaxes his grip on the barbell. You may need to provide support until he can sit and rest.

- As he tires, he's likely to drop his gaze from the spot on the wall he needs to be looking at. If this happens, his head will drop and his upper back will begin to round. A simple verbal reminder, "eyes up," will usually correct this potential problem.

Two Add-on Exercises

The exercises in the previous chapter aren't specifically geared to work the biceps and triceps, although several multi-joint exercises provide a good workout for these muscles.

Following are descriptions of exercises for the biceps and the triceps muscles. Feel free to add them into your SE's training sessions whenever he seems interested in working harder on his arm strength.

The Biceps Muscles—The Dumbbell Curl

The biceps muscles provide a pulling motion that is highly useful in everyday life. Any time your SE picks up something, he's using his biceps. If he picks up something heavy, he's using them even more—sacks of groceries, grandchildren, bags of books. If he's walking down the hall holding something heavy close to his chest, he's using his biceps.

The biceps is exercised by flexing (bending) the arm at the elbow. This curling motion is popular from childhood through old age for demonstrating strength: "Show me your muscles!"

There are many variations for the curling exercise—seated or standing, with dumbbells or barbells, using a wide grip or a narrow grip, lifting straight up or across the body, and so on.

Note that the seated and standing band rows also work the biceps. Therefore, if you run short of time in a training session or your SE tires early, you can omit a specific biceps exercise. Most people like this exercise and may ask to do it. The basic dumbbell curl starts with the correct position.

Preparation

Ask your SE to do the following:

- Stand straight and tall with his arms approximately shoulder width apart.

- Take the universal stance.

- Grasp the dumbbells which you hold out to him and let them hang down at his sides with his palms turned inward toward his thighs, as Jack does in Figure 6-7.

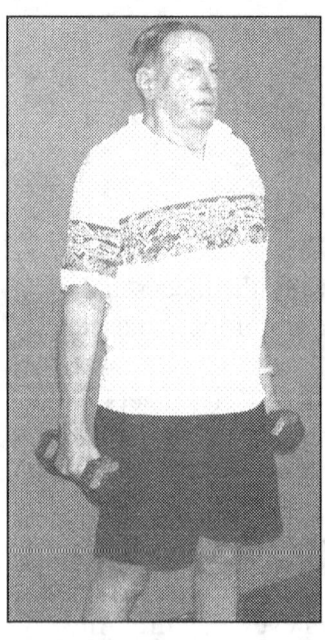

Figure 6-7. Jack gets ready.

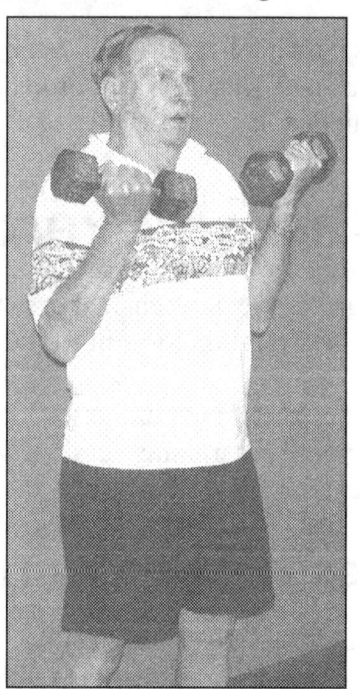

Figure 6-8. He curls 15 pounds in each hand.

Performance

Ask your SE to do the following:

- Inhale.

- While exhaling, bring both hands up near his chest but below his clavicle, rotating the wrists to the palms-up or supinated position as he does so. See Figure 6-8.

- Inhale and lower his hands on a count of two or three, rotating the wrists back to the original palms-in position.

- Repeat for 8-12 reps.

- Rest for a minute.

Finer Points

Everyone likes to curl a lot of weight. It feels good. It's a classic muscle-making pose. As a result, even the most ethical people tend to cheat on this exercise, usually without realizing it. Ensure that you ask your SE to do the following:

- Maintain good posture.

- Keep his elbows down and at his sides. If he brings his elbows forward, the front shoulder muscles come into active play. Remind him that this is a biceps exercise.

- Keep his shoulder blades down and back—depressed and retracted.

As he gets tired, he will want to:

- Lock out his knees and lean back.

- Swing the weights backward on the down stroke to get momentum to lift again instead of being still for a second at the bottom of the arc.

None of these are critical errors unless he's too tired or tries to lift too much. Just remind him gently about good technique.

If your SE prefers or needs to sit, he can still curl with good technique. Because of an injury to her right shoulder, Anna Fay in Figure 6-9 holds three pounds in her right hand and five pounds in her left.

You can make similar adjustments with your SE after a temporary injury or for a permanent condition.

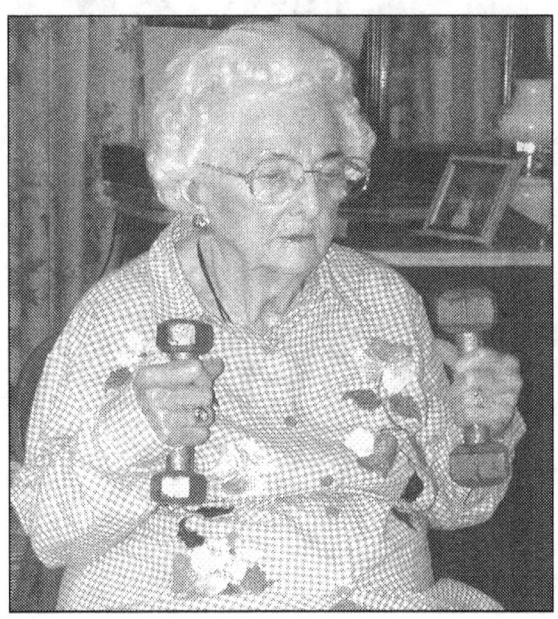

Figure 6-9. Anna Faye performs the seated curl.

The Triceps Exercise—The Armchair Dip

Many triceps exercises require equipment, but this one uses only a sturdy armchair or Mary's locked wheelchair in Figures 6-9 and 6-10. The exercise does a good job of strengthening and firming the backs of the upper arms. For that reason, women are especially interested in it because it helps get rid of the Bingo Wave, also called the Hi, Janes.

Preparation

Ask your SE to do the following:

- Sit at the front edge of his chair with erect posture and both feet on the floor. Remind him about the athletic seated posture on page 70.

- Grasp the arms of the chair with each hand with the knuckles facing as far forward as comfort allows.

- Point the elbows to the back instead of out to the side.

- Keep his shoulder blades retracted and depressed.

- Maintain excellent posture.

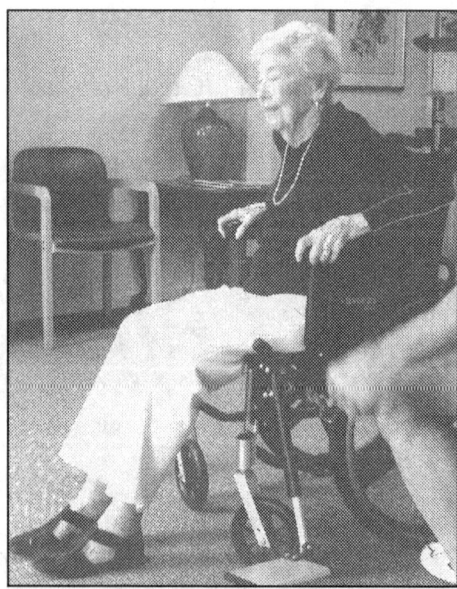

Figure 6-10. Mary prepares for the armchair dip.

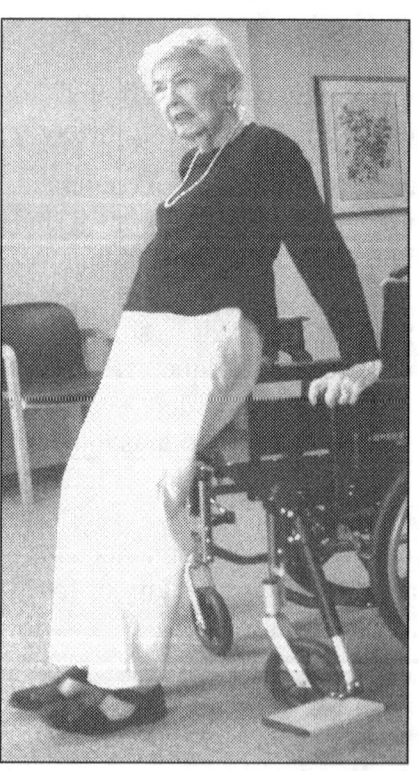

Figure 6-11. Mary performs the armchair dip.

Performance

Ask your SE to do the following:

- Inhale and push up, using only his arms, so that both arms are fully extended, elbows straight. His feet will remain on the floor, his knees will be partially bent, and his hips will come off the chair. Remind him not to use his leg strength for this exercise.

- Exhale and lower his hips back onto the chair by slowly bending his elbows.

- Repeat for 8-12 reps.

- Rest for a minute.

Finer points

Once he has a feel for this exercise, ask him not to settle his hips when they touch the chair, but rather to let his hips touch the chair lightly, and then extend his elbows again. Another way to make this exercise more challenging is to ask him to move his feet a few inches forward before he begins lifting his body. This adjustment increases the body weight that his triceps are required to lift—a good progression.

The main error in technique with the armchair dip is to spread the shoulder blades and round the shoulders. This is a costly error because it places the rotator cuff muscles in a position of danger. Sore muscles or even an injury can result from incorrect technique.

Seven Supplemental Exercises

These seven exercises are included to help you provide variety and greater attention to a specific muscle group if needed. For example, if your SE dislikes or can't perform one of the exercises in the previous chapter, you can substitute one of these for the corresponding muscle group. Also, if he wants to work harder on his legs, for example, you can add some of these leg exercises to help ensure mobility and prevent falls.

The Abdominal Muscles—Two Exercises

The abdominal muscles are so important for older people that you might consider adding these two exercises to your SE's training sessions, if he's interested, instead of replacing the exercises in the previous chapter with these. The manual trunk rotation and crunches offer great benefits and are easy to add into his training sessions as you have the time and interest.

Remember that with any manual exercise, you are the machine.

Manual Trunk Rotations

Manual trunk rotations target the external and internal oblique muscles, which, in addition to supporting the spine, help to rotate the torso. The abs are also involved, and the taller your SE sits the more involved they are. Remind him to sit straight and tall.

Preparation

Sit in a chair facing your SE but don't sit directly in front of him. Offset your chair enough that the outer edge of your right thigh is touching the outer edge of his right thigh. Make sure that, when you lean forward, your left hand can touch his back at the right shoulder blade. Ask him to do the following:

- Sit on the front edge of the chair as upright as possible.

- Pull his shoulder blades down and together and lengthen his spine.

Place the palm of your left hand on his right shoulder blade and the palm of your right hand on the front of his right shoulder to provide resistance—very light at first.

Performance

Ask your SE to do the following:

- Inhale. Rotate his upper torso, head, and shoulders as far as possible to his left side.

- Exhale. Slowly return to the starting position without using his hands.

- Do 8-12 on the left side and then, after you move your chair, do 8-12 on the right side, reversing the procedure.

- Rest for 30 seconds to one minute.

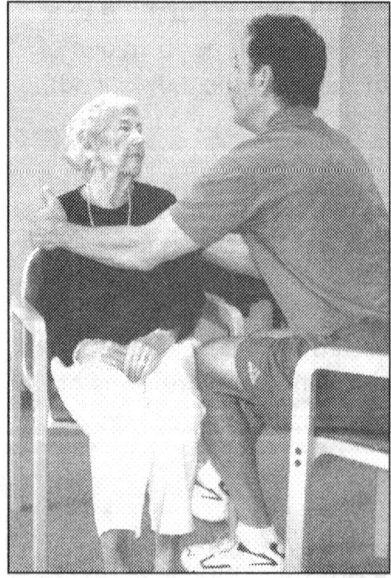

Figure 6-12. Mary prepares for trunk rotations.

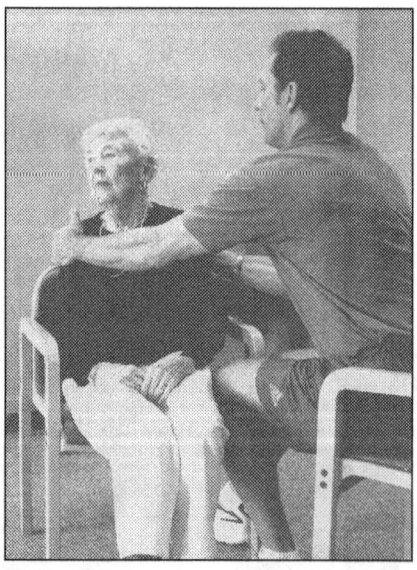

Figure 6-13. Mary rotates her torso.

Finer Points

Go light at first as it's easy to overdo this exercise. Watch carefully to ensure that he is doing the following:

- Keeping his back flat and vertical.

- Keeping his head and neck in alignment with his torso and letting them turn with his torso.

- Pushing steadily and not jerking to the left or the right.

- Using the muscles in his trunk and not pushing with his legs and feet.

Crunches

If your SE can easily get up and down from the floor or a bench, you can introduce crunches into his training sessions as soon as you both want to. The seated push and chair crunches in the previous chapter are good ab exercises, but the crunch is superior. The idea of doing the same exercise that younger people perform may appeal to him.

Preparation

Ask your SE to do the following:

- Lie flat on his back on the mat or on the bench.

- Lace his hands behind his head. The hands form a hammock to support his head and neck. Remind him not to pull his head up by using his hands. If he is unable to cradle his head in his hands, ask him to place them across his chest.

- Lift his feet from the bench so that his thighs are perpendicular to the bench. See Figure 6-14 below.

Performance

Ask your SE to do the following:

- Inhale. Then exhale as he lifts his head and shoulders as high as he can from the bench or mat without jerking or yanking.

- At the same time, bring his knees as close to his chest as possible.

- Exhale as he slowly lowers his head and shoulders. Return the upper legs to vertical.

- Repeat for 8-12 reps.

- Rest for 30 seconds to one minute.

Finer Points

A common technique error is to lead with the chin, thereby straining the neck muscles. Remind him to start the motion in his abdominal muscles and to keep his neck relaxed. Also, remind him to go up slowly because yanking or jerking can cause injury or muscle strain to his lower back. Another common error occurs if he uses his hands and arms to pull his head and neck up, thus failing to engage the ab muscles.

For some older people, the most difficult thing about this exercise is getting down onto the mat or getting flat on the bench because getting up is hard for them. You may need to give him a hand up.

In Figure 6-14, Esther, 92, brings her knees and shoulders close together with her hands on her chest. Note that a weightlifting bench is not designed for crunches, so if your SE is large, make sure he is well centered and balanced. Prevent him from falling off. In Figure 6-15, Kathleen performs an advanced version of the crunch.

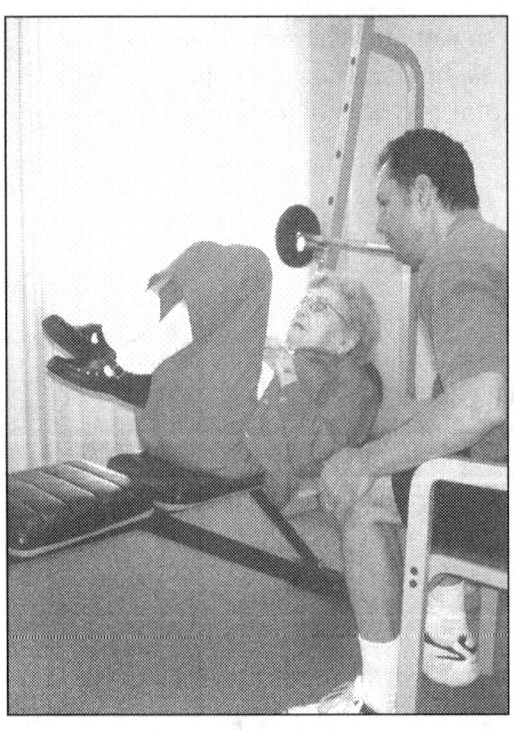

Figure 6-14. Esther crunches.

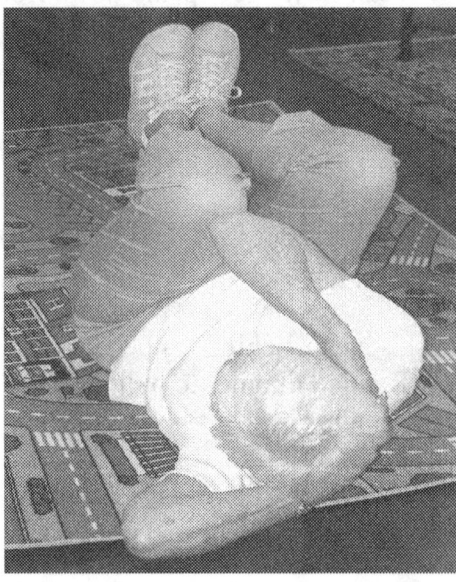

Figure 6-15. Kathleen touches elbow to knee.

The Leg Muscles—Four Exercises

Since mobility is so important for a feeling of independence, this chapter contains four manual exercises for the leg muscles. Instead of expensive machines, you will use your strength to provide resistance in the manual abductor, manual adductor, manual leg curl, and manual leg extension exercises. As with the manual trunk rotation, you are the machine.

The abductor muscles work the lateral hip muscles, principally the gluteus medius. The adductor muscles work the inner thighs. Exercises for these muscles are important for assistance in walking a straight line, standing, and balancing. These muscles prevent the wobbles. Older people with weak abductors and adductors tend to veer left or right when they try to walk straight ahead.

Manual Abductor Exercise

The basic exercise for the abductor muscles is simple and requires only the use of two sturdy armchairs and a little bit of your own strength.

Preparation

Ask your SE to do the following:

- Sit in the chair with his back and hips firmly against the back of the chair.

- Take a firm grip on the arms of the chair.

Sit in another chair facing him. Leave about three feet between the two chairs.

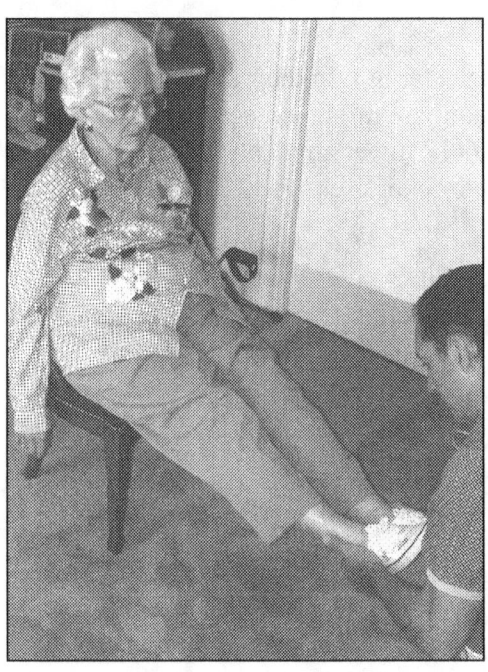

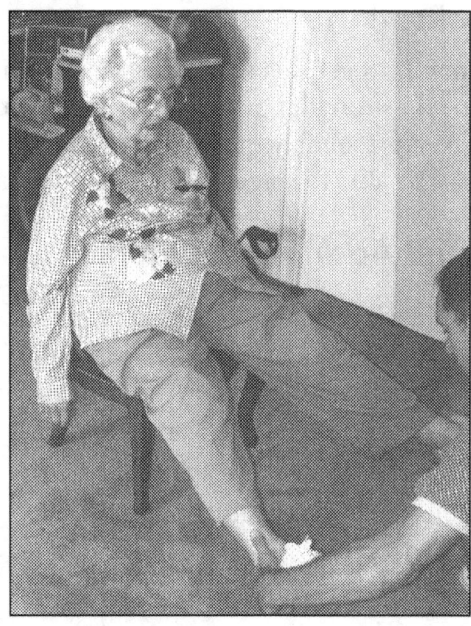

Figure 6-17. Anna Fay works the abductors.

Figure 6-16. Anna Fay gets ready.

Performance

Ask your SE to do the following:

- Extend both legs out straight in front, parallel to the floor, with the ankles together, as in Figure 6-16.

- Inhale.

- As you hold and push the ankles together to provide resistance, have him try to spread his legs as far apart as possible while keeping his legs parallel to the floor. Give enough support under his heels that he doesn't have to expend any energy holding his legs up. Ask him to exhale as he spreads his legs.

- Return slowly to the starting position with the ankles together.

- Repeat for 8-12 reps.

- Rest for 30 seconds to one minute.

Finer Points

In general, John finds that older people don't have much strength in their abductors before they begin strength training. Start light, even lighter than you might expect. But you can anticipate reasonably quick improvement. See Figure 6-17 to get an idea of how far your SE may be able to spread his legs in the manual abductor exercise.

Manual Adductor Exercise

The basic exercise for the adductor muscles works the inner thighs and looks like the abductor exercise in reverse. It's also simple and requires only the use of two sturdy armchairs and a little bit of your own strength.

Preparation

Ask your SE to do the following:

- Sit in the chair with his back and hips firmly against the back of the chair.

- Take a firm grip on the arms of the chair.

Sit in another chair facing him. Leave about three feet between the two chairs.

Performance

Ask your SE to do the following:

- Extend both legs out straight in front, parallel to the floor.

- Spread his legs as far apart as possible as Faye does in Figure 6-18 below.

- Inhale.

- As you hold and pull his ankles apart to provide resistance, have him try to bring his legs together until his knees touch, still keeping his legs parallel to the floor. Give enough support under his heels that he doesn't have to expend any energy holding his legs up.

- Return slowly to the starting position.

- Repeat for 8-12 reps.

- Rest for 30 seconds to one minute.

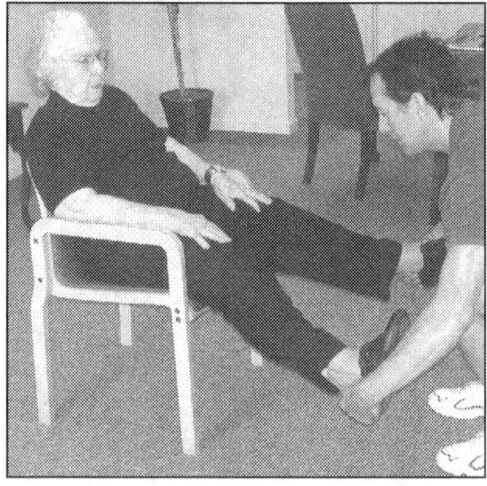

Figure 6-18. Faye prepares for the adductor exercise.

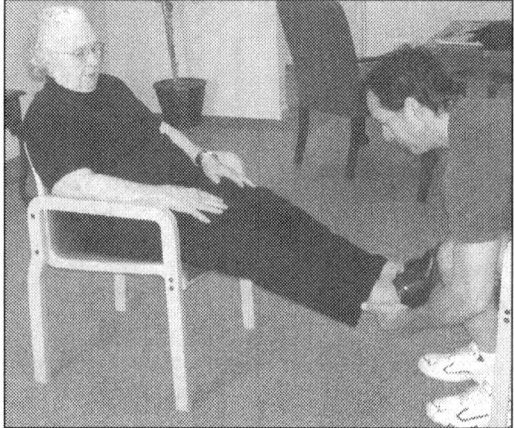

Figure 6-19. Faye works the adductors.

Finer Points

Expect his strength to be substantially greater here than for the abductor exercise above. More muscle mass is at work. If his adductors aren't substantially stronger than his abductors, ask him to perform two sets of adductors for each set of abductor exercises until he achieves better muscle balance. For both the abductor and adductor exercises, you can increase the difficulty as his strength improves by providing a lesser amount of resistance for the motion during which he returns to the starting position.

Manual Leg Extension

This exercise provides the same benefit to the quads as the exercise on a machine that Jack performs in Figure 6-20. The manual part comes about when you are the machine as John is with Faye in Figure 6-21.

Preparation

Ask your SE to do the following;

- Sit back in the chair.

161

- Brace himself with the armrests so that his back is firmly against the back of the chair and both feet are firmly on the floor.

- Raise his left knee so that his left foot is six inches from the floor after you get in place.

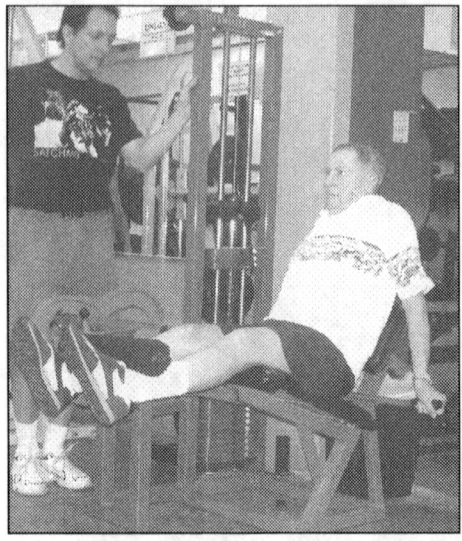

Figure 6-20. Jack uses a leg extension machine.

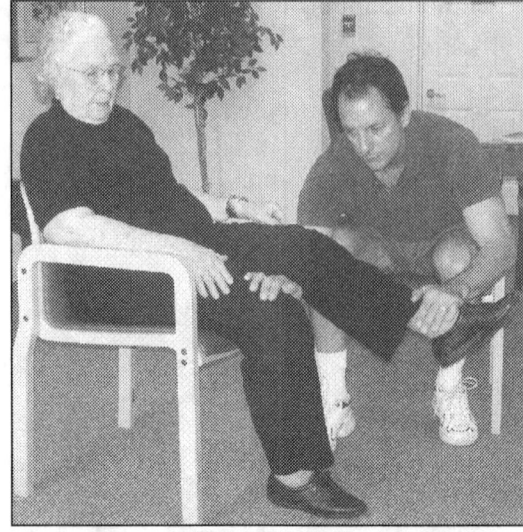

Figure 6-21. Faye does the manual leg extension.

To provide the manual resistance, do the following:

- Sit with your chair at a right angle to his chair on his right side and your knees about six inches from his.

- Put your right forearm under his left knee and rest your right palm on his right knee as pictured in Figure 6-21.

- Then put your left palm on the top of his left ankle.

Performance

Ask your SE to:

- Inhale.

- Extend his left leg out straight against the resistance of your left hand as he exhales.

- Return slowly to the starting position by flexing or bending his right leg.

- Repeat 8-12 times on the left side and 8-12 times on the right side after you move your chair and take the opposite hand positions.

- Rest for 30 seconds to one minute.

Finer Points

As he extends or straightens his left leg, apply firm resistance to his ankle with your left hand. Then as he slowly flexes or bends his left leg back to the starting position, continue to apply light resistance.

Manual Leg Curl

Leg curls strengthen the hamstring muscles of the posterior thigh. Instead of lying on his stomach to use a leg curl machine in a gym, your SE remains seated but gets the same benefit as he would from the machine.

Preparation

Ask your SE to the same thing he did for the manual leg extension:

- Sit back in the chair.

- Brace himself with the armrests so that his back is firmly against the back of the chair, and both feet are firmly on the floor.

- Raise his left knee up so that his foot is six inches from the floor after you get in place.

To prepare for providing the manual resistance, you will do the following:

- Sit with your chair at a right angle to his on the left side with your knees about six inches from his.

- Place your right forearm under his left knee and rest your palm on his right knee.

- Ask your SE to extend his left leg out straight.

- Then reach out with your left hand over the top of his left ankle and grasp his left heel.

So far the two of you look similar to John and Faye in Figure 6-21 except that your hand is under his heel instead of on top of his ankle. See Figure 6-22 below.

Performance

Ask your SE to do the following:

- Inhale. As he exhales, flex or bend his knee, pulling his heel underneath him. Ask him to try to touch the underside of the chair with his foot.

- Return slowly to the starting position by extending or straightening his leg.

To provide the manual resistance, you will:

- Apply upward pressure to his left heel as he flexes or bends his knee downward.

- Repeat 8-12 times on the left side and 8-12 times on the right side after you move your chair and take the opposite hand positions.

- Rest for 30 seconds to one minute.

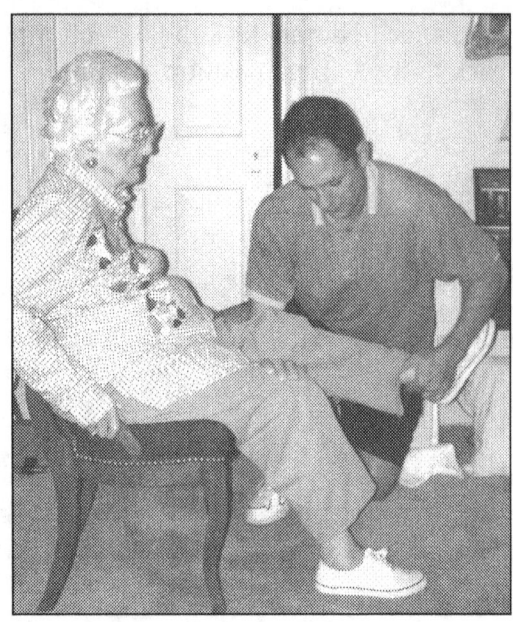

Figure 6-22. Anna Fay prepares for the leg curl.

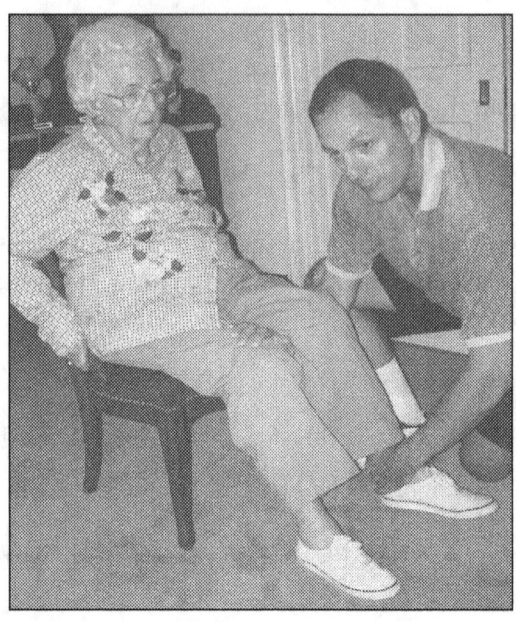

Figure 6-23. Anna Fay pushes down.

Finer Points

You may find that you can't provide enough resistance while you are seated. If so, then half-crouch, as John does for demonstration purposes in Figure 6-23. Place your right knee on the floor beside your SE so you can reach his extended ankle. If necessary, support your left forearm on your left knee while you apply resistance. As he extends his leg on the return motion, continue to apply resistance but make it lighter. Expect a lot of jerky movement until he learns to complete the return smoothly.

The Shoulder Muscles—The Dumbbell Press

The dumbbell press is the same as the presses you will see in any gym. The only difference is that you will stand close to your SE in order to provide support if he loses his balance. If he can't complete the lift, you will need to grab the dumbbells.

> When your SE holds a steel weight over his head, use extra caution.

Raising a barbell or dumbbells overhead with both arms is constricting and difficult for many older people. Before you introduce this exercise, make sure your SE can easily raise his arms overhead within 20 degrees of vertical without pain and stiffness. He will probably find it easier to manage two dumbbells than a barbell, so start with dumbbells. If he's able to perform the exercise well with dumbbells, then later on you can try increasing the difficulty by using a barbell. His flexibility is likely to be better with dumbbells, and his balance is usually better with a barbell.

If your SE can't raise both hands nearly vertically overhead, do not perform this exercise. Instead, continue using the lateral raise described in the previous chapter.

Preparation

Ask your SE to do the following:

- Take the universal stance on page 69.

- Hold a pair of dumbbells loosely at his sides. Start with one-pound dumbbells or no weight at all for teaching purposes because technique is important in this exercise.

Performance

Ask your SE to do the following:

- Bring both dumbbells up to shoulder level so that they are near the outer edges of his shoulders with the dumbbells perpendicular to his body.

- Turn the palms facing forward so that the dumbbells are in line with his shoulders. If this position causes shoulder discomfort, he can keep his palms facing inward.

- Inhale.

- On a count of one, while exhaling extend the arms overhead so that the dumbbells nearly, but not quite, touch.

- Try not to straighten the knees completely.

- As he exhales, lower the dumbbells to the shoulders on a count of two.

- Repeat for 8-12 reps.

- Rest for one minute.

As the Spotter or Strength Coach, you need to place your open hands near his wrists, ready to assist if his strength or balance falters. Although Jack can press 15 pounds in each hand without assistance in Figures 6-24 and 25, you need to stand in front of your SE to support his elbows in case of trouble.

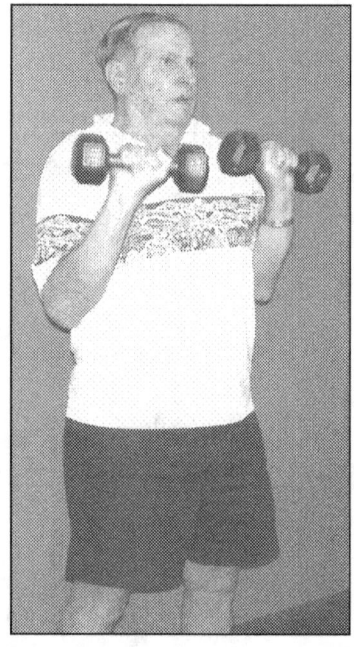

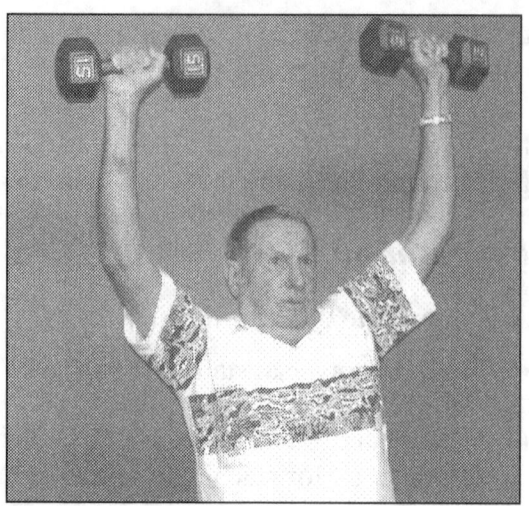

Figure 6-25. Jack presses 30 pounds.

Figure 6-24. Jack takes the ready position.

Finer Points

You might want to start out for teaching purposes with your SE seated on a chair or bench. The press can seem awkward and unbalanced, and sitting removes any fear—yours or his—of toppling over. He needs to keep his back firm and flat or slightly arched, his head up, and his feet flat on the floor. Encourage him not to lean back as he does this exercise. Note that the shoulder strength required for this exercise is greater when sitting than when standing, so use light weights.

For your SE, the motion of the overhead press may feel as if he is bringing the dumbbells behind his head, but he isn't. Anybody over the age of 70 who can get the dumbbells straight over head has good range of motion indeed. How far overhead to lift depends upon your SE, but someone who can't come within 20 degrees of vertical should not do this exercise. Ideally, your SE will be able to lift the dumbbells right over the crown of his head.

A final point is to make sure that he doesn't cock his wrists forward or backward. The wrists are in a vulnerable position with this exercise, and they need to be in the same line with the forearms and locked into place.

A Note on Shoulder Range of Motion and Safety

If you work out yourself, you probably perform several varieties of shoulder exercises and don't worry at all about safety or about the range of motion that you put your shoulders through. You can complete the shoulder tests in the Appendix without a second thought.

166

For your SE, however, you may need to work on increasing his overhead range of motion by using the following techniques:

- Ask him to stand as you take a position close behind him.

- Ask him to lift his arms as high as he can.

- Assist by placing your hands lightly on his elbows and gently helping him to lift his arms a little higher. Stop at the first sign of discomfort—don't wait for pain.

- Hold him in this position for 5-10 seconds.

Over several weeks, you may be able to increase his range of motion to the point that he can raise both hands with assistance to within 20 degrees of vertical. If he is able to do this without weights, try a pair of one-pound dumbbells.

The Cool-down/Calm-down

Use the cool-down/calm-down described on page 135. Even if your SE trains for years, don't neglect this important aspect of the training session. Returning to normal is especially important after a particularly taxing workout.

A Note to Certified Personal Trainers

If you don't have much experience with older clients, you will want to use the readiness indicators or methods of your own devising to ensure that your older clients are able—today—to perform the exercises in this chapter. If you train someone over 85, use particular caution to make these exercises truly safe.

You have probably taught the bench press, the dumbbell press, and the dead lift for years without mishap and without excessive concern for safety. However, with older clients, you really do need to take the precautions described in each additional note on safety. The strength and health of older people fluctuates more than that of younger people, and a normally strong client may suffer a momentary weakness or period of dizziness with little to no warning.

John advises using the warm-up before each training session as a diagnostic tool for checking on the client's state of health and strength. Remember:

- Be prepared at all times to substitute less taxing exercises, fewer reps, and fewer sets if needed.

- The focus is always on safety.

Summary of the Main Points

This chapter shows you how to do additional exercises with your SE. The main points to remember include the following:

- Take particular care with safety for the bench press, dead lift, crunch, and dumbbell press.

- If your SE can't perform a particular exercise, continue with the exercise for the corresponding muscle group described in the previous chapter.

- Introduce change gradually into his training sessions and only when he's interested.

- He will probably enjoy the new exercises for the biceps and triceps muscles.

- If your SE shows good flexibility and aptitude, introduce the exercises in this chapter as early in his training sessions as you both desire.

- Since the advanced exercises are more subject to injuries, make sure that you practice excellent safety precautions.

- Be especially careful with his shoulder range of motion.

- *Always* have him warm up and cool down.

What's Next?

The next chapter shows you how to ensure that your SE isn't sabotaging his strength training sessions by eating and resting sub-optimally. The suggestions are practical and are based on common sense.

Chapter 7. Food and Rest

If You Are What You Eat, You're Also How You Rest

"Squats, collards, and a good night's sleep—the not-so-secret basics of the good life."
  John Payne, 54

Important Points for Advocates: To improve your Significant Elder's eating and sleeping habits, ask for help from the support group you have set up, as recommended in Chapter 2. Family members and friends who live nearby, including her personal trainer, are in a better position to check on her meals and to ask how she slept last night. You can make some inquiries by phone and on visits, but the support group will need to help you handle the day-to-day contact with your SE.

Introduction

What do food and rest have to do with strength training? Indeed, what do they have to do with each other?

Here's the connection—good nutrition and adequate recovery are two of the three physical prerequisites for strength training.[28] A Significant Elder who seldom eats right or sleeps well can't do a great deal to increase her strength on a consistent basis, even if she looks healthy enough. She is battling herself—trying to build a stronger body while failing to refuel and recover adequately.

However, someone who gets good nutrition and adequate rest can indeed become stronger through strength training, even if she is over 80 and has medical problems (such as those listed in "Handling Health Issues Safely" on page 87.

> Your SE has been eating and sleeping a certain way for 70,
> 80, or 90 years and has survived. Be gentle with changes.

How can you even talk with your SE about improving her food and rest? Admittedly, it's not easy to bring up the subject. Consider what it might take for you to give up alcohol,

---

[28] The third, being "too frail" for physical activity, we discussed in Chapter 1. Recall that attitude is more important than physical condition and that most frail older people can take up strength training provided the trainer or Strength Coach is experienced in working with the frail.

caffeine, nicotine, chocolate, and sugar or, perhaps even harder, to go to bed at 8:00 PM and wake up at 4:00 AM every day, including weekends, for the rest of your life. Your objections would be endless.

Further, if you are a parent, you can recall how difficult it may have been to introduce new foods to your four-year-old or to get him to eat anything at meal times. Recall how hard it was to get your teenager to bed at a reasonable hour and how difficult to wake him up in the mornings.

Changing long-held habits, especially such intimate habits as eating and sleeping, isn't easy. Fortunately, you don't have to worry about changing everything in your SE's food and rest practices. Just as you start with baby steps in strength training, you also start with baby steps in nutrition and recovery.

The goal of this chapter is not to help you reform your SE. That's impossible and it's not your job. A total make-over probably isn't even necessary because, to reach her advanced age, she's certainly doing something right if only having been born with good genes.

Instead, the goal of this chapter is to show you a few changes you can encourage your SE to adopt and to present a few steps for helping her make these changes. A few small changes in her eating and sleeping habits can improve your SE's life for all of her activities, not just strength training. It's likely that both of you will be surprised at the difference a few little improvements can make in the quality of her life.

Food

We discuss three main areas associated with nutrition: determining the general guidelines to follow, finding out whether your SE could use some nutritional improvements, and implementing a few specific techniques to help her achieve better nutrition.

The purpose of these small changes isn't necessarily to help her lose weight, if she could stand to shed a few pounds, but instead to make sure she isn't sabotaging her success at strength training with less-than-healthy eating. She will need good nutrition in order to be successful because food, along with water and good breathing, provides fuel for the body to use in strength training as well as everything else she does.

Determining Some General Guidelines

Ideas about *dieting* and *diet* are finally converging to provide sensible guidelines on nutrition. Dieting, defined as following an eating plan to lose or gain weight, now closely resembles the daily diet, defined as an eating plan to maintain current weight. We focus on the daily diet as nutritional maintenance for strength and health, not dieting as a way to gain or lose weight, for several reasons:

• Your SE probably needs and will respond more positively to minor adjustments rather than major changes to her eating habits even if she doesn't always eat nutritiously.

- Americans, especially women, already know quite a bit about dieting to lose weight, as evidenced by the best-seller status of many diet books.

- There are only three macro-nutrients—carbohydrates, fat, and protein. If we eliminate any of these three from our diet, we eventually die. Therefore, the only arguments are those related to proportion and quality. Today's popular diets for weight loss, such as Atkins, South Beach, Weight Watchers, and the Zone, ask you to reduce the amount of carbohydrate and fat you eat. Most dietitians agree that active people need more protein than inactive people do.

USDA Guidelines

The food pyramid developed by the U.S. Department of Agriculture is perhaps today's most widely circulated and well-known guideline for eating. Until the April 2005 revision, however, a person of average size was allowed to eat 11 slices of bread a day, which clearly provides too much carbohydrate for most people.

Nutritional guidelines in the U.S. have always been based on "preventing nutritional deficiencies," according to Alice Lichtenstein, who also notes that today a need to "prevent chronic diseases" has driven the first complete revision of the USDA Food Guide Pyramid since 1992 and the first update since 1996.[29]

Note that many Americans seem to have ignored the recommended serving size for carbohydrates. For example, a serving size is 1/2 cup of pasta or rice, one ounce of cereal, 4 small plain crackers, or 1 slice of bread. Many Americans eat far larger portions. They may have taken to heart the idea that they don't need to measure the size of their servings because the booklet that accompanies the Food Guide Pyramid contains the following question and answer:

> Do I need to measure servings?
> No. Use servings only as a general guide.

To some people, this statement was a license to carbo-load, even if they led sedentary lives, as three-fifths of Americans do today. Clearly, people today are eating too much and getting too little exercise. The media report that 66% of Americans are somewhat or severely overweight. If the trend continues, by 2030 nearly all Americans will be overweight. Food scientists and the U.S. Department of Agriculture are no doubt doing their best to provide good guidelines, but it may be several years before the revised Food Guide Pyramid makes an impact on the American public.

The new Food Guide Pyramid, published in April 2005, provides better guidance and includes recommendations for exercise. The only difficulty is that it was first published

---

[29] Gershoff Professor of Nutrition Science and Policy at Tufts University, as cited in *Harvard Public Health Now*, October 2003 (email newsletter at http://www.hsph.harvard.edu/now/oct3/forum.html).

online (at www.mypyramid.gov), and your SE needed a computer to access it. For your convenience, we provide the new pyramid in, Figure 7-1 and explain the vertical stripes and exercise recommendations. The tables that follow show the types and quantities of food for women and men over age 50.

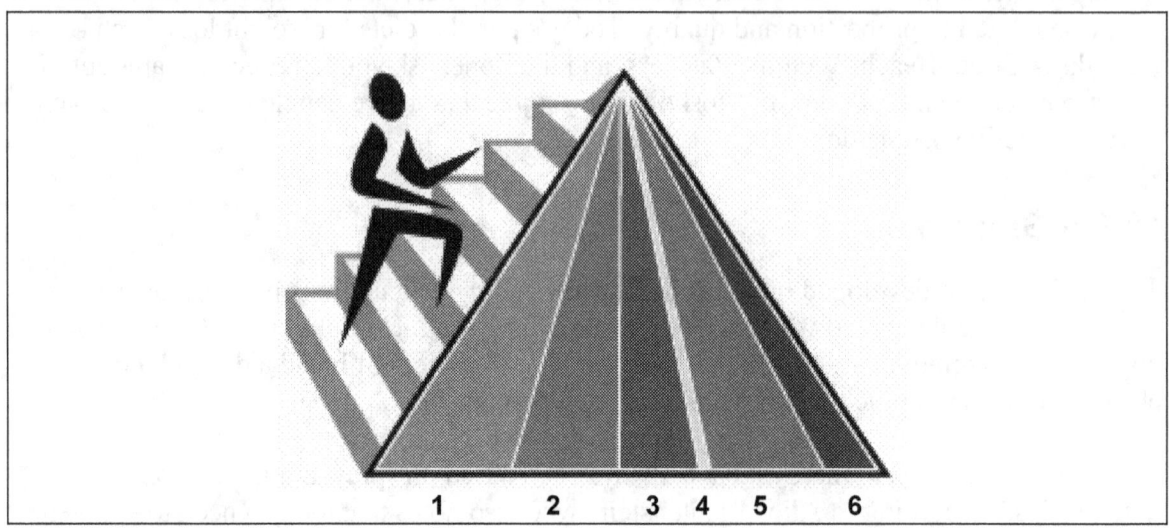

Figure 7-1 The 2005 Food Guide Pyramid

The new guidelines encourage 30 minutes a day of exercise beyond your usual daily activities. The food allowances in Table 7-1 and Table 7-2 are based on getting up to 30 minutes of exercise. If you exercise 30 to 60 minutes a day, you can increase the portions very slightly.

Women

Stripe Number	Daily Food Allowances for Women Age 51+
1	Grains: Five ounces, three of which should be whole grains.
2	Vegetables: Two cups. Eat dark leafy greens three times a week, orange vegetables twice a week, and peas and beans three times a week.
3	Fruits: One and one-half cups but go easy on fruit juices. Enjoy fresh, frozen, canned, or dried fruit.
4	Oils: Five teaspoons. Eat more fish, nuts, and vegetable oils but limit butter, mayonnaise, shortening, and lard.
5	Milk: Three cups. Use low-fat and fat-free milk, cheese, yogurt, and milk-based desserts like pudding and ice milk.
6	Meat and beans: Five ounces. Use low-fat and lean meat and poultry. Bake, broil, or grill it. Use a variety of fish, beans, peas, nuts, eggs, and seeds.

Table 7-1. USDA Recommendations for Women 51 and over

Men

Stripe Number	Daily Food Allowances for Men Age 51+
1	Grains: Six ounces, three of which should be whole grains.
2	Vegetables: Two and a half cups. Eat dark leafy greens three times a week, orange vegetables twice a week, and peas and beans three times a week.
3	Fruits: Two cups but go easy on fruit juices. Enjoy fresh, frozen, canned, or dried fruit.
4	Oils: Six teaspoons. Eat more fish, nuts, and vegetable oils but limit butter, mayonnaise, shortening, and lard.
5	Milk: Three cups. Use low-fat and fat-free milk, cheese, yogurt, and milk-based desserts like pudding and ice milk.
6	Meat and beans: Five and a half ounces. Use low-fat and lean meat and poultry. Bake, broil, or grill it. Use a variety of fish, beans, peas, nuts, eggs, and seeds.

Table 7-2. USDA Recommendations for Men 51 and over

Comments on the Changes

The new pyramid places men and women between 51 and 115 in the same category. If you are an adult child between 51 and 64, you may feel that the next revision of the pyramid should acknowledge that you are stronger and better able to exercise than your 80-year-old SE and, therefore, able to eat a little more. However, the metabolism slows with age, and you and your SE might find yourselves following the same daily diet.

Some improvements in the new pyramid are the more specific measurements (one cup instead of one serving) and the reduction in quantities. Grains, for example, are limited to five or six ounces, not six to eleven servings. The new pyramid also links exercise to the amount of food you can eat, although there is little guidance for those 51 and over who exercise more than one hour per day.

How can you best help your SE get the right food for strength training?
The answer, of course, is to take a sensible, incremental approach.

Sensible Tips

Following are some tried-and-true nutritional guidelines that you and your SE can believe in:

- Take all things in moderation. Don't follow the latest fad diets because they all have a hidden price to pay.

- Always eat breakfast.

- Eat lots and lots of leafy greens, especially dark green vegetables like spinach, collard greens, mustard greens, turnip greens, kale, and cabbage. If your SE claims not to like these foods, you can find ways to make them acceptable, if not eagerly anticipated. After all, they are great for you, low in calories, inexpensive, and delicious if prepared well.

- Don't consume huge meals—ever. At a restaurant, encourage your SE to take home a doggie bag. At home or at a friend's house, eat moderate portions and don't go back for seconds.

- Know your own and your SE's nutritional vices. They are mostly starches and sweets— ice cream, chocolate, high-fat cheese, pasta, baked goods—all of the tasty stuff.

- Skip dessert if you can. If you must have some birthday cake, take a tiny piece.

- Get a balance of carbohydrates, proteins, and fat at every meal, even breakfast. Avoid the low-calorie, low-fat, high-starch style of eating.

- Get a little more protein than usual on the days that you work out because protein repairs, maintains, and strengthens the muscles.

- Never skip a meal before a workout and have the meal or a light snack an hour before the session starts.

- Always drink some water and eat a little something that's nutritious after a workout, preferably something with a little protein, such as half a turkey sandwich.

- Eat before you are hungry and quit before you are full.

- Investigate whether three small meals and two or three very small snacks per day would work in your SE's schedule.

- When you grocery shop with your SE, stick to the perimeter of the store and avoid the prepared foods and pre-packaged items along the interior rows.

- When you can't account for a weight gain, it may be due to alcohol or other carbohydrates. Alcohol metabolizes in the body as sugar, which is a carbohydrate.

Even if your SE lives in a retirement facility that provides three meals a day, you still need to take an interest in her nutrition. Chefs at even the most expensive facilities seldom specialize in nutrition for older people and very few have a registered dietitian on staff.

Examining Your Significant Elder's Eating Habits

Because you grew up eating what Mom served at the table, you may believe you know her eating habits. You probably do know her public habits—what she eats when other people are around—but you may not know her private habits—what she eats when alone.

If there's no difference between public and private eating, your SE is to be congratulated. However, all Americans who lived through the Depression and World War II remember food shortages and rationing. The habit of hoarding food for a rainy day may still influence your SE's thinking. Every retirement facility in the country has its cadre of octogenarians armed with plastic bags that they use for taking home leftovers.

Daisy

Someone we will call Daisy, who is in her 80s, always brings home rolls and muffins and stores them in her otherwise unused oven. Fortunately, she forgets to eat them. They go stale, and eventually she tosses them out. But she still brings them back to her apartment. "I might need them!" she protests whenever her family members point out the ironies of the situation. Psychologically, she probably does. For her nutritional needs, it's good that she doesn't remember she has them.

Hidden Habits

One private, or hidden, eating habit that often interferes with the nutrition of many an older person who still cooks is tasting or sampling what she cooks. Even if it's just a smidgen, a half-teaspoon of chocolate fudge not only contains fat and calories but can also diminish the feeling of hunger. She may not feel hungry enough to go to the dining room for lunch or dinner if she's in a retirement facility or to prepare a nutritious meal if she has her own kitchen. Later in the day, she may consume food with far less nutrition and far more calories than she would have at her regularly scheduled meal.

Another private habit is unconsciously snacking while reading or watching TV alone. Your SE may recall eating only a couple of cookies and potato chips and drinking only one cola, yet her trash may be full of empty bags and cans, and her grocery list always contains both items.

Johnnie Lou

For example, someone we will call Johnnie Lou, in her late 80s, gets anxious when she opens the last six-pack of her favorite cola. Whenever possible, she gets her sodas by the case and is always surprised when they are all gone. The sugar and the caffeine provide too many empty calories in her diet, but she remains unaware of how many she drinks. She claims not to know why she can't lose weight and why she doesn't sleep well at night.

John's Clients

Nearly all of John's older clients express a desire to lose weight. "I tell them that they can do it and I can help them. Then I explain the changes in their eating habits that losing weight will require. I say, 'I'm working with you two hours a week. The other 166 hours, you're on your own.' This gives them a realistic perspective that's quite different from expecting the pounds to melt away just by doing what I ask of them twice a week."

Most of John's clients have modified their eating habits at least a little, starting with being more aware of what and how much they eat. This awareness is the first step toward better nutrition. Not many, however, have gone on to shed the pounds they say they want to lose.

Food psychology experiments indicate that when people have ample food on hand, they tend to eat more, especially if the food is in plain sight.[30] Therefore, a very simple way to help your SE cut down on empty calories is to put these items into cabinets and cupboards—out of sight, out of mind, at least for a while.

Documenting Your Significant Elder's Eating Habits

You don't need to feel like a snoop or a Big Brother character when you examine your SE's eating habits. After all, you are trying to help. The main points to make about documenting your SE's eating habits are the following:

- Gather evidence and keep records. Don't call attention to your activities, but do them in person. Eat meals with her and see with your own eyes how much and what she consumes. Take her to the grocery store and see what she buys.

- Don't always believe what she tells you about how nutritiously she eats, but never scold her for her choices. Never judge her. Just observe for yourself. Write it down and then add comments about whether you believe she exaggerates or minimizes anything about her eating habits.

- Enlist the assistance of her doctors by discussing the results of her blood work. Remember that older people in general are greatly influenced by medical opinion, as much as they may gripe about their doctors. If your SE has a high triglyceride level, high cholesterol, or other indicators of less-than-ideal nutrition, enlist the doctor's help in making just a few changes to her eating habits.

- Recognize that it's a rare person over 65 who routinely keeps track of what she eats.

- Since food allergies can develop at any age, be alert to any allergies that she may have and help her to plan around them. Wheat, dairy products, and peanuts are common offenders.

---

[30] Center for Science in the Public Interest, "See More, Eat More," *Nutrition Action Newsletter*, Vol. 30, No. 2, March 2003, p.8.

- Watch for several specific concerns that affect many older people: lactose intolerance, irritable bowel syndrome (frequent upset stomach, bloating, gas, indigestion, and so on), and frequent diarrhea or constipation.

- Be sensitive to various problems that may make eating difficult for your SE and do your best to make improvements for these conditions:

  - Poorly fitting dentures.

  - Hand tremors.

  - Various conditions of the mouth and jaw that make drooling all too easy.

  - Diminished sense of smell and taste.

  - Impaired vision.

  - Having to eat alone but not liking it.

  - Having to cook for herself but being unable or unwilling to do so.

In short, learn or re-learn her nutritional downfalls, her less-than-ideal habits, and her attitudes toward the food she consumes, as well as any problems she may have with eating nutritiously.

Elspeth

Poorly fitting dentures pained someone we will call Elspeth, 84. She lost weight steadily over the course of a year to the point that her friends and family became concerned. It finally emerged that her dentures caused painful ulcers in her mouth, and chewing had become next to impossible. Yet Elspeth seldom or never complained. After she heeded her friends' urgings, a skillful dentist was able to solve the problem, and her new dentures have helped her enjoy eating again.

Watching Out for the Underweight

Note that most of this chapter and virtually all diet books focus on the overweight person who wants to lose weight. When addressing an older population, however, we regularly run across individuals with the opposite problem—how to keep on the weight they have. A fairly common problem is developing wasting syndrome, in which too many nutrients are burned for fuel and too few are stored as muscle building material.[31]

Frailty and wasting syndrome are a deadly duo.

---

[31] Connelly, A. Scott, M.D. *Body Rx*. (New York, Berkley Books: 2001), pp. 34-35.

Being too thin, which is defined as having a Body Mass Index (BMI) below 19, poses a separate set of health hazards from being overweight or obese.[32] An underweight older person has limited resources to call upon in a physical crisis, be it a fall, an infection, surgery, or an emotionally distressing period.

Physical energy is the root source of all other energy. When our supplies run too low, when there isn't enough meat on our bones, our resistance, our ability to cope with stress of any kind—physical, mental, or emotional—may be quickly and dangerously compromised.

Maude

Someone we will call Maude was underweight and didn't have the physical resources to ward off a massive intestinal infection that wasn't detected until it was too late to save her. It's impossible to say whether a few extra pounds would have kept her alive, but being of normal weight couldn't have hurt.

Darlene and Ted

One of the best ways to help the underweight is to have someone who lovingly provides food and encourages eating. A couple we will call Darlene and Ted attended a picnic at their retirement facility even though Darlene had to wheel Ted from the nursing home wing out to poolside. He was quite weak and not aware of much around him.

To observers, Ted seemed unresponsive to the decorations, the food, the music, and the people who stopped by their table to visit. From time to time, Marlene offered a bite of food, always identifying it: "This is potato salad. You like potato salad, and this is very good."

Ted would open his mouth and take the food without uttering a sound. After Darlene had finished feeding him, she sat holding his left hand and keeping time with the music. Ted's right hand lay stiff and motionless except for the fingers which extended over the edge of the chair arm. These he moved gently to the beat of the music.

When the music stopped, this apparently unconscious man slowly took his wife's hand in both of his. With great effort, he lifted her hand to his lips and kissed it.

Techniques for Changing Eating Habits

Dieting is a multi-billion-dollar industry in the United States, partly because it's hard to give up the foods we love and partly because most of us are all too eager to embrace an alleged quick fix. If your SE is fairly young, she may have kept up with nutritional research

---

[32] To calculate your Significant Elder's BMI, divide her weight in pounds by the sum of her height in inches squared. Then divide this result by 703. For example, a woman weighing 90 pounds and standing 5' 4" tall (64" x 64" = 4096) has a BMI of 15.44 (15.44= 90 / 4096 x 703), which indicates that she is seriously underweight. A normal BMI ranges from 19 to 24. A BMI between 25 and 29.9 is considered overweight, and 30 or more is considered obese.

as reported in the media. However, if she's older, she may have missed or dismissed some of the recent sensible recommendations on nutrition and may still be eating the same foods she did as a teen-ager. If she has kept up with science and has moderated her eating habits as she has aged, she's to be congratulated because she's one of the few, at least in our experience.

Adding Nutritious Foods

The best technique for change is to start by adding something to her diet rather than trying to take something away. Following are some examples to think about trying if they seem appropriate:

- If she skips breakfast, take her out on a weekend morning and show her how great breakfast can be. Encourage her to start eating breakfast every day. Tell her that skipping breakfast isn't helping her lose or maintain weight and that it may sabotage her strength training efforts. And remember—no breakfast, no training.

- If she always eats cereal for breakfast with very little milk, encourage her to add a piece of cheese toast or some Canadian bacon, yogurt, or cottage cheese in order to increase her protein.

- If she complains about constipation, encourage her to add dark green leafy vegetables as well as other vegetables and whole grains, such as steel-cut oatmeal, to provide roughage or fiber.

- If you are aware that she hates vegetables and fruits and seldom or never eats them, you can consider encouraging her to add a multivitamin tablet to her daily routine. No vitamin pill can increase her strength and energy, but you may feel better knowing that she isn't suffering from nutritional deficiencies.

- Cook some dark green leafy vegetables using a gourmet recipe and take her several servings. If the greens are delicious enough, she may enjoy them.

- Encourage her to drink a lot of water during the course of her day. Many older people don't seem to sense when they are thirsty, yet even mild dehydration can cause problems, such as headaches and mental confusion. Adequate hydration is especially important for people with heart disease or diabetes.

- If she gets hungry between meals or in the evenings, encourage her to enjoy a small snack:
    - A few berries or bits of dried fruit and a few nuts, especially almonds.
    - A couple of bites of cheese and three or four crackers.
    - A teaspoon of peanut butter on half a banana.
    - A tablespoon of cottage cheese on a stalk of celery.
    - A hard-boiled egg and half a piece of toast.

- A piece of string cheese and half of an apple.

- Half a cup of yogurt and a small slice of cantaloupe.

Athletes of any age need a little more protein than couch potatoes do.

One of the main principles behind adding nutritious foods into her diet, of course, is to increase her protein since many older people don't seem to consume enough. Another reason is to decrease her appetite for junk food between meals.

In John's experience, most of his older clients know the general idea of good nutrition, but it's the specifics for each individual that cause them trouble. Knowing when to stop eating is a particular problem for overweight people. They may have forgotten how to tell when they are full and have had enough food for now.

If you can at least help your overweight SE to eat more slowly, you will have made a great start. It takes 20 minutes or so for the brain to get the message that the stomach is no longer empty. The slower she eats, the better.

Substituting Nutritious Foods for Empty Calories

The next step after adding nutritious foods is trying to substitute healthier foods for the junk food she may be consuming in private. Following are some substitutions to think about trying if they fit your situation:

- **Potato chips**. Some varieties of baked potato chips contain less fat and sometimes less salt than regular potato chips. Experiment to find a brand that she likes and encourage her to make the switch.

- **Colas**. Since many popular soft drinks come in a sugar-free and sometimes a caffeine-free variety, help her to find a brand that she likes. Over time, she may come to prefer the healthier choice.

- **Bread**. If she loves bread, muffins, and similar foods, encourage her to substitute whole-grain products for those made with white, refined flour. The same principle is true for rice, oatmeal, cereal, and similar foods—whole grains, long-cooking oatmeal, and brown rice provide better nutrition than the overly refined versions of these foods.

- **Salt**. If she uses too much salt and has high blood pressure, you can suggest some of the flavored salt substitutes that give almost the same taste as salt. Over time, she may get used to the difference and her health may improve.

- **Sugar**. If she has a sweet tooth, bake her some brownies or her favorite dessert using a sugar substitute. Over a period of time, she may find that she doesn't miss the sugar.

- **Ice cream**. If she loves ice cream and has to have it every day, try an occasional substitution of sugar-free ice milk, low-fat ice cream, sugar-free sherbet, or a similar product.

- **Whole milk**. Gradually introduce 2% and then 1% milk before going all the way to non-fat milk.

- **High-fructose fruit drinks**. Perhaps the only thing wrong with orange juice is the tendency to drink too much of it, but you can try helping her substitute a whole orange for a big glass of juice. She will not only save calories but will also get more fiber from the whole orange. Encourage her to make similar substitutions wherever possible, and apple for apple juice, for example.

Cutting Back on Less Nutritious Foods

Only after you have helped her add and substitute more nutritious foods can you even think of suggesting that she give up anything that isn't so good for her but that she loves to eat. In fact, you can't expect her to cut out these foods completely. The most you can hope for is that she will moderate her consumption of them.

Note, however, that if she's been successful in adding and substituting nutritious foods, she will probably admit that she feels better than she used to. She may then be more willing to go along with a few cutbacks and additional substitutions.

> If you are your SE's Spotter or Strength Coach, you can readily
> tie her performance in strength training to her nutritional practices.

Remind her frequently that if she eats right and sleeps well, she will train right. As a result she will grow stronger, remain mobile, and feel good.

Overcoming Dependencies and Addictions

If your Significant Elder thinks she needs sweets or caffeine or feels addicted to nicotine, pain pills, or alcohol, she may talk about giving them up, but doing so will take a lot more than talk. Sometimes, it takes a major health crisis, an automobile crash, or a doctor's orders to motivate the dependent or addicted person to take action. Even then, your SE will need more support than you can supply by yourself.

Until your SE is *ready* to cut back on or cut out these substances, you can't do much to help. However, you can set up a support network for your SE, do your research on methods of quitting, and remain alert to opportunities to start the dialogue with her. It may break your heart to watch her destroying her health, but with time and patience, you may be able to exert more influence over her daily habits than you realize.

Ann

John's mother Ann is a self-professed choco-holic. John recalls, "She didn't used to be, and I don't remember when it happened. Maybe it was after she had her back-to-back heart attacks and had to give up smoking. She eats chocolate probably every day and always has three or four kinds at hand. She doesn't talk about it much, but she doesn't hide it either. I've even given her chocolate for Christmas.

> The point to ponder is what I should tell her. She's 91, she's in excellent shape for her age, and she leads an otherwise healthy lifestyle. She looks great except for the tummy she has acquired since moving to Austin. What I choose to do is this: I ask her frequently what she's had to eat in the last 24 hours. If she doesn't mention chocolate, I ask her directly: "Did you have any chocolate?" Depending on her answer, I make a comment. "Wow, you really ate well" or "You had great nutrition except for the chocolate" or "You know, that's the fourth time this week you've had chocolate." And then I shut up.

If your SE is serious about becoming healthier, she will take steps on her own to moderate her intake of chocolate and other sweets and to use sugar substitutes. If she's not serious, there aren't any easy steps you can take to help her except to keep on showing interest in her nutrition. Over time, she may start practicing better self-care. If she develops Type II or adult-onset diabetes, she will have to give up most sweets or else risk disability or death. Her doctor can be your greatest ally.

Louise, Faye, and Birthday Cakes

Every Significant Elder, like every other human being, needs a treat now and then. Faye is an excellent cook and baker and loves to give away homemade goodies. When her friend Louise turned 100, Faye baked a birthday cake for her. As she was thanking Faye, Louise said: "And I will bake you a cake on your one-hundredth birthday."

"Then take good care of yourself. You've got the job," Faye said.

"Well, hurry up and get to 100!" Louise shared the cake with several friends and pronounced it one of the best she had ever had. Faye isn't certain she will ever get that cake from Louise, but there's always hope.

John's Advice on Talking about Food

"How are you?" is a very common greeting, and "Fine," "So-So," or "Not bad" are typical answers. In general, the question really means are you okay? In general, no one expects or wants a long answer or a negative one. John always asks his clients, "How do you feel?"

> I ask them at the beginning of the session at the same time that I ask them how they slept last night and what they had for breakfast. They have learned that these are

serious questions and that I expect and need considered answers. Usually, they tell me the general state of their physical health, and this is what I most need to know. If they feel poorly or have pain, I mentally begin to scale back the workout. Likewise, if they tell me that they are "drinking from the saucer"—their cup runneth over—I will probably push them a little. Perceived state of health is very important.

Often, I'll get more than a report on physical health. A quarrel with a loved one, a worry about a pet, money concerns, the blues, the blahs, a spiritual anxiety—all can be and are part of the answer to "How do you feel?" In general, they just want to voice that feeling; externalize it, and it's easier to bear. And that's a good thing.

If they want to say more, I encourage them, and I'm happy to listen. Sometimes I offer an opinion, sometimes not. The point is that the somewhat formal setting of the training session makes my clients comfortable enough to reveal to me the true answer to the question. A discussion of physical health can lead naturally to a discussion of mental, emotional, and even spiritual health. I consider this a huge advantage professionally. The better I know the person, the more I can help. Plus, they are all my friends, and listening is something you do for your friends. And by the way, it works both ways. I have benefited from their sage advice, experience, and observations to get through some of my own rough times.

Rest and Sleep

Rest is a large and important topic, and so is sleep, even though it's a subset of rest. The purpose of both is to enhance recovery after exertion so that good health and additional activities are possible. The purpose of this section is to help you understand the importance of rest in your SE's life and to assist her in achieving the type of rest and sleep that will enhance her health and strength.

Rest

In our time-obsessed society, it's easy to lose sight of the purpose of rest and sleep—to recover from the physical, emotional, and mental demands of our daily activities. You know you have to sleep, but people of all ages resist going to bed in time to get enough restful sleep to see them through their days. For many adults, the idea of taking a rest is anathema, and in our culture napping is only for the very young and the very old.

Even a human dynamo has the right to a few days off when she needs to rest.

Without good rest and recovery, your SE won't enjoy the best success in strength training. Rest includes time periods ranging from 30 seconds during a workout to eight or ten hours or more at night. During strength training sessions, your SE needs from 30 seconds to two or three minutes between sets for recovery time. After a strength training session, she may need to rest for half an hour or longer as she eats a nutritious snack or meal. At night, she needs a restful sleep for the number of hours that will allow her to wake up feeling refreshed. When she's not feeling well, she probably needs to take it easy for a couple of days or longer to give her body time to recuperate from whatever feeling of illness, pain, or weakness she's having. However, her doctor can best advise her on resting while she's ill. Our only recommendation is that she not force herself to carry on with her usual activities if she doesn't feel like it.

It's a well-known maxim among young weightlifters that more muscle growth occurs at the dinner table and in the bedroom than in the gym itself. Lifting causes micro-tears in the muscles, and sufficient rest is necessary for these tears to heal and the muscle to grow stronger. Recovery periods are vital to young and old alike. Rest for your SE, however, promotes recovery that enables her to keep on strength training even late in life. She won't gain bulging muscles through good nutrition and rest, but she will remain strong enough to work out for as long as she wants to, barring major illness or injury.

Rest is so important for all exercisers, especially older people, that we break the concept into its smallest parts and work outward to the larger sections. Your job as Spotter or Strength Coach is to become fluent in your SE's body language so that you can determine when she needs a rest. Your job is especially important if she's the type of older person who says she's "fine, just fine" through clenched teeth and will never admit to being tired.

Rest during a Set

Normally, your SE will be able to complete a set of 8-15 reps without a break. If you see her struggling during a set, you might feel that you must stop after the rep on which you notice the struggle. However, you may want to try asking her to pause for a couple of seconds, take a deep breath, and do one or two additional reps. The deep breath is a mini-rest that may enable her to finish or nearly finish the set.

If the pause for a deep breath restores her strength and determination, you can ask her to group the remaining reps into sub-sets. For example, if she has been doing 12 reps on the bench press for several weeks, but one day she tires during reps 7 and 8, then you can try asking her to do the following while still holding the bar in position:

- Pause for a couple of seconds after rep 8 and take an extra breath.

- Perform reps 9 and 10.

- Pause after rep 10 and take an extra breath.

- If she feels well, perform reps 11 and 12.

- Then take a longer-than-usual rest before the next exercise.

The mini-rests and deep breaths may help her to perform the complete set and will give her a sense of achievement. Communication is the key, however, and you will never want to push your SE beyond her abilities or her willingness to work out. If she needs to stop the set after rep 8, praise her for what she accomplished and tell her a funny story.

Rest between Sets

As you saw in "Rest Intervals" on page 58, the rest interval between sets ranges from 30 seconds to two minutes or more, depending upon difficulty and evident fatigue. As a general rule, your SE will need slightly more rest between two sets of the same exercise than between sets of different exercises. The reason is that doing the same exercise continually will fatigue the same set of muscles.

During the rest just before you switch to a different exercise, you can use the time to talk up the next set. Help your SE recall past successes with the upcoming exercise. If it's the most difficult exercise of the session, such as chair squats, you will want to prepare her for the exertion at the same time that you express confidence that she can do the work. As always, take your cues about rest from your SE's body language, especially her breathing patterns. If she's unfocused or breathing hard, give her a little extra time to recover.

Rest between Training Sessions

The same rule for young weightlifters applies to older exercisers: Give the muscles 48 hours of rest between heavy training sessions. On rare occasions, an older person may work up to a split routine four days week. On Mondays and Thursdays, for example, she will work the back, legs, and biceps, while on Tuesdays and Fridays, she will work the chest, shoulders, and triceps (the "push-pull" split). On this plan, she will still rest each body part for 48 hours or more before stressing it again.

Since the majority of older exercisers will work all of the body parts during the same session, you can be sure that she gets plenty of rest between sessions. Early in her training, your SE may need the do-nothing type of rest days in between her training sessions, but later on you can encourage the do-something type of rest days.

Do-Nothing Rest Days

This type of rest is almost completely inactive, and many older people take right to it, especially if they have been largely sedentary before starting strength training. Right after a training session, your SE may even stretch out in her recliner chair and take a nap. If so, encourage her to drink some water and eat a small but nutritious snack first.

If she trains two days a week, she may be completely inactive on the other five days. At first, you can encourage her to get all the rest she needs because she's at least getting two good workouts a week. Just make sure that she doesn't stack the training sessions back to back. When or if she adds a third session to her week, enforce a day of rest in between each session. Later on, you can try to encourage some light activity on rest days.

Do-Something Rest Days

This type of rest is a little more active than do-nothing rest, but it shouldn't tax the same muscles that your SE stressed the previous day. Instead, your SE can do 20-30 minutes of walking or a similar mildly aerobic activity during her off days between training sessions.

Some older people strenuously resist the do-something rest days, feeling that they deserve to just sit and rock. It may take a long time to interest someone like this in the more active type of rest days. Others, however, welcome the chance to increase their activity levels without fear of muscle soreness or injury. If your SE is strong and healthy enough, there's nothing wrong with two or three 20-minute walks or swims per day. If she's always been fairly active, she will probably enjoy the do-something rest days.

Faye

Faye is John's only client over 80 who fully participates in active recovery. She trains with him only once a week, but at least four other days of the week, she performs a routine that features walking on the treadmill, doing ab exercises, and working her leg muscles lightly. She developed this routine on her own at age 89 and is continuing it at age 90. She feels better, sleeps better, and burns more calories. "I finally realized that I can work out by myself," she reports, "and I'll keep on until I can't do it any more. Sure, there are times when I just don't feel like going to the exercise room, but what gets me there is the absolute certainty that I'll feel better afterwards."

Longer Rest Periods

One of the most common reasons for taking four or five days off between training sessions is an older person's fear that she's coming down with something. While many younger people ignore a headache, a runny nose, or a scratchy throat and work out anyway, your SE may have learned that she needs to attack these potential problems by getting some extra rest. If she feels that the need to skip a training session or two, you can try encouraging her to walk for 10 minutes every day. Also, review Chapter 4 for some recommendations on rest during illnesses or injuries.

Sleep

We discuss three main areas associated with sleep—determining the general guidelines to follow, finding out whether your SE could use some improvements in her sleep habits, and implementing a few specific techniques to help her achieve a good night's sleep night after night. But first, let's take a quick look at the results of a 2003 poll[33] for some important information on sleep and older people:

---

[33] Conducted by the National Sleep Foundation. See http://www.sleepfoundation.org/_content/hottopics/2003SleepPollExecSumm.pdf.

- Two-thirds of older adults report frequent sleep problems. However, only a small fraction, one in eight, can report that those problems have been diagnosed. Seldom do their doctors inquire about their sleep habits.

- Insomnia is the most common sleep problem with about one half of older adults reporting that they frequently experience at least one symptom.

- The more medical conditions an older person reports, the more sleep problems are likely to occur. Sleep problems are reported by:

  - 82% of those diagnosed with depression.

  - 81% of those who have suffered a stroke.

  - 76% of those being treated for heart disease.

  - 75% of those diagnosed with lung disease.

  - 72% of those being treated for diabetes or arthritis.

  - 71% of those diagnosed with hypertension.

- Poor sleep is also associated with bodily pain, excess weight, and ambulatory limitations:

  - More than three-quarters (77%) of those having frequent pain also report at least one sleep problem.

  - Sleep problems are common among older adults who are classified as obese (77%) and are linked with almost two-thirds (64%) of those considered overweight.

  - The majority of older people with ambulatory limitations are likely to report a sleep problem (84%) or to experience a symptom of insomnia (66%). Ambulatory limitations are defined as difficulty or inability to walk one-half mile or to walk up and down a flight of stairs without help.

If your SE has a great deal of trouble sleeping, take her complaints seriously and ask her to talk with her doctor about them.

Determining Some General Sleep Guidelines

Everyone knows that most people need to sleep for seven to nine hours per night, more if they perform heavy physical labor or strenuous training. And yet sleep deprivation is one of the most common health problems in the U.S. It hits older people especially hard. About 60% of older Americans don't get enough sleep, at least occasionally.

If sleeplessness becomes chronic, your SE will be shortchanging her body and possibly accelerating the aging process. Yet sleep is an absolutely vital component of good health. Adequate sleep actually enhances your health. In fact, sleeping seven to eight hours nightly is one of the chief health habits shared by people who stay fit well into their old age.

Examining Your Significant Elder's Sleep Habits

Your SE's sleep habits will usually be much less familiar to you than her eating habits, so you will have to do a bit more investigating to learn about them. Listen closely when your SE complains about "tossing and turning all night long." Recall whether she has always had trouble sleeping or whether sleeplessness is something new for her. Every time you talk with her, start asking her how she slept last night, and keep an informal record or log of what she says.

The main points to make about documenting your SE's sleep habits are the following:

- Gather evidence and conduct a careful examination. Do it without fanfare but do it faithfully over a period of several weeks.

- Don't always believe what she tells you about how poorly she sleeps unless she seems quite fatigued during the day, but never scold her. Never judge. Just write down what she tells you. Then add comments about whether you believe she exaggerated or minimized her sleep status.

- When she reports a bad night, start asking questions like the following:
    - Did you take a nap yesterday?
    - Did you drink coffee, tea, or cola in the afternoon or evening?
    - Did you drink more alcohol than usual?
    - Did you stay up late watching an exciting movie or TV program?
    - Was your bedroom too hot or too cold?
    - Is your shoulder, knee, or other injury site still bothering you?
    - Did you have indigestion?
    - Was there too much light or noise in your bedroom?
    - Are you still worried about some problem or other, whether large or small?
    - Do you think you're getting a cold?

Techniques for Changing Sleep Habits

In trying to improve your SE's sleep habits, the best way to start is to remove sleep inhibitors from her routine. Later on, you can try adding and substituting things that may help.

Removing Sleep Inhibitors

After you talk with your SE about her sleeping problems over several weeks, you will be in a good position to analyze her sleep inhibitors. Some of these suggestions may seem patronizing or excessively intrusive. Can't Mom tell if she needs darker drapes? Yes, of course. But she may be so used to putting up with what she has that the thought of making improvements never occurs to her.

If her watchword is, "Use it up, wear it out, make do," then you can provide a real service by helping with the following inhibitors to good sleep:

- Too much light in her bedroom—Remove the old curtains and hang some light-blocking drapes.

- Too much noise in her bedroom—If a white noise machine doesn't help, look into such improvements as masking noisy plumbing, insulating the heating and cooling system, or perhaps soundproofing her bedroom.

- A snoring bed partner—Encourage your SE either to use ear plugs or ask the partner to go to the doctor for anti-snoring assistance.

- Multiple trips to the bathroom—Encourage your SE to drink a lot of water early in the day and to cut down on liquids after dinner. Provide a nightlight so she does not need to turn on the lights for bathroom trips. Low lighting will make it easier for her to get back to sleep. Just make sure that the route between the bed and the commode is as short as possible and completely free of obstructions.

- Conditions that a physician can help with:

  - Restless leg syndrome (a creepy-crawly feeling).

  - Leg cramps.

  - Sleep apnea.

  - Severe insomnia.

  - Medications that seem to interfere with a good night's sleep.

> If at all possible, go with your SE to the doctor and take along your records of her reported sleep problems.

Adding Sleep Aids

Consider taking your SE to her doctor for a sleeping aid prescription only after you have tried some of the following:

- Encourage her to take a 20- or 30-minute nap right after lunch every day. If she's afraid of sleeping all afternoon, encourage her to set an alarm or timer. This recommendation may seem counter-intuitive, but a nap can refresh her energy level enough to promote more activity, which in turn contributes to a good night's sleep. In general, the more active she becomes, the better she will sleep, and a short nap can do a lot to keep her moving well into the evening.

- Encourage her to establish a relaxation routine at bedtime, including any of the following that she doesn't already do:

  - Drink a small cup of sleep-promoting tea just before going to bed. Any caffeine-free tea will do, but something containing chamomile or valerian often works better.

  - Take a relaxing bath at night, complete with body oils and pleasant scents.

  - Go to bed at the same time every night.

  - Follow the same grooming rituals every evening.

  - Use a white noise machine or soothing music in the bedroom.

  - While lying in bed, use such relaxation techniques as mild stretching and releasing of the muscles starting with the toes and moving up to the forehead or crown.

  - Start using positive self-talk and visualization, especially for times when she wakes up in the middle of the night and can't get back to sleep. For more on these techniques, see Chapter 9.

- Encourage her to talk about whatever is on her mind that may be keeping her awake at night. You may think that your SE couldn't possibly have the kind of stress that keeps you awake at night, but if you listen, you will learn not only that she has problems but that talking about them helps decrease them so she can sleep.

Substituting Aids for Inhibitors

The final step is trying to substitute healthier habits for the sleep inhibitors she may be using. Following are some substitutions to consider and to try if they fit your situation:

- The first thing, of course, is to encourage her to substitute caffeine-free drinks for her usual coffee, tea, cola, or hot chocolate. If she's a heavy consumer of caffeine, encourage her to make the switch gradually to minimize withdrawal symptoms.

- Since alcohol can also interfere with sleep, encourage her to substitute non-alcoholic drinks in the evening. Watch for problem drinking and possible alcoholism so that you can get her some help for these serious problems.

- Consider encouraging her to substitute a small dinner for the main meal she may be consuming at 6:00 or 7:00 PM. It may be easier for her to sleep well if she eats less at night. Taking her main meal at noon would also promote the short nap recommended above.

- Encourage her to substitute a pleasant afternoon activity, such as walking, bowling with friends, or easy gardening, for some of the TV shows that she may have gotten used to watching in the afternoons. The news and the soaps can contain subject matter that may disturb her, whether she realizes the turmoil or not.

- Encourage her to substitute reading or listening to music for an hour or so before bedtime instead of watching the violence she may have become accustomed to on TV. She can stop the reading or the music at any time, while she may feel compelled to watch until the end of a TV show, no matter how upsetting the content.

- Since older skin is more sensitive than young skin, see whether you can make any improvements in her nightwear and bedding. Wrinkled sheets seem to contribute to a sub-optimum rest.

- If she hasn't bought a new bed in decades, encourage her to get rid of the old one and investigate some of the new sleep systems that promise more comfort at night. If you don't live nearby, it's worth a visit your SE to help her find the right bed.

A Note to Certified Personal Trainers

If you haven't worked with older clients very much, you will need to develop a sixth sense about their eating and resting habits. At the beginning of each training session, ask the following questions without fail:

- How do you feel today?

- When did you eat last and what did you have?

- How did you sleep last night?

Poor nutrition and rest show up in an older person's eyes, in the breathing, on the face, and sometimes in the speech. Scale the training session back if you see any of the following signs of fatigue:

- Glassy, unfocused eyes.

- Difficulty catching her breath.

- A sagging or even ashen look to the face.

- Rambling, disorganized comments that sometimes may seem irrational.

- Difficulty holding her head up as high as she does on good days.

Summary of the Main Points

Food and rest are vitally important to good health in general and successful strength training in particular. You can best help your SE with the following:

- Keep a food log and a sleep log of her habits over several months.

- Add good practices into her eating and sleeping habits.

- Substitute better practices for less successful ones.

- Encourage her to change habits that interfere with good nutrition and rest.

- Don't feel that food and rest are unimportant to your SE's health and strength.

What's Next?

Part III, "Getting Ahead," provides three types of motivation:

- Deriving inspiration from case studies of John's and Jody's mothers and two more of John's clients.

- Using the mind-body connection, visualization, and similar techniques to promote good health and strength.

- Employing current practices of empowerment and full engagement to improve the lives of older people.

PART III. GETTING AHEAD

"So, it looks as though I'm going to live—at least for another 50 years or more. But whenever I need to reassure myself of this, as I sometimes do, I go out to a place called Dead Man's Hole [...a large green mineral pond gouged out of a circular limestone cliff, so deep into the hill country of Texas that it's hardly got an address ...], and I stare down into it, and then, with firm intent, I strip off my shirt and I leap straight out into what you might call the great sublime."
       Lance Armstrong, winner of seven Tours de France[34]

Part III presents what you need to know to get ahead in strength training with your Significant Elder (or how to be truly supportive if you are the Advocate). You will learn:

- How to apply the inspirational stories of our four case studies to your SE.

- How to use the mind-body connection, visualization, and other techniques to keep you and your SE highly motivated.

- How to help empower and energize your SE by developing purposeful activity-recovery habits.

---

[34] *Every Second Counts*, with Sally Jenkins (New York: Broadway Books, 2003), p. 1.

Chapter 8. Inspirational Case Studies

Ann, Faye, Jack, and Lyn

"No young person, it matters not how intelligent, how sensitive, how educated, how loving he is, can understand what it feels like to be old."
     Faye, 90

Important Points for Advocates: Your SE may or may not have anything in common with our four case studies, but chances are good that you and he both will gain inspiration from something in this chapter. For example, one of Jody's friends said that a newspaper article featuring Ann and Faye had inspired her 70-something father to take up strength training because, as he put it, "I can't have a couple of 90-year-old ladies kicking my butt."[35]

Introduction

Four of John's clients have agreed to serve as case studies. Two are the authors' mothers, Ann Payne, 91, and Faye Kelly, 90. Two others are much younger, but both have special needs, Jack Lewis, 74, and Lyn Byer, 73. We describe who they are as people, discuss their strength and health before and after strength training, and provide a table of their physical abilities at five points in their training:

- Day 1.
- Month 1.
- Month 6.
- Best ever.
- Typical current workout.

We also provide comments from Faye and Jack in their own words, since both enjoy writing, as well as extensive analyses that John has made over his years of working with these four extraordinary people. To each of them, we are deeply grateful not only for permission to feature them but also for the example they set for athletes of all ages and conditions.

Ann, Faye, Jack, and Lyn are heroes to their families and friends.

---

[35] LeBlanc, Pamela, "Worth the Weight: These Women Prove It's Never Too Late to Pump Iron," *Austin American-Statesman*, March 28, 2005, pp. E1, E8.

Ann Platt Payne

Ann called herself an old maid high school English teacher in Monroe, Louisiana, before she married at age 26 and devoted her life to bringing up her five children in Shreveport. She was always an avid reader and member of in-depth reading seminars. She also devoted much time and energy to state-wide Episcopal Church activities and to her home, where she lived for 62 years.

Ann's husband, Francis Cameron Payne, was an All-American football player at Tulane University who excelled as a stockbroker at Merrill Lynch, where he became a national vice president. He died of cancer in 1976 at age 64.

Before Strength Training

Before she began strength training, Ann, 91, had smoked for 68 years. She smoked Chesterfield unfiltered cigarettes until about age 50, then switched to filtered, and wound up smoking about four ultra-light cigarettes a day until age 88. Then she had her first heart attack and stopped cold turkey.

She also enjoyed one or two highballs on most days of the week and never drank more than three. Her daily caffeine intake has always been about six ounces of very strong Louisiana coffee spread out over three demitasse cups. She consumed sweets moderately until she stopped smoking. Now she consumes too many sweets.

Ann had never played golf, tennis, or any other organized sport, but she walked nearly every day. Sometimes she covered a mile or more. Even today, she walks up to half a mile daily. She has always had excellent posture and an athletic stride.

Her medical conditions include pronounced macular degeneration and hearing loss, some short-term memory loss, peripheral neuropathy (tingling and aching in the feet and fingers), mild arthritis in both shoulders, nagging hip pain that would occasionally prevent her daily walks, and occasional digestive problems (but she refuses to consider giving up coffee).

After Strength Training

Today, after three years of strength training, the hip pain is virtually gone. In fact, it disappeared after just two months of chair squats. She still walks up to half a mile per day. Her shoulders are still an unpredictable source of pain but only during exercise. She also has excellent posture, which she attributes to her two older brothers, Jack and Layton, who used to grab her shoulders from behind, press a knee into her upper back, and say, "Don't slouch!"

Her workouts went well from the beginning even though she had little confidence about her physical capabilities. Her main difficulty is that she was inexperienced at thinking about anything that she was doing with her body. She had never played sports. Her strength training instructions were so basic that John had to move her arms, shoulders, and legs for her, in the direction that they needed to go.

Her dietary vices include two ounces of strong coffee three times a day at 7:30 AM, 10:30 AM, and 3:00 PM. She also craves sweets, especially chocolate, and has gained a few pounds since moving to Austin. However, her BMI is not classified as obese by any means. Her vision, hearing, and memory continue to decline, and she takes six prescription medications a day to help her heart, to lower her cholesterol, and to thin her blood.

At 91, she lives in the retirement, or independent living, section of her residential facility and has no plans to move to the assisted living section, where residents engage a companion to help them bathe, dress, eat, remember their medications, and so on. Like virtually all residents there, she hates the thought of moving to assisted living only a little less than she hates and fears the idea of moving into the nursing home section, euphemistically termed the Health Care Unit. She states, "John, if they ever tell me I have to go to Health Care, do me a favor and just shoot me in the head!"

Ann's Workouts at Five Points

Exercise	Day 1 Lbs x Reps	Month 1 Lbs x Reps	Month 6 Lbs x Reps	Best Ever Lbs x Reps	Current Lbs x Reps
Upper Back Exercise: Lat Pull	15 x 10	20 x 12	22 x 14	40 x 8	40 x 8
Chest Exercise: Bench Press Wall Chest Press	10 x 10	15 x 8	**Note 1** below Wall x 12	Wall x 12	Wall x 12
Leg Exercise: Chair Squats	Self x 8	1 x 10	4 x 8	8 x 10	8 x 10
Shoulder Exercise: **Note 2**					
Lower Back Exercise: Dead Lift	**Note 3**			40 x 8	35 x 8
Biceps Exercise: Curls	5 x 8	6 x 10	8 x 8	8 x 10	6 x 8
Triceps Exercise: Pushdowns	10 x 10	12 x 12	12 x 10	17 x 8	15 x 8

Table 8-1. Workout Sheet for Ann Payne

Notes:

1. We substituted the wall chest press for the bench press due to shoulder pain.

2. We immediately discontinued shoulder exercises because the pain was too great.

3. We were able to incorporate dead lifts after six months of training.

More about Ann

"Well, I'm deaf, blind, and a little bit cuckoo. Otherwise, I feel great." John adds that she misses her home, misses her hometown, misses driving, and misses her few remaining old friends. Her first year in Austin wasn't terrible, but it wasn't easy. She was easily confused and easily discouraged. She felt lonely a lot of the time. What worked best was helping her establish new routines.

John notes, "The routines we established together were working out and visiting after I finished my daily work at her residence facility to drink her wonderfully strong Louisiana coffee and chat about anything and everything. Mostly light, mostly funny."

Ann's dog also provided an excellent transition from Louisiana to Texas, and Ann walks Mitsy several times a day, just as she did back home. The companionship and the sense of responsibility also contribute to Ann's wellbeing.

John found out things about his mother that he had never known before. You will find out things about your SE too.

John told his mother the same thing he tells his other clients: "Most of what I know I can teach you in an hour. Training you to do it without thinking takes a while longer." With patience from both, Ann slowly progressed, slowly learned the motions, slowly learned the exercises and the breathing.

John's father was very athletic—all-American football player, track star, champion badminton player, and so on. He and his siblings assumed that they inherited any physical prowess they had from their father. John soon discovered that his mother was a diamond in the rough. She had some essential tools, namely excellent posture and reasonable strength in nearly all of her muscles. She was an athlete waiting to happen. It took a while to convince her of that.

Faye Lucius Kelly

Faye was a tenured full professor of English at The American University in Washington, D.C., until her retirement in 1976. After marrying at age 22 and teaching high school English while bringing up two children, she took the opportunity of going to graduate school at the University of Florida, where she earned her Ph.D. in 1964, writing her dissertation on Shakespeare.

Faye's husband, Bruce William Kelly, served as an artillery officer in World War II. After earning his Ph.D. in economics at the University of Florida, he rose to the top of the civil service as a mathematical statistician at the U.S. Department of Agriculture. He died of cancer in 1985 at age 75.

Before Strength Training

In August of 1996 when she moved to Austin at age 82, Faye felt tired, weak, and dependent because she was still recovering from the serious case of pneumonia that had hospitalized her the previous March. Every winter for decades, she had contracted bronchitis or another respiratory illness, but she had always bounced back. This time, it took much longer. For almost the first time in her life, she needed assistance with the activities of daily life, and she wasn't happy about it.

Faye became an athlete in her 80s, proving that it's never too late.

She had always had many interests, although she was never athletic, and wanted to resume her independent life. Giving up her many interests was not an option. She wonders whether contracting malaria in her youth may have contributed to her later bronchial troubles. Her only other major health problem was developing breast cancer at age 75, but the surgery produced good results and there has been no further incidence of cancer.

A physical advantage she has always had is good to excellent flexibility in all her joints. Up through middle age, she could bend over at the waist and place the palms of both hands on the floor without bending her knees. Even now, she can raise both arms straight overhead and out to the side, which none of John's other older clients can do without experiencing pain. Another advantage for her general health is that she never smoked, although she enjoyed a drink before and wine with dinner.

Health drawbacks include being overweight since her 50s and developing a BMI in the obese range during her 70s. She's an excellent cook and loves to cook and bake, always providing banana bread and Kahlua cake for meetings of her writing group and family get-togethers. Her self-care practices have been limited to taking daily vitamins and switching from coffee to decaf in recent years.

Faye has profound macular degeneration, which classifies her as legally blind, though she can still make out shapes well enough to enjoy live theatre. When she became unable to hear people at the far end of the dining table, she got digital hearing aids right away. Her short-term and long-term memory faculties are still excellent.

After Strength Training

Today, after six years of strength training, Faye has regained her natural vitality and has considerable stamina for someone of her size and age. Using the assistance of a laundry cart, she walks hundreds and hundreds of yards every month to deliver books to fellow residents who participate in the monthly book club meetings, although she can no longer drive to the library to check out the books. She now uses books on tape.

She takes only one prescription medication for blood pressure. Shortly after her move to Austin, a physician prescribed seven additional medications for her, but the drug regimen made absolutely no sense to her, and she found another doctor who listened to her and agreed that she needed only the one ongoing medication.

Faye's Workouts at Five Points

Exercise	Day 1 Lbs x Reps	Month 1 Lbs x Reps	Month 6 Lbs x Reps	Best Ever Lbs x Reps	Current Lbs x Reps
Upper Back Exercise: Lat Pull	15 x 10	20 x 10	25 x 12	45 x 10	40 x 10

Chest Exercise:
   Bench Press
   Flye
	15 x 8	15 x 15	20 x 10	30 x 8	**Note 1**
					8 x 10

Leg Exercise: Chair Squat	Self x 6	Self x 12	3 x 12	10 x 10	5 x 8
Shoulder Exercise: Dumbbell Press	3 x 8	5 x 12	5 x 12	8 x 5	5 x 10
Lower Back Exercise: **Note 2**					
Biceps Exercise: Curls	5 x 10	8 x 10	10 x 8	12 x 10	10 x 10
Triceps Exercise: Pushdown	**Note 3**	10 x 10	15 x 10	20 x 10	16 x 10

Table 8-2. Workout Sheet for Faye Kelly

Notes:

1. We discontinued working on the flat bench because her pulmonary problems worsened in the supine position. We substituted the manual seated bench press using a dowel and the butterfly.

2. We don't do lower back exercises because of breathing problems.

3. We started with the triceps pushdown as soon as we acquired the apparatus.

More about Faye in Her Own Words

Faye wrote an article for the July 1999 issue of *The Focus*, a newsletter written by and for the residents at her retirement facility. With her permission, we reprint it here.

This Could Be You and Me

By Faye Kelly

Until the Older Women's Legacy Circle suggested that we write about our bodies, ourselves, the idea had never occurred to me. Since then, I have done some research on the subject of the aging body. It seems that we are now at the beginning of a wave of research into what can be done to slow the aging process of the human body. One thing for sure is that we are all given at birth a body uniquely our own until we die. It accompanies us always and everywhere and makes everything we do possible.

Research has shown that with age and inactivity, the body gradually loses its range of motion and its muscular strength. But at any age the body has amazing capacity for recovering lost flexibility and strength if a regular program of fitness is followed. The course of action recommended by specialists in the field is to combine stretching exercises with strength training such as weight lifting. As a teacher for many years, I spent years of relative inactivity. About twenty-five years ago, I started half-heartedly on a walking program which I increased and became more consistent with after retirement. I then discovered water aerobics and added this exercise to my program.

After coming to Austin, I added Tai Chi, which more than almost any other exercise helps to maintain balance. A loss of balance causes most falls. I frequently, in jest, refer to our residence facility as the "house of fallen women" because almost every week one of us falls and breaks an arm, a hip, or a wrist. A few months ago I had a fall, which forced me to try to get myself fit enough that my chance of falling would be lessened. Although I did not break any bones, I did injure the muscles and tendons in my upper right arm. I did not have enough flexibility to comb my hair. After much massage therapy and exercise, I regained normal flexibility. Now I am working on strength.

My daughter had often suggested that I employ a personal trainer. I secretly hooted at the idea. At my age, and the expense! As a survivor of the Depression, I have never been accustomed to spending money on unnecessary things, particularly on myself. While I was pondering the possibility, I happened on a PBS program on "Women's Bodies, Women's Minds," by Christiane Northrup, a physician who operates a health clinic for women in Maine. One sentence she said clicked in my mind. She said, "Anything you spend to improve your body is not self-indulgence; it is self-preservation." That convinced me.

In fear and trembling, I took my daughter's advice and employed a personal weight trainer. I am the first elderly person he has ever worked with, but he is very understanding and helpful in every way. The many reports I have read saying that weight training is the very best means of keeping your bones strong is encouraging. One study reported that a group of post-menopausal women increased bone density in the lumber spine and lean body mass after high intensity strength training. This has direct implications for preventing osteoporosis and physical frailty.

I had considered myself in pretty good physical shape for my age, after my water aerobics and Tai Chi, but the weight training program has found muscles I did not know I had. After just three months on the program, I have already experienced a pronounced gain in my strength and energy. Almost without my realizing it, physical capabilities are returning. The other day I walked up the steps to my apartment with a heavy sack of groceries in each hand. Three months ago, I had to hold on to a railing to walk up and down steps carrying nothing.

I realize there is no guarantee that I will not fall. But if weight training will decrease my chances of falling and increase the enjoyment of my remaining years, it is worth the time, the effort, the money, and even the sore muscles. If you are interested, my trainer is John Payne."

John adds the following comments.

Faye is my patron saint for training older people. If it weren't for her, I probably never would have gotten into the residence facility where she lives. After learning from Jody that Faye might be interested in working with me, we met for lunch in March of 1999. She was skeptical, but as I learned later, she always likes to try new things. Even though she said, "Don't get your hopes up," Faye always had the right attitude about working out, especially about an older person working out. She said, "I just want to keep doing all the things I like to do, as long as I feel like doing them."

Faye soon discovered to her delight that not only was she pretty adept at lifting weights, she also enjoyed it, and she felt the change in her the energy level within just a few sessions. She started with just a few simple dumbbells, but at a certain point, she realized that we needed better and more equipment. She got a lukewarm reception from the management at her residence facility when she asked them to buy the equipment. So she said, "John, you choose it. I will pay for it. Let's do it." I went to a sports equipment resale shop and selected three items. One Saturday afternoon, we and Faye drove to the shop, where she tried out each piece of equipment. Faye was my guinea pig, and we had a good time.

If your SE does a strength training exercise pretty well, she will enjoy it and stick with it. She will also get a great deal of good from doing the exercise.

Faye's best exercise has always been lat pull downs. Many times over the years, she has come to a training session tired, low on energy, and not feeling especially well. Sometimes she's had a bad knee, and other times she's had various respiratory and stomach complaints. But if she does anything at all, she gets on the lat pull down machine, and it always makes her feel a bit better. Why? Because it makes her breathe deeply. It doesn't hurt that she can sit down to do it. On a good day, she can pull 40 to 45 pounds 8 to 12 times in two or three sets.

John continues, "I consider Faye a pioneer proto-feminist. As a university professor, she made her way in a man's world and is very used to having been discriminated against. As a result she's tough, can be quite confrontational, and is often combative and blunt. She is also fiercely loyal to those she approves of. She has a very strong sense of justice and she rather likes the underdog. Faye doesn't intend to let anything or anyone stop her from doing what she's decided she wants to do."

Jack Lewis

Jack was a U. S. Marine in the years between World War II and the Korean Conflict and worked as a petroleum geologist with Phillips (now ConocoPhillips) for over 30 years. His career took him for lengthy periods to Africa, Australia, and England. Shortly after retiring, he moved into a retirement facility in 1994 at age 67. He now lives in an apartment attached to his daughter's house but visits his friends at the retirement facility often.

Before Strength Training

Now 74, Jack has always been active and was in good shape for a man of his age, which was 71 when he started strength training. He had good flexibility and strength and took a minimum number of medications, though he suffered nosebleeds during training sessions if his head went lower than his heart.

His major medical problem was an inherited blood disorder or auto-immune anemia called telangiectasia, which caused chronic gastrointestinal bleeding and required him to receive frequent blood transfusions, sometimes as often as once a week. Despite this condition, he remained quite active and was only slightly overweight.

Jack's goal was "to tone up my muscles, and strength training did that very well."

After Strength Training

The main point about Jack's health is that strength training did not worsen his disorder and may possibly have helped, although we have no scientific proof. His doctor, however, has confirmed that the frequency of his transfusions has gone down to one every three or four months, which has made an important difference in the quality of his life.

Jack is John's only client over age 70 whose progress in strength training resembles that of a much younger person. Like a 30-year-old, he made large, steady gains in both strength and endurance. There is no exercise he can't do. His only problems in strength training have been twisting his knee a couple of times and having to focus on upper body strength while his knee healed.

> Jack can dead lift 100 pounds, squat 100 pounds, and bench press 75 pounds. Men decades younger can't lift these weights, men without a life-threatening blood disorder.

Jack enjoyed everything about strength training and regretted giving it up when he moved to his daughter's house from the residence facility where John trains his older clients. "I was always glad when a session was over because I was tired, but I always enjoyed working out," he says.

Jack's Workout at Five Points

Exercise	Day 1 Lbs x Reps	Month 1 Lbs x Reps	Month 6 Lbs x Reps	Best Ever Lbs x Reps	Current Lbs x Reps
Upper Back Exercise: Lat Pull	10 x 15	45 x 8	33 x 12	65 x 8	62 x 12
Chest Exercise: Bench Press	12 x 15	40 x 12	30 x 12	65 x 8	57 x 12
Leg Exercise: Chair Squat Real Squat	Self x 10 	 16 x 8	 Self x 12	 55 x 8	 30 x 12
Shoulder Exercise: Dumbbell Press	12 x 15	25 x 8	16 x 12	42 x 10	35 x 12
Lower Back Exercise: Dead Lift	12 x 10	40 x 8	30 x 12	85 x 8	70 x 12
Biceps Exercise: Curls	15 x 15	30 x 12	24 x 10	45 x 10	45 x 10
Triceps Exercise: Pushdowns	10 x 15	20 x 12	12 x 12	27 x 8	22 x 12

Table 8-3. Workout Sheet for Jack Lewis

Note: Unlike the other case studies, Jack has no limitations on his physical abilities and made steady, consistent progress, often doubling or tripling his strength on a particular exercise.

More about Jack in His Own Words

Jack wrote the following essay on March 11, 2002, in the "Tell Me a Tale" writing class, which is offered through the Austin Institute of Lifetime Learning. Austin Community College journalism professor Anita Howard teaches the class. We print Jack's essay here with his permission.

Personal Training

By Jack Lewis

Some years ago I read magazine stories of famous people in the entertainment field who had physical trainers come to their homes to direct them in exercises. Another example of extreme extravagance by the super wealthy, I thought then. The real, everyday people I know who worked out, as formal exercising was called, did their thing at a gym. They paid a fee to join and use the exercise equipment there, sharing with many others. Instructors were usually available to advise people, but they were not considered personal trainers.

About three years ago a Summit resident took her daughter's advice to start an exercise program, working with a personal trainer who came to The Summit to work with her on a regular schedule. This resident believed she benefited enormously from these sessions. She felt stronger, had better balance, and acquired more endurance. She even wrote an article about this for our newsletter, thus acquainting me with a solution for a poor condition I was just beginning to recognize.

As a result, about two years ago I began two one-hour sessions each week with the same trainer, who by then had several other clients at The Summit. When he asked for my goals, I told him I wanted to regain muscle tone and lose my big, round belly. He tested me with various weights and exercises to find my strength level and then began a program that let me regain strength in arms, legs, back, and abdomen. As for my belly concern, he said that was for me to take charge of—aerobic exercise to burn calories and a more strict diet would reduce the belly. That was my responsibility to execute, but he designed a walking schedule and specified types of food to eat and/or avoid.

So I now have one of those personal trainers that I once thought extravagant, coming right to my residence to direct my own strength exercises. During the two years of this regular exercise, I must have doubled my strength in handling weights. Only rarely now do I have the sore muscles afterward that usually were a feature of my early sessions. If I do develop a tender joint now, my trainer allows a week or more of rest for the sore spot, concentrating on other areas.

For example, if I have a catch and click in a knee joint, I can tell him about it on order to avoid the exhausting "squats" and "dead lift" exercises which really pull the energy from legs and back. Some days he may wonder if I really have a sore joint or muscle, thinking I am trying to get him to give me easier exercises. But so far he accepts my word on this. I sure hope he doesn't think it would occur to me to make up such soreness.

My goal now is to do some serious work on belly reduction. A more selective eating practice and a regular walking program are both in my immediate future. Outside walking will be enjoyable for the next few months, and inside walking on our long hallways is a popular pastime activity for many. No excuses there. I am rescheduling some of my activities so I can have more time for this. So if I can forego the cookies and ice cream while picking up on broccoli and spinach (ugh!), I should be a slimmer person when we meet in the fall.

John adds the following comments.

Jack Lewis worked out with me from August 1999 to October 2002. He has since moved away. When we started working together, we were very, very careful to see if anything happened with his condition: whether he lost blood more quickly, whether he had to get transfusions more frequently as a result, whether he felt faint, and so on. Happily, during most of the time we worked, the frequency of his transfusions dropped from a high of once every week or two to a low of every one to three months. I don't know whether working out helped his condition, but it certainly never seemed to exacerbate it.

In all his activities, Jack acts like anything but someone with a potentially fatal blood condition. A retired petroleum geologist, he has traveled quite extensively to Australia, England, and West Africa. He was extremely popular at his residence facility because he always volunteered to help with any problem, be it solving a computer problem, running projectors, running slide shows and videos, or delivering books to book club members. Much younger than most of the other residents, he made friends easily and still comes back to visit often.

In strength training, Jack is very strong and very focused. At 5 feet 6 inches and about 155 pounds, he had some extra weight around his middle, but he learned quickly and he learned well. He could do any exercise John threw at him. John calls him "my guinea pig for some of the more extreme programs I've used over the years."

One day when Jack couldn't lift as much as he had four days before, he said, "John, that was last week. You know I'm a lot older now."

Chronologically, Jack is young-old, but he doesn't seem old at all. He can do just about anything that anyone in the gym can do, young or old. His attitude was that of a young or middle-aged man and, says John, "He's a blast work with. Always laughing."

Marilyn Jeannette Byer

Lyn, as she is known to one and all, earned a doctorate in education from Syracuse University in 1965 and had a career as an educator. One of her main goals was training the general population to understand how to assist the handicapped. Despite her disability (cerebral palsy), she drove a car, swam, played tennis, traveled, and enjoyed an active social life, including gentleman friends.

An only child who never married, she is John's only client who has no family at all to call on for help. Her friends at the Episcopal Church she attends in Austin are her substitute family, as are several people in her retirement facility.

Lyn has had to form her own support network, and it serves her well.

Before Strength Training

Born with moderate cerebral palsy, she developed severe scoliosis, which caused major backaches and required surgery in 1996 to implant steel rods along her spine in order to provide stability and relieve the pain.

Lyn has also had a partial hip replacement about 1980, a hysterectomy for uterine cancer in 2003, and intestinal surgery in 2004. With two permanently dislocated shoulders and limited use of her legs, she could walk only a few feet and could not dress herself or lift her fork to her mouth.

After Strength Training

After four years of strength training, Lyn's backaches have gone away, she can walk alone for about 160 yards on a good day, and she is able to feed herself at the dinner table. Her quality of life has markedly improved.

Even though Ann, Faye, and Jack are very different in their capabilities and fitness levels, they all have reasonable entries in their respective charts. With Lyn, however, it's difficult and potentially misleading to present her progress in tabular form for several reasons:

- She performs many of her best resistance exercises using her body weight.

- She has had to abandon some exercises when her pain exceeds the perceived benefit, such as the bench press.

- No tabular representation of her progress in walking (distance, speed, and rest times) could begin to tell the full story.

   For example, we need to be aware of whether her knees are apart or hitting each other, whether her right leg is working or being carried, and whether she needs to pause due to loss of stamina, balance, technique, and so on.

   Nonetheless, we have included Lyn's representative charts, especially the ones using free weights. We ask you to read between the lines and to admire her progress.

Lyn's Workout at Five Points

Exercise	Day 1 Lbs x Reps	Month 1 Lbs x Reps	Month 6 Lbs x Reps	Best Ever Lbs x Reps	Current Lbs x Reps
Upper Back Exercise Manual Pull		**Note** 1	Self x 10	Self x 12	Self x 10
Chest Exercise: Bench Press		**Note 2**	10 x 8	15 x 10	
Leg Exercise: Chair Squat	1/8 Squat: Self x 10	1/2 Squat: 10 x 2	Full squat: 8 x 8	8 x 8	5 x 8 **Note 3**
Shoulder Exercise: **Note 4**					
Lower Back Exercise: Dead Lift	Partial (to knees): 10 x 10	10 x 10	Full Dead Lift: 25 x 8	40 x 8	30 x 8
Biceps Exercise: Curl	3 x 10	3 x 20	6 x 8	6 x 10	8 x 8
Triceps Exercise: Pushdown	12 x 8	12 x 10	12 x 10	14 x 10	10 x 12

Table 8-4. Workout Sheet for Lyn Byer

Notes:

1. We introduced the seated pull using a band after six months of training on the manual pull.

2. We introduced the bench press after six months of training but discontinued it because of unremitting shoulder pain from an injury.

3. As of this writing, Lyn is suffering from an as yet undefined condition in her hip and lower back which prevents her from bearing weight on her right leg. She is currently receiving trigger-point release injections and massage. Yet she still works out because she is indomitable.

4. We don't perform shoulder exercises since both of Lyn's shoulders are permanently dislocated.

More about Lyn

John has much admiration for Lyn. She has been the client he has been most worried and most triumphant about.

> Dr. Lyn Byer is a friend of mine. I met her in the summer of 1999. At that time she had just recovered from a 15-hour operation on her back to correct scoliosis. She was 69 years old and had just spent a year in the nursing home section of her residential facility, which she described as the worst year of her life. During surgery, she had had four steel rods inserted alongside her spine to give her some support. She wasn't sure if I could help her, and I certainly wasn't either. With this

understanding, we began training in the spirit of experimentation. That spirit has lasted to this day.

Cerebral palsy has kept Lyn from doing very few of the things she's wanted to do in life. She's charming and always ready for fun. She has a difficult life physically, but she has learned to deal with it and keep a smile on her face, even if it pains her. And often it does. Three times, she has had a prosthetic put in one shoulder. The tension of her muscles in opposition to each other has torn it out of the socket twice.

Like many Southern women of her generation Lyn is a steel magnolia. Whatever she says, good or bad, she has a smile on her face. In addition, like many handicapped people, she made the choice long ago to deal with her handicap, to accept it, and to provide an example to people that she can do anything she wants.

Despite her limitations, she has very high goals for herself in everything. An occupational hazard of this attitude is that she often feels that she should be doing better. She is constantly comparing herself to the self of a long time ago, almost always negatively. John needs to remind her on a regular basis of good things she's done and to remind her that her success is not always going to proceed in a linear fashion. Fortunately, she loves to argue. Fortunately, so does John.

As is the case with most of John's clients, the changes in Lyn began with the physical changes. Doing anything at all led to an improvement in her mood. And with the change in her mood came further changes in her physical capabilities. It's circular; the one feeds the other. The main goal she's always had is to walk without a cane or a walker. In general, this has not proved possible; however, she has succeeded in learning to walk without aid if she is very careful and very slow.

Her main problem with walking is that if she falls, she's unable to get up by herself. To date, her best practical success in walking is for her to walk arm in arm with another person. This enables her to move from a chair to a car, from a car to a restaurant, and from a taxi to a theater, which is a great improvement in her life. It makes her life easier, makes life easier for those taking her out, and gives her a great deal of self-confidence and self-esteem. It seems like a little thing. It's not.

Seemingly small improvements in strength can provide major benefits.

John continues,

>An unexpected and fantastic thing about working with Lyn is that her body is so different physically from that of other people I work with that I must continually experiment to find a way to improve her muscular strength. We've tried to use what I think of as a well-designed plan of trial-and-error to work all of her body parts. Our basic premise is, "If it hurts too much, don't do it." As a result of working with

her, I've developed a lot of new exercise techniques which are successful, not only with Lyn but with many other clients.

For example, it is very difficult to work the muscles of the upper back without using the muscles of the arms and shoulders or, specifically, without engaging the shoulder joint. As important as upper back exercise is, especially for posture, Lyn and I were unable to do anything for about a year and a half, possibly two years, because I reckoned that her shoulders simply could not stand the pain of pulling. One day, while holding her hands to assist her in doing heel raises for the calves, we found that she could lean back about six inches and pull herself forward.

This discovery slowly led us to develop the assisted body weight pull, an exercise I now use with nearly every single older client, at least until they've gotten the hang of independently retracting their shoulder blades. Lyn in the meantime has gotten strong enough to let herself back 18 inches or more from vertical. I really don't know how she manages to keep her shoulders in their sockets. I really don't know how she manages the pain required to pull her body weight up. What I tell her is, "Lyn, you have to be the judge. When it hurts too much, don't do it."

For Lyn, simple motions like an arm curl with the dumbbell are very difficult because her rotator cuff doesn't behave properly. Lyn has learned to perform dumbbell curls by sitting in a chair and holding the dumbbell at her side. With one hand, John holds her shoulder in its socket. With the other hand, he holds her elbow slightly away from her rib cage. Lyn uses her free hand to keep the dumbbell from pulling across her body. Then she curls. This one is really a victory.

Another example is machine triceps pushdowns. Lyn stands in front of the pushdown machine, leaning back directly against John's chest. He holds both of her elbows back and slightly away from her sides in proper position. She's able to stabilize her back against his chest and perform the exercise for triceps.

Another example is even more amazing—chair squats. She can squat 10 pounds in each hand. She weighs 108 and she's 74 years old. Like most people with cerebral palsy, her knees normally stay firmly pressed against each other. John kneels to her side slightly in front of her. He places his fist between her knees, forcing them apart. She squats, taps the seat with her buttocks, and stands back up.

John talks to her the entire time about how much pressure she's applying to his hand. He usually says something like, "Ouch! I still want to use those knuckles." She usually says something helpful like, "Go to hell." She has learned, much to her surprise, that she is able to slightly separate both knees. She had sworn that trying to do this was a waste of time. So this big improvement has enabled her to do the squats and has given her, as it gives everybody, a lot of extra strength in her quads, glutes, and hamstrings.

One more example is dead lifts. John uses nearly the same technique except that he places his fist between her knees from the back. They have the same brief conversation: "Keep

your head up. Lower your hips not your back. Ouch, that hurts." From her, "Go to hell."
But the result is this:

A 73-year-old woman with cerebral palsy and four steel rods implanted
near her spine can dead lift 40 pounds eight times. It's unbelievable.

John adds,
When I first began working with Lyn, her main complaint was terrible low back
pain. Naturally, I was very circumspect in any exercise that involved her lower
back. We began by doing the tiniest motion of good mornings. It became apparent
that she could do good mornings and she could do them pretty deep. The more she
did over several weeks, the less she complained of back pain.

Finally, on a hunch, I had her begin doing partial dead lifts or Romanian dead lifts.
To my delight—you know I love dead lifts—she did these well, the best of any of
my older clients. Eventually, she learned the entire dead lift motion. The key word
is eventually. We took it extremely carefully and extremely slowly. We started with
a wooden dowel. It took her sixteen months to build up to 40 pounds.

Using the Case Studies

We hope that your SE will be as inspiring as the four people who have graciously allowed
us to use them as case studies. If you can just get your SE started in strength training, he
will probably start feeling better right away and will continue to work out in order to feel
good. Your main obstacle may be to convince him that he needs to exercise. We hope these
case studies will help you motivate him to get started.

Use whatever motivations you can find to get your
Significant Elder into strength training.

If your SE is older and weaker or has more disabling conditions than these four people,
then you need to get expert medical advice for a strength program, perhaps starting with a
physical therapist before engaging a personal trainer. As the questionnaires in Chapter 1
demonstrate, however, almost anyone can work to get stronger and healthier.

Just a glance at the pictures of older people performing strength training activities may be
enough to overcome any remaining objections your SE may have. After all, he may not like
it if a couple of 90-year-old ladies can "kick his butt."

A Note to Certified Personal Trainers

You are already accustomed to tailoring a strength training program for each client you have, so the main differences in working with older people are to be more patient, progress more slowly, be more mindful of safety, use more ingenuity for accommodative exercises, and collaborate closely with them. Remember:

- Patience.

- Safety

- Ingenuity.

- Collaboration.

- Patience, patience, patience.

Summary of the Main Points

- Almost anyone can exercise, even people in their 90s and people who have a life-threatening condition or a major disability.

- Keep good records because the data will chart your SE's progress. The notes you take will give you a running commentary on his state of health.

- Maintain a good relationship with your SE.

What's Next?

The next chapter shows you how to take strength training for your Significant Elder beyond the purely physical. You can strengthen his motivation by enhancing the mind-body connection with half a dozen beneficial practices.

Chapter 9. Using the Mind-Body Connection

Turning Random Activities into Positive Habits

"The trouble with old age is that it takes twice as long to do half as much."
   Mary J., 80

Important Points for Advocates: This chapter gives you some motivational tools that you can use to help your SE stay committed to her strength program. Even from a distance, you can encourage her to strengthen the mind-body connection through massage, imagery, positive self-talk, water aerobics, Tai Chi, or yoga.

Full Disclosure: Neither author comes from a "woo-woo" background. We have lived our adult lives in states not well known for these pursuits—North Carolina, Louisiana, and Texas. Jody has also lived in Taiwan and Thailand but did not take advantage of the spiritual practices available there. Austin, Texas, where both authors live now, offers many resources. Both of us have experienced transformations in ourselves and in our mothers that border on the amazing, if not the miraculous. We invite you to set aside any skepticism you may have about applying these ideas to your SE and take a look at some highly practical activities that really work.[36] We and our mothers have received excellent benefits from one or more of the six methods that we recommend here.

Introduction

Whether you call it the mind-body connection, the bodymind, the psychosomatic phenomenon, the science of psychoneuroimmunology, the practice of mind-body medicine, or something else, considerable significant scientific interest in this area has developed over the past three decades. Note such statements as these, to select only a few:

---

[36] Such books as *The Mental Edge: Maximize Your Sports Potential with the Mind/Body Connection* by Ken Baum, Richard Trubo, and Kenneth Baum (Perigee: New York, 1999) and *Body, Mind, and Sport: The Mind-Body Guide to Lifelong Health, Fitness, and Your Personal Best* by John Douillard, Billie Jean King, and Martina Navratilova (Three Rivers Press: New York, 2001) show the effectiveness of enhancing the mind-body connection in sports.

- ...I use the words *psychosomatic* and *mindbody* interchangeably. They are synonymous and refer to the interaction between the brain and the body whereby psychological or mental processes induce either pathological or beneficial physical changes."[37]

- "Mind doesn't dominate body, it *becomes* body—body and mind are one."[38]

- "The body has a mind of its own."[39]

The research may be new, but the ideas have been around for a while. In our Significant Elders' generation, the idea that the mind, thoughts, or emotions influence the body, behavior, or health was present in such common expressions as these:

- Stiff upper lip!

- You're about as happy as you make up your mind to be.

- She died of a broken heart.

- Don't frown or your face will freeze like that.

Scientists have indeed proved that "molecules of emotion" circulate throughout the body. Further, some health care professionals find it viable to use visualization and other techniques to improve their patients' mental and physical health, sometimes even to help them achieve remission of disease. It's easy to see, however, that one of the main differences between the older expressions and today's findings is that many of the old sayings tended toward the negative, while today's practitioners focus on the positive.

> **Your SE is already familiar with the connection between mind and body.**
> **You can help best by making this connection a positive experience.**

The considerable strength, determination, and will power of those who triumphed over the Great Depression and World War II can now be channeled into self-care for the purpose of becoming and remaining strong and healthy.

The trick, however, is to be subtle and gentle in your approach. If your SE is unaccustomed to paying much attention to herself, she may not be comfortable with an approach that seems too touchy-feely or that strikes her as being selfish, the word some older people use for anything that turns the spotlight on themselves.

---

[37] Sarno, John E, M.D. *The Mindbody Prescription: Healing the Body, Healing the Pain.* (Warner Books, New York: 1998), p. 35.

[38] Pert, Candace B. *Molecules of Emotion: The Science behind Mind-Body Medicine*, by Candace B. Pert, Ph.D. (Scribner, New York: 1997), p. 187.

[39] Chopra, Deepak. *Quantum Healing: Exploring the Frontiers of Mind/Body Medicine.* (Bantam, New York: 1990), Chapter 2, pp. 19-34. Also see his *Perfect Health: The Complete Mind-Body Guide.* (Crown, New York: 2001).

You may have to help your SE redefine the negative term *selfish* as the positive term *self-care*. You will also need to help her recognize that self-care is one of her most important priorities. Anything that improves her quality of life is worth doing, and she deserves only the best.

Enhancing the Mind-Body Connection

Congratulations! You couldn't have chosen an easier way to start enhancing your SE's mind-body connection than helping her get into strength training. As she exercises, she *has* to become more aware of her body and of the interplay between mind and body. Reinforce the connection by asking how she feels at several points during a training session. Near the end of a typical session, she will feel better, more energetic, and possibly more optimistic than at the start. Encourage her to notice the improvement. Point out that she looks stronger than she did an hour ago, and ask, "Do you feel better than you did before we started working out today?"

We hope you are having great success: Your SE is becoming stronger and healthier, you are receiving many emotional rewards, such as pride in her accomplishments, and everything is working well. If so, don't change a thing. This chapter is intended to help with two situations that occur with older athletes, the first of which is quite common and the other, less so:

- **A motivational breakdown**. Your SE has lost her enthusiasm or simply stopped training and you need something to get her going again. If your own interest has flagged, you may also be able to use this chapter to get yourself back on track.

- **A desire to get a little more out of the program** than health and strength, though these are wonderful enough. Your SE may not know that there can be more, but if the circumstances become favorable, you can initiate a discussion, or at least implement the results, of some of the ideas presented in this chapter.

Note that there are many paths to enhancing the mind-body connection and many payoffs for doing so. Your own participation in these activities is not a requirement, but you might consider using the results of some of these non-material motivators or enhancements to promote a better life for your SE.

Many Paths

Many entry points are available for enhancing the mind-body connection. For example, if your SE knows a little about the human potential, personal growth, New Age, or consciousness movements of the last three decades, you can use this chapter as a review of the lessons learned from such movements. However, this knowledge is rare in those over 75 or 80, especially if they live outside New York, California, or a few other areas of the U.S. Instead of giving her the background on these lessons, just present them as ways to enhance her quality of life.

Whether or not she cares about lessons from these movements, chances are excellent that your SE has experienced personal growth and developed some positive habits or else she wouldn't have made it to a ripe old age. However, in the area of self-care, which includes strength and health, many older people range from somewhat to extremely neglectful of themselves.

Various random activities may have served your SE well from time to time during her life, but unless these haphazard interests become constant, positive forces, they won't reliably support her through the tough times. Such setbacks may include illnesses and injuries as well as discouragement, skipping sessions, and other manifestations of lost motivation. At the very least, your SE may from time to time experience a Withdrawal of Enthusiasm (WOE) phase, which causes a "Whoa!" or a slow-down in her progress.

Many Payoffs

Numerous positive results derive from enhancing the mind-body connection. It is one of the best ways to produce and solidify the positive habits that will make motivational concerns virtually unnecessary. Enhancing the mind-body connection is also an excellent way to improve anyone's life and, indeed, to empower your SE.

As she strengthens her body, she also strengthens the mind-body connection, and vice versa. When your SE is fully convinced that strength training helps her feel better and gives her more energy, she will suffer fewer motivational problems. When she spontaneously talks about *wanting* or *needing* to exercise, you will know that she is convinced of its value.

Six Mind-Body Methods to Explore

There are many aspects of the mind-body connection to explore, and all of them have the goal of cementing some of the helpful but largely unplanned self-care activities your SE might occasionally practice. In this chapter, we will include six of the tried-and-true activities that show the strongest promise of keeping your SE motivated.

The first three methods use a less active, largely individual approach through massage, imagery or visualization, and positive self-talk. The other three use a more active, group approach through water aerobics, Tai Chi, and yoga.

The main uniting factor among massage, imagery, and positive self-talk is that none of the methods requires much, if any, expenditure of energy. You can introduce these methods and encourage their use even if your SE is frail, discouraged, or less energetic than usual. Another connection is that all of these methods are fairly easy to implement and don't require an expert teacher—you can do it yourself. Finally, it's likely that your SE has already heard about them in some form or other.

How Massage Can Help

The easiest, most direct step in enhancing the mind-body connection may be to encourage your SE to get massages periodically. If she has ever had physical therapy for injuries, massage is just a hop and a skip away. If not, massage may still be fairly easy to sell to your SE because it feels good and helps relax sore muscles. Further, as mentioned in Chapter 3, many older people suffer from tactile deprivation, and massage relieves some of the stress of seldom or never being touched.

In terms of enhancing the mind-body connection, massage works extremely well. One of the first elements it provides is greater body awareness. As touched on in Chapters 3 and 4, many older people have never had the occasion to listen to their bodies in any specific way.

A good massage therapist can provide your SE with a vocabulary for talking about the aches and pains of the aging body. If Grandma says her shoulder hurts, the massage therapist can ask whether the pain throbs dully, slices like a needle or a knife, radiates from a point, feels a little like a burn inside her body, and so on.

The therapist can also ask about the quality and quantity of the pain, discomfort, or stiffness. From this vocabulary of physical pain, your SE can branch out to happier examples of body awareness—how empowering it feels to be able to pick up a great-grandchild or how good it feels to breathe deeply after chair squats.

Remind your SE periodically about the advantages of strength, independence, self-confidence, and good cooperation between the mind and the body. If necessary, make non-judgmental contrasts between any of her earlier episodes of weakness and despair and her later experiences with increased power and optimism.

It may be quite easy to interest your SE in massage therapy. If not, then watch for your chance when an inevitable muscle strain occurs. Note that a massage costs about the same as a strength training session. Even though insurance so far doesn't usually cover massage, as it does physical therapy, your SE can probably afford a few sessions and may well want to schedule massages regularly.

Let her know that most physicians approve of massage therapy because good results are well documented. To find the right massage therapist for your SE, take many of the same steps you took in Chapter 2 to select a certified personal trainer.

You and Massage

Just as you can more easily entice your SE into strength training if you do it yourself, so you can better recommend massages if you also enjoy them. You can speak from experience about such benefits as:

- Improving the circulation of blood throughout the body.

- Relaxing tense muscles.

- Preventing and caring for injuries.

- Improving lymphatic drainage.

- Flushing toxins out of the body.

Justine

One regular massage client, let's call her Justine, not only gets many physical benefits from massage but also uses her state of deep relaxation on the massage table to achieve breakthroughs in her writing projects. As a budding screen writer, she realizes that she can't be creative through sheer willpower. She has to let go of worry and become open to creativity.

Once when a particular creative writing project seemed to have only a middle but no suitable beginning or ending, she dreamed up just the right framing device during a massage. No words accompanied the idea, but she said, "A series of images flashed through my mind, and I just knew they were what I'd been looking for." When she returned to her computer, the images were easy to translate into the words that opened and concluded the story.

Your Significant Elder and Massage

Some older people take to massage as a dog takes to bacon. Others may feel uncomfortable being touched by a stranger. Whatever your SE's attitudes may be, you can encourage her to take advantage of this beneficial activity.

If Mom is too modest to think about taking off all her clothes, you can point out how fully covered she will be with the sheets that a massage therapist uses. An alternative is to ask for a fully clothed massage. If Grandpa worries that a massage may increase the pain of an injured shoulder, you can coach him on how to communicate with the massage therapist by simply saying, "That hurts!" The massage therapist can then take appropriate steps to treat the injury. If lying down on a massage table would worsen a respiratory condition, ask for a chair massage, which keeps the client upright and well supported by the chair.

Whatever objection she comes up with, you can reframe it in positive language. If all else fails, give a gift certificate for a free massage. Offer to be on the scene during the massage if your presence would make your SE feel more comfortable. Good massage therapists can accommodate most requests because they are in the business of helping people feel better.

How Imagery Can Help

Imagery[40], also known as mental rehearsal and visualization, is the practice of seeing yourself performing an activity in your mind's eye before you actually do it. Virtually all professional athletes and a majority of amateurs, all the way down to pre-school T-Ball players, are coached in using some form of this technique. You have probably used it yourself, consciously or unconsciously, before a performance review at work, on the golf course, or in almost any stressful situation for which you made mental preparations.

Using imagery can also help your SE turn her occasional successes into habitual triumphs in the strength training room. Here's how it works with the chair squat, for example. Before starting the exercise, ask Mom to:

- Sit upright and relax deeply, paying attention to her long, deep breaths.

- See in her mind's eye a photograph of her stance before she starts the exercise.

- Run a movie in her mind of the action she takes to lower herself to the chair.

- Take a quick snapshot of the tiny pause before she starts to rise.

- Run a movie in her mind of the action of raising herself back to the standing position.

- Take a photograph of her position at the end of the rep.

The imagery is even more effective if she can mentally hear the little grunt she gives as she starts back up, feel the steel dumbbells she holds in her hands, taste the sweat on her upper lip, and inhale the fragrance of her freshly laundered workout clothes.

After this mental and sensory preparation, she's guaranteed to perform a better chair squat than she would without it. If she has doubts about her ability to visualize the senses, you can at least encourage her to play Let's Pretend, as in, "Pretend you can feel the weight of the dumbbells as you think about holding them in your hands."

You and Imagery

Maybe you do mental rehearsals all the time, but if you have never practiced imagery as an adult, you will probably want to begin. Soon, you will see some remarkable benefits. Let's take a look at two of John's experiences with imagery, one that he did as a teenager and one that he engages in today.

As a kid, John loved playing basketball. It was his passion. On Sunday afternoons, he always watched the NBA Game of the Week. Throughout the first half of the game, he

---

[40] Also see *Mind & Muscle* by Blair Whitmarsh (Human Kinetics: Chicago, 2001) and *Imagery training in sports: A handbook for athletes, coaches, and sport psychologists* by Brent S. Rushall (Sports Science Association: New York, 1991).

absorbed every move the Boston Celtics made. At halftime, he grabbed his basketball and rushed out to the driveway, where he became the star, the fans, and the announcer all at once.

"Pandemonium reigns in Yellow Jacket Field House. Payne drives deep into the left corner, goes up, and releases that feather-light jumper … nothing but net!"

Seeing himself as the star player in front of thousands of screaming fans not only improved his game but also increased his motivation. The same phenomenon occurs today in his Olympic weightlifting sessions. Before he addresses the barbell for the Olympic lift known as the snatch, he plays his coach's words in his mind:

- *Feel it* reminds him to send his awareness to the muscle groups that he engages first.

- *Hear it* reminds him to listen for his intake of breath before he starts his lift, to notice the slight scratchy sound of the plates as they leave the mat, and to pay attention to the utterly quiet moment as the bar is weightless and motionless in mid air just before he catches it. He hears the sound of the catch itself as a tiny click.

- *See it* reminds him to run a stop-frame movie in his mind with a series of steps:

    - A snapshot of the starting position.

    - A movie of rising with the bar.

    - A snapshot of the instant at which he is absolutely extended with the bar at its highest point and perfectly balanced against the forces of gravity.

    - A snapshot after the successful snatch.

John has become so expert with imagery that he can run his mental movie from various camera angles and with sound.

Your Significant Elder and Imagery

The language of the mind-body connection is images. Words may or may not accompany the mental pictures. For example, some cancer patients receive coaching in visualization techniques. They are encouraged to picture their white blood cells chasing, capturing, and chewing up their cancer cells. Some patients become quite creative with their images of strong, armor-clad warrior cells fighting and defeating slimy enemy cancer cells.

Martin

"It's a battle for my body," states one patient we will call Martin. "And my warriors are winning."

In happier circumstances, you can help your SE apply positive imagery to her strength training routines. Recall that Chapter 3 advocates that you gently place your hand on your SE's upper back, for example, to reinforce the idea of retracting the shoulder blades in several of the exercises. You can gradually encourage your SE to "feel" the touch even when your hand isn't making contact.

Tweet

One of John's clients, Tweet, age 84, has a stronger self-image and is more willful than most of his older clients, some of whom have gradually lost their sense of purpose. Although physically self-aware and active, she was never really convinced of the benefit of strength training until her doctor informed her that she had osteoporosis and prescribed weight-bearing exercise.

Overnight, she became a chair squat fanatic and a poster child for good technique. Like everyone, however, she tends to falter and lose both her focus and her technique near the end of the set. John's admonitions, "Chest up, tight back," and so on were having no effect. Suddenly, John drew inspiration from her strong self-concept and said:

"Be Tweet. Just be Tweet."

Instantly, her posture, focus, and determination crystallized, and she finished the exercise stronger than she started it. Since then, "Be Tweet" has become very effective imagery for her, a short-hand way to achieve focus. It brings a shared smile to them both.

If your SE has strengths in some area of life, show her how to translate them into the exercise room. Remind her of who she really is—a valuable human being who is taking appropriate steps to remain strong and healthy. You will both be surprised at the positive results.

How Positive Self-Talk Can Help

Note that positive self-talk serves the same purpose as imagery, but it takes place in unspoken words rather than mental pictures. Even though positive self-talk works on the mind more than on the body, it's one more tool that you can use to keep your SE motivated in strength training.[41]

It's surprising how negatively some older people talk to themselves—some younger ones too, of course. A constant stream of self-criticism runs through their minds. They say such phrases as, "Not that way, you dummy!" or, "Idiot! I figured you'd mess that up."

---

[41] Books such as *Positive Self-Talk for Children: Teaching Self-Esteem Through Affirmations: A Guide For Parents, Teachers, And Counselors*, by Douglas Bloch (New York: Bantam, 1993) contain useful information that you can modify and apply to your Significant Elder.

Much of the time, the negative self-talk seems to be unconscious, but the self-criticism may come to the surface during the stress of a mistake in the exercise room. Be on the alert for your SE's disparaging comments so that you can restate them in a positive light.

For example, Ann isn't fond of the wall press and sometimes says so. John often reminds her of how well she performs the exercise and points out how much her efforts have improved her posture. She has no dowager's hump and easily takes an upright stance. After a bit of struggle, she now says this about the wall press, "Well, it's not my favorite exercise, but I do it anyhow."

If your SE displays a generally negative attitude toward the world, one of the best things you can do is to turn the critical comments into positive or even humorous expressions. Your SE may not even be aware of speaking so negatively. However, your job isn't to confront the negativity head-on. Instead, try some of the techniques discussed on page 222.

Providing positive feedback to your SE during strength training is a good way to encourage her to practice positive self-talk. She may come to rely on your positive comments as she becomes able to tell the difference between a good set and a not-so-good set.

For example, when Lyn performs extremely well but John neglects to provide enough praise, she will banter, "Wasn't that good? What am I, chopped liver?" He banters right back, "You're great, my dear. You're pâté de foie gras."

You and Positive Self-Talk

Unless you are one of those always-cheerful people who seem to have been born with self-confidence and positive thinking, it may be as hard for you as it is for your SE to see the need for positive self-talk. If you occasionally or frequently fall into negative thinking, you may think there's nothing you can do to become more positive and optimistic. But there is. And the benefits to you will be as great as they are for your SE

For example, Jody used to hold a generally pessimistic, largely negative view of the world, and her self-talk reflected that view. People who knew her well used to tell her that she was her own worst enemy because she habitually criticized herself and seldom or never celebrated victories. She thought the good things that came her way were just flukes. Even when friends invited her to parties, she might accept, but to herself, she would say, "Okay, I will go, but I won't enjoy it." Sure enough, parties weren't much fun. Life wasn't a barrel of laughs either.

Then she was forced into daily contact with several people who were even more negative. She soon realized that she had to do something to avoid being pulled into the emotional morass. Over a considerable period of time, she developed a number of self-talk strategies that worked. The first was, "Okay, he's an unhappy, judgmental person, but I don't have to be like that. I don't have to let him drag me down." As soon as she stopped reacting to the criticisms with defensive measures, the fun was gone, and the negative people gradually stopped making disparaging remarks.

The next step was a more positive example of self-talk: "I can take care of myself no matter how negative someone is." She was sometimes able to disconcert negative people by smiling and nodding during their outbursts. Finally, she achieved virtual nirvana when she could feel sympathy for them because they remained such unhappy people. She has not and will not try to change these folks overtly, but some of them are gradually changing themselves into somewhat less negative, judgmental people. And Jody is much happier in positive mode. Life is good.

John also practices the principles of the peaceful warrior[42] and uses kill-them-with-kindness techniques when appropriate. He realizes that negative, unhappy people are the ones who most need praise and positive feedback. A strength training session may be the only place where such a negative person can receive praise for doing something she intended to do anyway. Such approval can become a strong motivating force for keeping this person coming back. Over time, the increase in endorphins may help her achieve a more positive outlook.

Your Significant Elder and Positive Self-Talk

Positive self-talk or positive thinking is not a wild and crazy idea to your SE's generation. In fact, Norman Vincent Peale (1898-1993), popularized it.[43] Your SE can't have escaped contact with this idea unless she was completely isolated from American culture in the 1950s and early 1960s. If your SE has a positive impression of Peale, you can refer to the techniques in this section as examples of positive thinking. If she has a negative attitude toward Peale, then refer to them as examples of positive self-talk. In either case, you can tap into ideas that your SE is already familiar with.

One common example you can use is peer comparison. Notice what happens when your SE sees someone whose posture is poor and who looks much older than she herself does. Her typical response will be to throw her shoulders back and stand as straight as she can. Watch for an opportunity such as this to compliment her posture, using the catch-her-doing-something-right principle of management. Then you can go on to encourage her to talk about the negative people she knows. Point out how much happier and more positive she is than they are, and note how much strength training has contributed to her more positive emotional life.

Using Prayer or Meditation

Encourage your SE to use prayer if appropriate, especially contemplative rather than intercessory or supplicative prayer. In contemplative prayer, practitioners surrender themselves to inner silence and open themselves to contact with God. During one or two twenty-minute sessions per day, they merely note the passing of thoughts through their minds and attempt to quiet those thoughts in order to experience the presence of God.

---

[42] See *The Way of the Peaceful Warrior*, 20th Anniversary Edition, by Dan Milman (New York, H.J. Kramer: 2000).
[43] *The Power of Positive Thinking,* first published in 1952, is available today in the 1996 reissue edition from Ballantine Books.

Sometimes, they focus on a sacred word to help them with the experience. This practice resembles meditating with a mantra, but prayer may be more acceptable than meditation to members of your SE's generation. Both, however, can reinforce the connection between intention and action, that is, between mind and body.

If your SE has an active prayer life, you can also encourage prayer centered on viewing the body as the temple of the soul. You can point out that the meet-your-maker event has not happened yet and that God must have some purpose for keeping her alive. She may as well stay as strong and healthy as she can for her remaining years because this seems to be God's plan for her. As one of John's clients says, "God must love little old ladies because He sure makes a lot of them."

Using Positive Affirmations

Instead of or in addition to prayer or meditation, you can consider helping your SE develop some positive affirmations to use. Encourage her to say, "I can do this" or "I can do the chair squat" either sub-vocally or aloud. Her exercise routine will go more smoothly and she will feel more successful than if she tells herself, "I can't do this" or "I can't do the chair squat." Other positive affirmations that may work include the following:

- I'm good at the lat pull (or some other exercise).

- I'm getting stronger.

- I'm taking charge of my health and strength.

- I'm doing just fine.

- I'm glad to be exercising.

- I feel good.

- I feel better now than I did when I first got here today.

Affirmations, like prayer and meditation, can help make the connection between what she thinks and what she does, that is, between mind and body.

Expressing Gratitude

Encourage your SE to express gratitude in general. This statement doesn't mean that she needs to say thank you all day long. Instead, it means that you can encourage her to feel grateful to be alive and grateful to be getting stronger. If you have any familiarity at all with 12-step recovery programs, you know that members of these programs are taught and encouraged to express their thankfulness for each tiny step away from addiction because it's a tiny step toward living an addiction-free life.

When a member of a 12-step group endlessly whines and complains in a meeting, someone longer in sobriety is sure to ask, "How's your gratitude?" This expression immediately encourages people at the meeting to start counting their blessings. Some may have to "fake it till they make it," but even those in the greatest pain can often find some little something to be grateful for.

Older people who are grateful are much less likely to dwell in the negative emotions. One connection that you can make is that the sedentary lifestyle of so many Americans of all ages has its addictive qualities.

> Any activity that gets your SE away from the sofa and the TV set is a victory worthy of gratitude and celebration.

After each training session, you can reinforce your SE's gratitude by saying things like, "You inspire me. I hope I'm lucky enough to live to your age and be able to work out as hard as you do. I'm thankful that you're still able to do so much. I will bet you're grateful, too."

It's entirely appropriate to be glad about any part of an aging body that still functions.

Using the Five Senses

Since negative self-talk takes place in the mind, you can make your SE's thoughts more positive by helping her pay more attention to enjoying her senses. A good place to start is to support experiences such as watching birds building a nest, listening to the spray of a fountain, sniffing the early morning air after a rainfall, stroking the soft ears of a dog, or tasting a bite of Indian curry. If you are with her, remain calm and silent during these times to encourage her to experience them fully.

It's a good idea to talk about these experiences afterwards, however, to reinforce the connection between the five senses and the mental appreciation of them. Even people with diminished vision, poor hearing, or the inability to smell or taste well can still use their memories and their remaining senses to enhance the mind-body connection.

Reframing

Simple reframing is the technique of turning a statement around or giving it a different context for the purpose of making it sound more positive. An example is changing the *glass is half empty* to the *glass is half full*. But it's more than just a wording change.

> The habit of reframing the negative into the positive can make a big improvement in your SE's outlook on life.

Be alert for opportunities to move your SE's words toward the positive. At first, if negative comments pop out like firecrackers, you will have to ignore all but the most flagrant. During strength training sessions, watch for complaints like, "I just hate dead lifts."

Respond with, "But I know dead lifts love you. Just look what they've done for you. Since you started doing them, your lower back doesn't hurt any more."

Never ever confront one negative with another negative.

Review the section on banter on page 65, and use humor or at least a light-hearted phrase wherever possible. In short, don't let your SE's despair get you down. Be prepared with a good come-back. Some useful reframing techniques include the following:

- Change the subject suddenly, even if the change feels forced. If you are a parent, you have probably used this technique to distract a child away from a dangerous or unwanted behavior.

- After noting some of your SE's typical negative phrases, think up some positive responses and be prepared to use them. For example, if she always says, "I just don't have any energy any more," but you know that the statement is an exaggeration, you can say, "I think you have more now than you did a year ago." You know that strength training produces energy rather than draining it.

- If you know of another older person who does strength training, you can tell your SE about some of the benefits her peer has seen. Better yet, introduce the two of them.

- Perhaps a visit to your own gym would help so that she won't think strength training is such an odd thing to do. Take her at a time when older members usually work out.

- Use reverse psychology in the form of taking your SE to visit someone who's too frail to walk. Point out that your SE has the opportunity to get stronger and to prevent frailty.

There are many ways to reframe a negative into a positive. It's in your best interest to find ways that work with your SE because a positive outlook produces many positive physical results. Both of you will be happier for the effort.

How Water Aerobics Can Help

Water aerobics, Tai Chi, and yoga require some expenditure of energy, although less than strength training. These methods first engage the body and then the mind. If your SE is frail, discouraged, or less energetic than usual, you can still recommend these methods even though they are a little harder to implement than the less active ones.

For these activities, it's probably better to look for a group setting and a well-trained leader to conduct the classes unless you practice these methods yourself and feel comfortable teaching your SE. Depending on her experience, she may or may not be interested in them. They can be a little harder to promote, especially if she has never tried them and doesn't like to do anything new and different. They will prove worth the effort, however, if you can find a way to convince her to give them a try.

Taking a water aerobics class can help anyone of any age. For your SE, such a class is especially beneficial because it places no strain on the joints, it provides a good combination of light cardiovascular activity and light strength exercise, and it's fun for most people.

Exercising in water is a great way to support the body because the buoyancy of water neutralizes some of the effects of gravity. Water makes you feel lighter. It doesn't cause joint, muscle, and bone injuries. Since water is much denser than air, it provides much greater resistance. Doing nothing more than walking in chest-deep water makes a pretty good workout. Further, in warm weather, people who run or walk tend to sweat, but water exercisers don't, or at least they don't feel the sweat because they can duck down and cool off.

In Figure 9-1, Weldon, 92, enjoys the pool because he can hold on and press his feet against the side of the pool in a modified horizontal squat. He explains, "I can't do real squats, but this exercise makes me feel good."

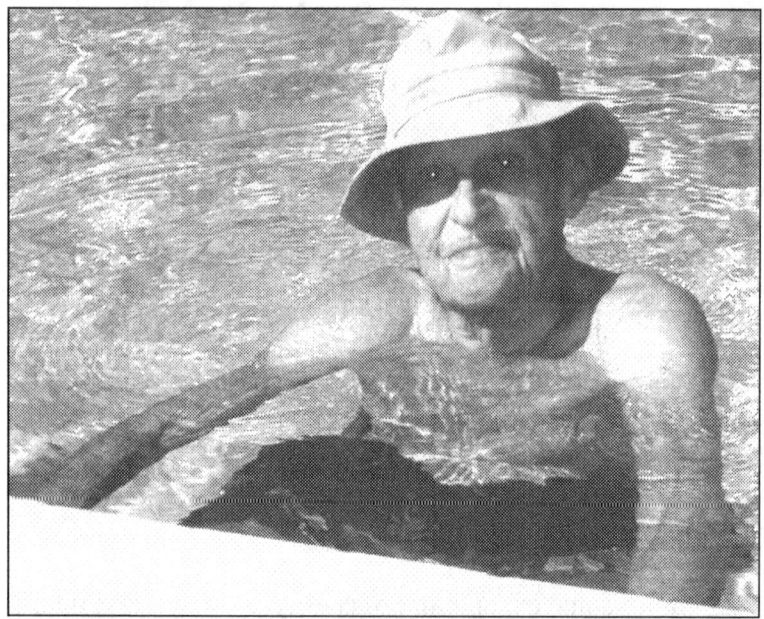

Figure 9-1. Weldon pushes against the side of the pool.

There's something quite refreshing about getting in a pool. Many adults feel like kids again in the water, especially if they use kick boards, water noodles, diving boards, and other enjoyable equipment.

In Figure 9-2 below, Carl, 86, uses floating dumbbells for a fitness routine that a personal trainer at his health club developed for him. He exercises nearly every day to keep his arms and legs strong.

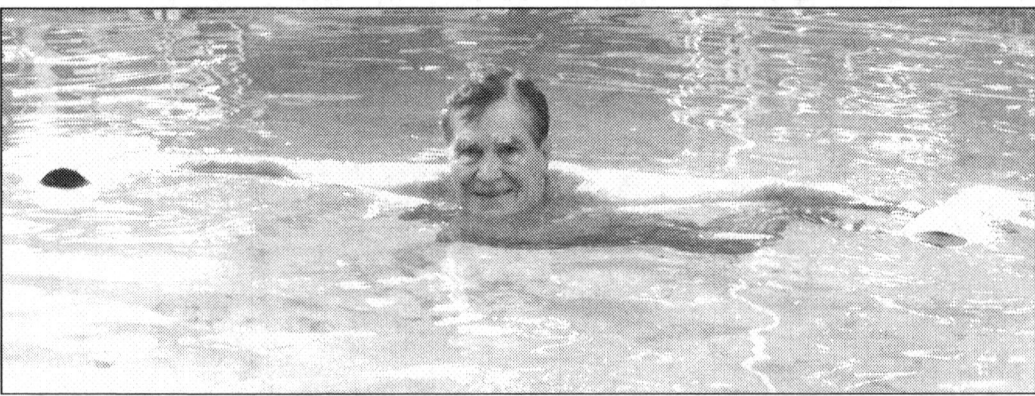

Figure 9-2. Carl exercises with floating dumbbells.

You and Water Aerobics

Every time you swim laps, you do an advanced and highly specialized version of water aerobics. "Once a swimmer, always a swimmer," says Jen, 53, who was a varsity long-distance swimmer in college. She doesn't feel like herself unless she gets to a pool frequently. Formerly an occupational therapist in skilled nursing facilities, she is well aware of the benefits of pool workouts to older clients as well as to her own health.

If you are an ardent swimmer who has never tried water aerobics, you may wonder whether it's real exercise. Participating in just one class might convince you that it is.
Also recall that aquatic physical therapy is an excellent and well-known method of rehabilitating injuries. It can also strengthen and condition the muscles. Your SE will perform a version of water aerobics that's appropriate to her age and condition but will receive benefits similar to those you get with a good swim.

Your Significant Elder and Water Aerobics

Although nearly everyone enjoys getting into a pool, your SE might have various types of objections to water aerobics. You need to be prepared with information to counteract any negative statements.

For example, if Mom is embarrassed about her appearance, you can help her find an attractive bathing suit, beach towel, beach coat or jazzy bathrobe, and some aqua shoes. She may be more willing to give it a try if she has the right equipment. You can also find a class designed for older people, where all the members look 70 or 80 because they *are* 70 or 80.

If Dad worries that he might be the only man in the class, you can try to enlist a male friend to go with him. You can also assure him that the women go to class for the exercise and not to chase men. Challenge him to work hard to keep up with them in an ongoing class. A little competition may be just the thing to motivate him. In Figure 9-3, John and Kathy, both 81 and married for almost 60 years, motivate each other to swim and do pool exercises.

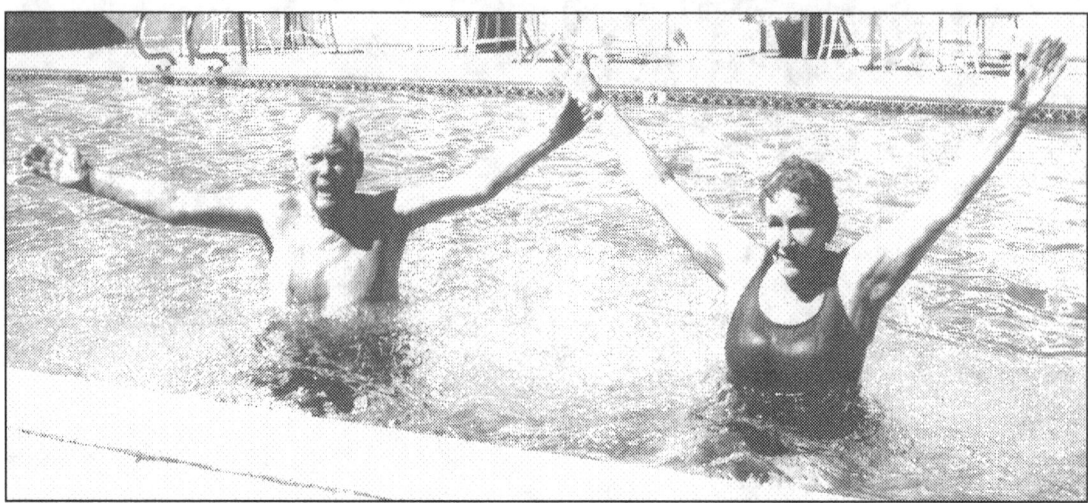

Figure 9-3. John and Kathy exercise in the pool.

Use whatever works. Once your SE starts attending, you probably won't be able to keep her away from the pool. For example, Faye has enjoyed water aerobics for a dozen years. She can't wait for spring to come each year so she can get back in the outdoor pool at her retirement facility. "This spring, I really need to work on my left knee," she says. "I'm tired of wearing a knee brace, and I know water aerobics will help me strengthen my leg muscles. Right now, the strength training exercises are just too painful, but soon I will be able to do them again." She has her boom box, her water aerobics tape, and a friend or two to go with her. That's the spirit!

The residential facility where Ann and Faye live offers a water aerobics class twice a week. Few attend, however, because the modest cost of the class seems too expensive for these very frugal people. They didn't get through the Great Depression nor amass the assets it takes to live in an upscale facility by spending their money on frivolous luxuries. $10.00 per class seems exorbitant to many.

If your SE enjoys a comfortable financial situation, your main job may be to convince her to spend money on herself instead of saving every nickle for you and your siblings. Do your best, though, because it's the right thing to do.

How Tai Chi Can Help

Throughout the Far East and many parts of South Asia, the parks and gardens are full of older people performing Tai Chi first thing every morning. For about an hour, people work through dozens of graceful moves that don't look very strenuous. When they finish the entire set of motions, however, they realize that they have had a gentle workout. In particular, Tai Chi improves the posture and sense of balance and provides excellent stretches without taxing the aging body. Because it requires a lengthy sequence of motions,

Tai Chi also encourages use of the short-term memory during class because practitioners need to anticipate the next action in a sequence of 80 or more moves. Tai Chi strengthens the mind-body connection by encouraging participants to think about and get an image of the motions before and during the performance of those motions.

Tai Chi is becoming fairly widespread in the United States, although most participants stay indoors and not many perform the sequence at 6:00 AM. If you can't find a class for your SE, you can certainly buy video tapes to give as gifts. However, you will probably find that you have to do Tai Chi *with* your SE instead of expecting her to do it on her own with just a video tape. Fortunately, Tai Chi can be good for both of you.

You and Tai Chi

You may not want to study Tai Chi yourself until you are in your 70s or 80s, but it wouldn't hurt to watch a tape, observe a class, or participate in a class once or twice so you can discuss what Tai Chi feels like. If you need to perform Tai Chi with your SE, you can certainly practice first. Like anything worthwhile, Tai Chi can take a long time to learn.

A few years ago Jody took a Tai Chi class once a week for two months until a change in her work schedule made it impossible to continue. Just as well. Although enjoying the motions, Jody was too much into competition and perfectionism to get the full benefit of the class, and two months was nowhere near enough time.

The instructor, Karen, 74, tried to convince Jody to relax and just let the motions happen organically, but Jody was determined to do them correctly and better than she had performed them the previous week. She remained stiff, tense, and awkward for the entire two months. She plans to try again when she's older and hopes that she will be better able to relax into the motions and just let them happen. "It's nice to have a challenge waiting for me," she says.

Your Significant Elder and Tai Chi

Your SE might really enjoy Tai Chi. Faye certainly does. For several years, an instructor came to her retirement facility once a week to teach a class. Despite how beneficial Tai Chi is, however, the class never had more than a dozen members among the 170 or so residents.

When the instructor moved out of state, he suggested that Faye take over as the instructor since she knew the sequence of motions extremely well, had a great deal of teaching experience, and could demonstrate the moves quite well. She was happy to keep the class going because she enjoyed it so much. She also knew that the weight-shifting motions strengthened her legs, helped her balance her weight in various positions, and gave her confidence that she could catch herself if she ever felt that she was about to fall down. "No more falls" is her watchword.

Participation in the Tai Chi class dwindled when several students moved away, passed away, or became too ill to participate. No new students could be persuaded to join the class.

She and Rae continue to meet. They faithfully go through two short forms in about 30 minutes. When Rae is ill or out of town, Faye performs Tai Chi by herself. "I wish a few more people would come," she says.

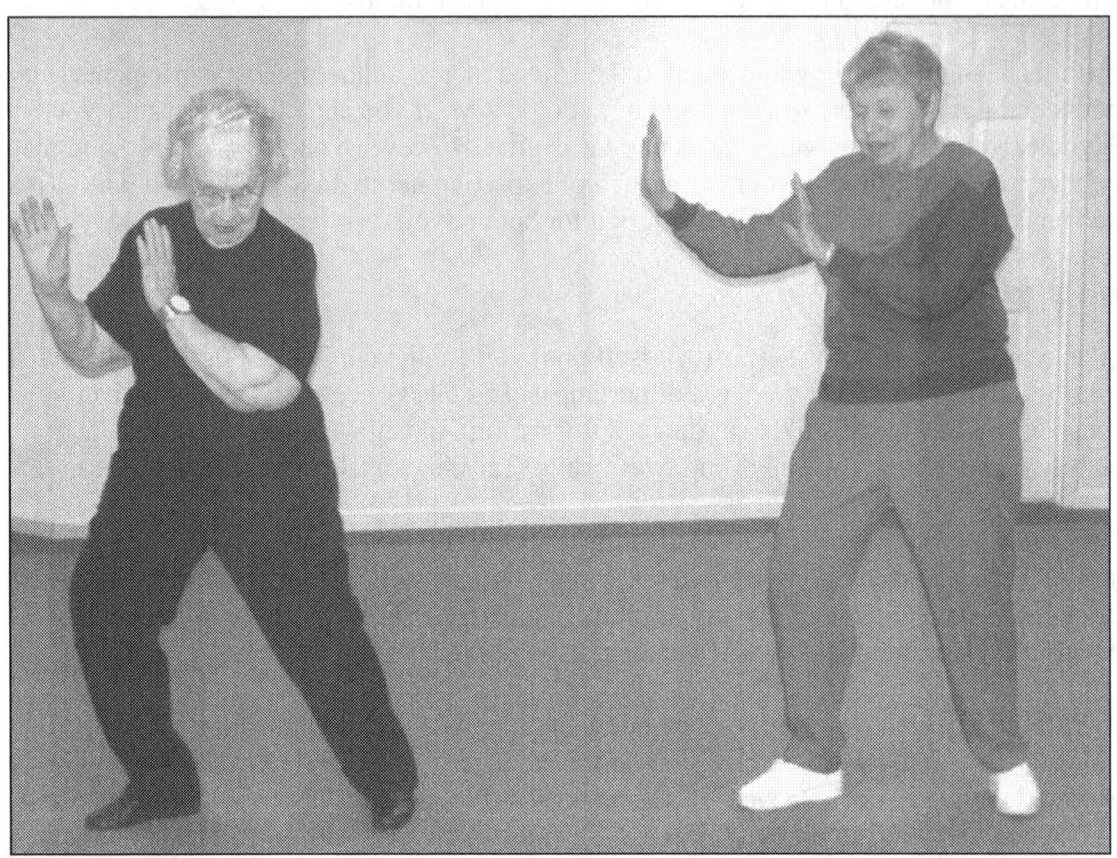

Figure 9-4. Faye and Rae have their weekly Tai Chi class.

How Yoga Can Help

Yoga is already helping your SE if she's doing the warm-up routine recommended in Chapter 3. The Triangle pose and the Sun Salutation at the end of the warm-up are yoga poses that promote presence of mind, a key concept in yoga. It can be quite worthwhile for your SE to learn more about attention, focus, awareness, mindfulness, concentration, alertness, or whatever you want to call it because this mental faculty offers improvements in every aspect of her life, not just in strength training. Yoga certainly paid off for John.

You and Yoga

If you practice yoga, it may be quite easy to encourage your SE to take it up. There are modified classes to accommodate almost any type of physical limitations. If you don't practice yoga, however, you can benefit vicariously from John's experience. Cite his words when you are trying to interest your SE in going beyond the Triangle and Sun Salutation poses.

During his first twenty years of recreational weightlifting, John enjoyed the exercises very much but had little consciousness of his actual performance. As soon as he began his first set, his mind would go on automatic pilot, so to speak, until he woke up an hour later in the shower.

Far from being rare, this experience is quite common among recreational lifters and many other kinds of solo athletes, especially long-distance runners, swimmers, and cyclists. The conscious mind seems to grow bored when a somewhat repetitive physical activity extends beyond 10 or 20 minutes, so it turns off. You have probably experienced this phenomenon yourself during a long drive, while cutting the grass, when rocking the baby, or while filing papers.

About 10 years ago, a big change came into John's life and, later, into his lifting routines. His wife, Bernadette, encouraged him to come to her yoga classes. After he realized that striving and competition were not pertinent to yoga, he began enjoying the stretches, poses, and breathing exercises. The guided relaxations at the end of every session were especially useful because he realized that yoga class was the only time during his busy day that he didn't have to make decisions and deal with stressful situations.

Over several years of practice, John became quite comfortable with the idea of going inside his body to pay attention to each muscle group as it stretched and contracted. He came to understand how the focus on breathing promotes self-awareness and was able to consciously enhance his state of being through yoga. However, his lifting routines remained largely unconscious.

John's "Aha!" moment came when he connected yogic breathing with using the breath as fuel in his lifting. As a lifter, he had always breathed correctly—exhaling on the concentric motion, which does the main work of the lift, and inhaling on the eccentric motion, which returns the weight to its original position after the lift. But he had never carried over this mind-body connection from yoga class to the gym.

Then, suddenly, he found himself paying attention to his breathing during lifting and, thus, remaining conscious and present during the entire session. This change was a revelation, and within just a few weeks lifting became a much different activity for him.

Now, he feels much more rooted in the moment, more graceful, and more in tune with the rhythms of his mind and body. He also gets better results. When he works out alone, the exercises resemble meditations. Further, his strength continues to increase as he improves his personal bests from time to time, even at the age of 54.

Your Significant Elder and Yoga

Since your SE is already performing two yoga poses in the warm-up, you can probably convince her that she can perform other poses. She may even enjoy a yoga class if one is available. In the retirement facility where Ann and Faye live, a yoga teacher who lives there conducts the class when she can. Helen is as lithe and flexible as someone 40 years younger.

Neither Ann nor Faye takes the class, partly because both feel it's beyond their abilities and partly because both are already doing so much. They *are* doing a lot for their health ad strength, and we don't press them. We are grateful they are so strong and healthy.

Maybe your SE will have the time and interest for yoga. If she has difficulty getting down on the floor and, especially, getting up again, look for a class that uses only the standing poses or that permits students to sit in chairs instead of on the floor. Many yoga studios are able to accommodate a wide variety of physical limitations. And most yoga teachers encourage students to do what is right for *their* bodies.

It's perfectly all right if your SE never achieves a full lotus position because there are many other poses that provide gentle stretches, improve the sense of balance, and enhance the connection between the mind and the body. At the very least, she will experience an hour of good deep breathing, which produces beneficial results all by itself.

Conclusions about the Mind-Body Connection

Enhancing the mind-body connection is one of the best not-so-secret reasons to perform physical activities of any kind at any age. People who have done so believe that linking the mind and the body has paid off brilliantly in all aspects of their lives. It leads to strength, health, happiness, integrity, personal power, trustworthiness, and many more benefits.

The reasons why you need to work on strengthening your SE's mind-body connection are many: her strength training will improve, her attitude will become more positive, and her whole life will see improvements.

If you want a short-cut way to improve your SE's quality of life, work on her mind-body connection.

The six methods provided in this chapter range from a passive experience, simply lying on a massage table, to a strenuous activity, yoga, which taxes the strongest of the strong in its most advanced poses. One or more of these methods can provide additional motivation for your SE to continue focusing on her health and strength. To show that a positive attitude is a great thing to develop, consider the story of Marie.

Marie

One of John's clients, whom we will call Marie, 85, is a classic hypochondriac, complete with imaginary illnesses and feelings of depression about them. She knows she's overly anxious about her health and sometimes jokes about it, so she has some lighter moments that alleviate her negative view of the world. She took up strength training only because her doctor insisted that she do so. Marie faithfully showed up for sessions, but she seemed resolute in her worries and negativity, despite all of the positive techniques John tried with her.

A turning point came after she experienced severe fibrillation at dinner with her children one Friday night. Her family called an ambulance, got her to the hospital immediately, and called John to cancel her strength training sessions for the following week. She had a pacemaker put in on Saturday.

On Monday morning, John phoned Marie to express his sympathy and to see how she was doing. He asked her to find out when her doctor would let her resume working out. He was delighted to discover that Marie had already asked this question. She was pleased with herself for taking such a positive step, and so was John.

Originally slated to go home in a week, she beat the schedule and returned home the same Monday John called. One week later, she resumed walking and light stretching. A week after that, she was back to strength training with the approval of her doctor.

Now, her instinct still leans toward the negative, but she has learned to lighten up a bit. The sessions are more fun for both of them and Marie appears to understand that a positive outlook is better for her health than her formerly negative attitude.

A Note to Certified Personal Trainers

You can use the same mind-body techniques that you use with your younger clients, but allow far more time and pay far more attention to your older clients. Remember:

- Be professional when you are with negative clients. Don't try to straighten them out.

- Accept them wherever they are on the emotional landscape. Change will be very gradual.

- Keep yourself positive, no matter how negative an older client may sometimes be.

- Use whatever techniques you are comfortable with in order to improve the mind-body connection in your older clients.

Summary of the Main Points

- Enhancing the mind-body connection is a great motivational tool.

- Try some of the following to keep your SE fit and motivated:

    - Massage

    - Imagery

    - Positive self-talk

    - Water aerobics

    - Tai Chi

    - Yoga

- These and other activities promote a positive attitude, something everyone needs.

What's Next?

In the next chapter, we apply current theories of empowerment and full engagement to improve the lives of older people. We offer several practical recommendations for developing or strengthening the spiritual or purposeful aspects of your Significant Elder's life. These recommendations are not religious, although your SE may incorporate some of them into her religious practices if desired.

Chapter 10. Empowering Your Significant Elder

Using the Energy of Positive Activity-Recovery Habits

"I have no purpose in life. My children grew up, my husband died, and I haven't known what to do with myself ever since. My sons and daughters-in-law are all wonderful, but I know they don't need me any more. I just feel useless."
        Frances, age 84

Important Points for Advocates: This chapter shows you how to improve the quality of life for your Significant Elder *through your own efforts*. A personal trainer can certainly help your SE physically, but you are better able to help him in the emotional, mental, and spiritual or values-based aspects of his life, no matter how far away you live. And you can handle much of it by phone. To be most effective, read the Loehr and Schwartz book, *The Power of Full Engagement*, on which this chapter is based. Then look for even more ways than we have found to help your elder feel truly significant.

Introduction

If your Significant Elder is as strong, happy, alert, and purposeful as he ever was, then you probably have few concerns about him. But most adult children or other caregivers worry about the health and happiness of their aging parents.

It's good news that you can help postpone or prevent most of the physical frailty too often associated with old age. Even better, you can help your SE carry over his increased physical strength into additional aspects of his life. *How*, you ask. Here's how:

You can help to empower your SE not only physically
but also emotionally, mentally, and spiritually.

To guide you in empowering your SE, we build upon Jim Loehr and Tony Schwartz's book, *The Power of Full Engagement: Managing Energy, Not Time, Is the Key to High Performance and Personal Renewal.*[44] Full engagement has applications far beyond the "corporate athlete" paradigm and training program they developed. We apply their progression from the physical, to the emotional, to the mental, and to the spiritual or

---

[44] Free Press: New York, 2003.

purposeful dimension in the lives of older people. As Loehr and Schwartz point out, spiritual energy is greatest in "he who has a why to live." (p. 110) Loehr and Schwartz do not use *spiritual* to mean *religious*, and neither do we, although you may easily bring religion or faith into the picture at any point if your SE would welcome it.

> The key to success in the physical, emotional, mental, and spiritual
> areas is to encourage your SE to develop excellent habits of *activity*,
> defined as expending energy, and *recovery*, defined as regaining energy.

Too often, older people and many younger ones as well, remain unaware of the power derived from planning for cycles of maximum effort and planning for truly restorative rest periods that refresh the body, heart, mind, and spirit.

At first, developing positive activity-recovery habits may feel like a lot of work. Over time, however, these habitual practices can greatly enrich the life of your SE, as well as your own. You are in the unique position of helping your SE to enjoy a higher quality of life than he would without your involvement. Then, when you reach old age yourself, you will be well positioned to apply these positive activity-recovery habits to your own quality of life.

Understanding Loss

To understand your SE's situation, you first need to see just how disenfranchised he may feel. It doesn't matter whether your SE has always been relatively powerless or once had great power at work, in the family, in the community, or in the larger world. He may feel "old," as in Table 10-1.

The young may be or feel...	The old may be or feel...
Able to see and read anything	Unable to read without assistive devices
Able to hear everything	Unable to hear without hearing aids (if at all)
Able to live in their own home and to live wherever they choose	Unable to live independently
Able to drive anywhere	Dependent upon others for transportation
Strong and healthy	Weak, ill, frail, or in pain
Happy and optimistic	Sad, depressed, or pessimistic
Mentally sharp	Unfocused or forgetful
Confident, able to decide for themselves	Fearful or worried, unable to make decisions
Living life to the hilt	Waiting to die
Useful, hopeful, full of potential	Useless, hopeless, empty, used up
Significant, important, valuable	Insignificant, unimportant, without value
"I'm somebody."	"I'm nobody."

Table 10-1. A few contrasts between the young and the old

Note that any one or two of the preceding losses or withdrawals would be enough to enrage or depress almost anyone at any age. Both the meek and the mighty who live into old age can and usually do feel deprived in many ways. Just think of the things that have been taken away from them or that they have had to give up, willingly or not.

Many older people experience more than one major loss. Late in life, such losses and other deprivations are daily reminders of the biggest loss of all, which for many older people is not death itself.

> **The most serious loss for older people may be giving up their sense of potential, their future, their hopes and dreams—in short, a reason to live.**

How can death be any worse than living without strength, optimism, focus, or purpose? For those without a sense of purpose, death may come as a relief.

As one of the people most dedicated to the welfare of your SE, you have a unique opportunity not only to help *him* but also to prepare for the quality of life that *you* will experience in your own future. Learning how to exert control over whatever is controllable can only help you live your life to the fullest as you age. You will find that your SE can learn to regain control over a great deal.

Selma

"If I'd known I was going to live this long, I'd have taken better care of myself," said someone we will call Selma, 84, who feels that she has no purpose in life. She also implies that she might have planned better for the non-physical aspects of her life. A relative newcomer to strength training, she is beginning to see the carry-over effects from the physical to the emotional and seems calmer than she did before she started working out twice a week.

> **Given a choice, most aging people would want to be fully engaged at 88 than half alive at 65. Your job is to give your SE that choice.**

Understanding Full Engagement

Loehr and Schwartz contend that life is a series of sprints, not a marathon. They show that world-class athletes and top corporate executives, in particular, can achieve the highest performance levels by *planning* for cycles of expending and replenishing energy. Loehr and Schwartz use the progressive resistance paradigm of pushing yourself a little farther than you are accustomed to and then recovering. They have developed this pattern for four intertwined and progressive levels:

- Physical.
- Emotional.
- Mental.
- Spiritual.

By engaging in cycles of activity and rest in these same four dimensions, older people can also achieve better performance, that is, a higher quality of life in their last years. Although it's possible to start with the emotional, mental, or spiritual dimension, we center everything in the physical because it can literally provide the engine for the other levels. Also, it may be easier for you and your SE to access the other three levels through the physical.

> When you help to re-empower your Significant Elder,
> he will feel *significant* in every sense of the word.

Using the Physical as the Basis of Empowerment

The main reason to attack physical frailty first is that strength provides the most rapid and straightforward results for your SE. The pathway is very clear and well traveled, and the results will be quite visible to you and your SE.

Within two to four weeks of starting a strength training program, your SE will feel better physically. Within one to three months, he will exhibit improved posture and will be measurably stronger. He will also feel more energetic and will notice that he has more energy.

Within six to 12 months, the training leaves the conscious mind and becomes automatic. Within 12 to 18 months, nearly all newly active elders will have doubled or tripled their muscular strength. At some point during the process, you may notice that your SE seems more mellow than he used to, perhaps even a bit happier.

> Physical strength comes first.

Accessing the Emotional through the Physical

The emotional dimension grows directly from the physical dimension. Working out produces endorphins and increases the heart and respiratory rates. These changes work at the cellular level. Within the first half-hour of a strength training session, even a worried or grumpy SE may perk up and feel a positive mood shift.

In addition to feeling better, he may possibly become more cheerful, in spite of himself. As a result of feeling positive, happy, or lighthearted at least some of the time, especially on workout days, your SE may begin to develop greater degrees of self-awareness and self-confidence as well as a more positive body image.

Approaching the Mental through the Physical

The mental dimension grows out of the physical and emotional dimensions. By getting more blood and oxygen to the brain through exercise, your SE may experience the mental boost of stronger optimism and enhanced focus, which may improve his ability to make decisions and solve problems—to take some of his power back.

Within just a few weeks, you may also notice that your SE has greater powers of concentration because he consciously or unconsciously trains himself to pay close attention during the strength training exercises. If he doesn't notice his greater ability to focus, you can use the improvement to give him some great positive feedback.

Virtually all people who exercise over the long term know that one of the best ways to banish not only malaise but also unfocused thinking is to work out strenuously. The same can hold true for your SE. Feeling stronger physically, being happier emotionally, and becoming sharper mentally will afford him the energy with which to revisit his most deeply held values.

Many of John's clients, for example, regain a purpose in life, even though their newly found intentions might be quite modestly stated: "I just don't want to be a burden to my children, and now that I'm stronger I don't think I will be."

Attaining the Spiritual through the Physical

The spiritual dimension, the "why of life," builds upon the preceding three dimensions. For many older people, it takes a kind of self-confident introspection to bring about a renewed sense of self, a larger awareness of the world, and a powerful realization of that connection between self and world—the expression of your SE's deepest values. He may also be able to examine the meaning of his life and to achieve a deep philosophical acceptance of who he is.

Your SE will be most truly himself when he has physical strength, emotional buoyancy, and clear-headed mental focus. He will then be in a position to share himself, his wisdom, and his highest values. He may also be able to articulate the things that mean the most to him. It's possible that he will seldom or never express these ideas to you, but you will know by his improved physical, emotional, and mental state that he has reached an integrated and enriched enjoyment of life.

Many members of the World War II generation have practiced the "why of life" by using prayer, church work, volunteerism, and similar activities as driving forces in their lives. When or if the body begins to falter, you may be able to help your SE tap into these lifelong altruistic tendencies. Spiritual considerations can motivate him to strengthen his body and can give him additional reasons to treat the body as the temple of the soul.

Starting with the Physical Dimension

Initially, exercise will give your SE the most benefit for the effort expended. It's the most accessible and most direct method of starting an empowerment process based on alternating cycles of challenging and recharging the body. Strength training, in particular, has a built-in cycle of spending and recovering energy—the exercises and the rest intervals. Your SE makes progress in strength training with planned, recurring periods of progressively harder work followed by rest or recovery periods.

> Frailty is frustrating enough all by itself, but it also eats away at emotional resiliency, attenuates mental acuity, and diminishes spiritual vigor.

As Loehr and Schwartz point out, recovery "serves not just health and happiness but also performance" (p. 28). Achieving a good balance between effort and ease is the secret to managing energy. "When we expend energy, we draw down our reservoir. When we recover energy, we fill it back up" (p. 29).

On some level, every human being knows about this cycle of depletion and replenishment, especially with physical activity. People in their twenties may think they can party hearty all night and work hard all day, but eventually even they run out of steam and crash. Many middle-aged people know they should start being more careful, but not as many know how to plan for their hourly, daily, weekly, monthly, and yearly rest cycles.

Full Steam Ahead vs. Dead in the Water

For your SE, especially if he survived the Great Depression and World War II, the concept of actually planning for rest periods may be new. Some older people have only two speeds—full steam ahead or dead in the water, the go-go/no-go syndrome. Recall the story of J. C. on page 93. His desire to work hard without rest periods during a training session is fairly common. So is the result—extreme fatigue.

One of your main tasks may be to convince someone who has such a strong work ethic that recovery is a vital component of managing energy levels. It's much better for him to go a little, rest a little, and go again each day. Periodically, he may need to rest all day once or twice a week. This lesson can be a hard one to learn. It took Jody's mother, Faye, a long time.

Faye

All of her life, Faye got up in the morning, dressed, and went about her business, no matter how bad she might have felt on occasion. "Even if I don't feel good, I can usually work it off," she has always said. She never rested or took it easy until her late 80s. Finally, she realized that "a little nap is a wonderful thing." On major holidays when the whole family gets together for the better part of a day, she wants to participate in family life as much as she can, so she talks with everyone for a while and then retires to a back bedroom to rest. When she feels refreshed, she returns to the assembly and visits some more. She systematically replenishes her energy.

If your SE wants only to sit and rock, however, your main task may be to promote the idea of expending effort. You may have to convince someone like this that it's not good just to sit all day reading, playing cards, or watching TV. Even though people who have worked hard all their lives may want to do absolutely nothing late in life, you must make a strong case for the benefits of strength training and its well-earned rest periods.

Using Routines for Physical Growth and Recovery

To manage the go-go/no-go extremes and every flavor in between, you can help your SE to set up rituals or routines for spending and recovering energy. As Loehr and Schwartz explain, a ritual is a "carefully defined, highly structured behavior" that we do "largely on automatic pilot, without much conscious effort or intention." A positive ritual is "a behavior that becomes automatic over time—fueled by some deeply held value" (p. 14). As an extended example, note this passage from their book:

> The more exacting the challenge, the more rigorous our rituals need to be. The preparation of soldiers for combat is a good example. The rituals of basic training are so exacting—especially in the Marines—that soft, fearful and slovenly teenagers can be transformed into lean, confident, mission-driven soldiers in just eight to twelve weeks. Recruits are compelled to build rituals in every dimension of their lives—how they walk and how they talk; what time they go to bed and wake up; when and what they eat; how they take care of their bodies and how they think and act under pressure. This code of conduct makes it possible for them to do the right thing at the right time even in the face of the most severe of all stresses—the threat of death (p.171).

John's Recovery Rituals

Recovery rituals should be highly individual. "Whatever works" is the mantra. The rituals don't have to be very fancy. They just have to become almost automatic to assist in the job of recovery time after time.

John fell in love with Olympic weightlifting at age 52. In these workouts, he has developed very effective techniques for his recovery periods. At the end of each set, he puts down the weights, picks up his bottle of water, takes a sip, and walks a few steps over to a leg extension machine. As he sits and enjoys the comfort of the padded seat and back rest, he takes another sip of water and waits 30-60 seconds for his heart rate to return to normal.

Mentally, he revisits the feeling of power and satisfaction he enjoyed during the recently completed set. He also anticipates the fun of accomplishing the next set. He visualizes the next repetition using specific imagery. One advantage of a simple but effective routine like John's is that he doesn't have to think or worry or wonder what to do next. The oscillation between exertion and recovery is built into his training sessions. It works—he snatched 154 pounds at age 54. For the snatch, he lifts the loaded barbell explosively from the floor to a balanced overhead position in less than two seconds.

The Physical Mission

Your SE isn't facing the threat of death like soldiers, but he may feel he is facing the imminence of death in the near future. Your mission is to help your SE make the most of his remaining years. Applying the idea of rituals to your SE, you will find that strength training is the perfect vehicle for forming excellent habits of spending and recovering energy.

The exercises are highly structured, require consistent repetition over time, are interspersed with structured rest periods, and become progressively more difficult. A common recovery ritual for many of John's older clients is similar to his own. His mother Ann, for example, takes a sip of water, catches her breath, enjoys a moment of light conversation, waits until her heart rate has dropped from the high point of maximum energy expenditure, and previews the next exercise. John reminds each client to spread the feet, keep the head up, keep the shoulders back, and use the breath as fuel. With long-time clients, he may need to say only, "Universal stance. Resistance breathing," as described on page 69.

From the micro-level of one repetition to the meso- or middle level of one workout to the macro-level of an on-going, long-term strength training program, you can and should encourage structure and consistency. Over time, your SE will feel better physically, and you will be able to move on to building emotional resiliency as well.

Engaging the Emotional Dimension

With a good physical program in place to empower your Significant Elder's body, you can now turn to the task of strengthening his emotional outlook. Deep-seated personality characteristics are hard or impossible to change, and you won't want to try. However, you can encourage every positive experience you observe. You can read back to him the satisfaction that you see when he completes a difficult exercise. Reframe negative talk into positive expression. Keep him smiling and laughing.

> Laughter keeps you feeling alive. Depression can kill.

Always listen for opportunities to congratulate him on difficult exercises, on achieving personal bests, and sometimes just on showing up for a training session when he would prefer to lie on the sofa. Recall the old watchword: Take care of the little things—technique, safety, rest, praise—and the big things—body, heart, mind, soul—will take care of themselves.

Loehr and Schwartz advocate using positive emotions such as "enjoyment, challenge, adventure and opportunity" in order to "transform threat into challenge." They point out that "emotions that arise out of threat or deficit—fear, frustration, anger, sadness—have a decidedly toxic feel to them and are associated with the release of specific stress hormones, most notably cortisol." (p. 72) Stress hormones can contribute to high blood pressure, diabetes, and other medical conditions and metabolic diseases.

Emotional resiliency, on the other hand, is the ability to bounce back from disappointment, loss, pain, fear, worry, and the like. It's the hallmark of emotional strength. Your SE may always have been able to regain his emotional footing after an upset. If not, or if it seems to take him longer now that he is older, you can help him a great deal.

Building Emotional Resiliency

Joy, delight, pleasure, fun, satisfaction—how many times does your SE use these words in a typical conversation with you? How often does he laugh and smile? If seldom or never, then you can and should look for opportunities to encourage positive expressions. Starting with the quantifiable exercises of strength training, you can help him take pride in each victory, no matter how small.

> Each step of physical progress is an opportunity
> to give positive emotional feedback.

Sometimes just showing up for a session is a major accomplishment on days when he doesn't feel as well as usual. When he performs a personal best, help him celebrate with a hug, a congratulatory handshake, a brief shoulder rub, a big smile, or something similar. If you are a long-distance Advocate, use your weekly phone calls to build his reservoir of positive experiences.

In the everyday life of your SE, you can also build his emotional strength by including him in the ups and downs of family life. Many of us with aging parents start sparing them the details of problems with the job, the kids, or the in-laws, partly because we don't want to worry them unnecessarily. However, we need to take a look at the possibility that we are selling them short.

Most Significant Elders don't live to old age by fainting in the face of emotional challenges. As long as they remain interested in the family, which usually lasts until death, it would be wise to continue sharing personal problems with them. Even if Sonny drove drunk and ran over someone, Great-Gramps can probably take the news straight without a lot of spin. He may even be able to offer words of wisdom and comfort, and he deserves the opportunity to contribute to the lives of the people he loves.

Miriam

"I'm a tough old bird," said one tough old bird we will call Miriam. "I shouldn't always be the last to know what's going on in the family. So spill, already."

_____

You may expect older people to drop dead at any moment, but they seldom do. Medical intervention, drug therapies, and the will to live may keep them going far beyond your expectations. For example, when John helped his mother move to Austin three years ago after her heart attacks, neither he nor the rest of the family expected her to survive to 91, let alone become as strong and healthy as she is today. Similarly, when Jody's mother moved to Austin eight years ago, the unspoken assumption in the whole family was that she might have a short stay. She thrived and surprised everyone, including herself.

Tools for Emotional Growth and Recovery

The methods people use to recover from emotional onslaughts are, of course, highly personal. What works for you may not work for your SE. In fact, he may not be consciously aware of doing anything to take care of himself during and after periods of emotional stress. The most he may allow himself is a little extra sleep, a few tears in private, hugs with whatever young children or pets are available, or a few more cookies than usual.

Taking time to soothe their ruffled sensitivities may be even rarer among older people than among the rest of us. People today who are over age 75 were called upon to make so many sacrifices for their country that the experiences made them "tough as hell and twice as ornery," as one octogenarian puts it.

The downside is that some have never learned how to express their tender feelings, even toward themselves. Some can't even acknowledge the presence of those emotions in their lives. Without necessarily participating in those feelings, you can help your SE enormously by encouraging him to acknowledge times of emotional stress and plan for recovery periods.

How does one recover from emotional stress? Vegging in front of the TV comes quickly to mind for many people, old and young alike. According to Loehr and Schwartz, television "is one of the primary means by which most people relax and recover. For the most part, however, watching television is the mental and emotional equivalent of eating junk food. It may provide a temporary form of recovery, but it is rarely nutritious and it is easy to consume too much" (p. 76).

Instead of TV, these tools might work for your SE:

- Keeping a journal or joining a memoir writing class.

- Continuing in some long-term role in the family, such as saying grace at family get-togethers, leading the Seder, taking the Christmas snapshots, hiding the Easter eggs, lighting the Fourth of July sparklers, or carving the Thanksgiving turkey. Any activity will work as long as people count on him to perform the role.

- Talking out his concerns with a sympathetic friend or family member.

- Revisiting a place or an experience that gave him great pleasure earlier in life or that meant something important to him, such as a World War II battlefield.

- Using prayer, meditation, contemplation, or philosophy.

- Laughing a lot, viewing comedies, participating in the laughter of small children, telling or listening to jokes, and the like.

- Going to therapy if a problem becomes acute.

- Considering anti-depressant or anti-anxiety drugs for extreme cases.

Since many older people are inexperienced in showing their emotions, not many would be able to use their feelings as the entry point to improving their quality of life and attaining empowerment. People like this might do better to take up the mental and spiritual dimensions after engaging the physical.

The most reliable way we have found to access empowerment is the physical route. Working out is never the shortest or the least difficult way to get in touch with happiness, but it's probably the most reliable over time.

**Exercise produces endorphins. Endorphins make you feel better.
Feeling better leads to emotional buoyancy.**

Strength training works. You can trust it. You and your SE can learn to trust that each workout will provide benefits on many levels, not just the physical.

To present an extreme case of people completely out of touch with their emotions, let's take a look at an older couple we will call Frank and Barbara.

Frank and Barbara

Frank and Barbara never did anything physical because they didn't think exercise was important. Neither were the emotions, in their view. In fact, they had no vocabulary for discussing their emotions. Like many of their generation, they were taught to grin and bear it.

So they grinned and bore their travails right into multiple major illnesses and surgeries. Their signals to each other that something was emotionally amiss were always expressed as bodily complaints. If Frank said that he had "a little touch of diarrhea," Barbara knew to step lightly around his feelings for a couple of days. If Barbara "felt a little achy" one morning, Frank knew to give her a wide berth. Silence and distance usually got them through their worries, fears, and sorrows.

Expressing the emotions somatically was probably better for their emotional and mental health than ignoring their feelings completely, but one wonders how their lives might have improved if they had known how to communicate more directly and to talk out their problems. A statement like, "I'm upset that you didn't appreciate the nice thing I did for you this morning" never occurred to them. For them, it was forbidden to say, "I'm depressed," "I'm afraid," or "I'm angry."

When their children and grandchildren started using blunt talk to communicate with them, Frank and Barbara ignored the emotional content and reacted with denial: "You can't be afraid. Come on. Let me fix you a sandwich." Neither of them believed in psychology or psychotherapy, but both used food to make themselves and their loved ones feel better.

When major upsets happened, such as the death of a family member, a large financial loss, a new job, or a move to a new city, Frank and Barbara were ill-prepared to handle the stress. They drank too much, ate too much, bickered and sulked, and suffered such illnesses as headaches, sinus infections, backaches, high blood pressure, and cancer.
Frank died before his time, and Barbara sank into unacknowledged depression and anxiety until she started strength training.

After a few years of feeling better physically, she now seems much more content and focused. She's able to participate fully in the ups and downs of family life. Today, she expresses genuine sympathy for family members who have undergone psychotherapy, although she may never seek counseling for herself.

Sharpening the Mental Dimension

As Loehr and Schwartz point out, "nothing so interferes with performance and engagement as the inability to concentrate on the task at hand" (p. 94). They note that lack of mental capacity comes from such attitudes as negative thinking, rigidity, unfocused attention, and shrunken perspectives on the world and one's place in it. Thus, they advocate developing an attitude of "realistic optimism," which is "seeing the world as it is, but always working positively towards a desired outcome" (p. 108).

> Thinking, solving problems, and being creative don't have to slow down just because the body often does.

Your SE might feel he no longer has to use his mind, just as he may feel he no longer has to perform difficult physical tasks. You might feel the same way. You may think, "Why not let him vegetate physically, emotionally, mentally, and spiritually? Why not let him decline into death if that's what he wants to do?" Many older people and their grown children seem to make this decision, if only unconsciously. Maybe you have, too.

If you want to try something different, however, nothing will help focus the mind more than consistent workouts over long periods of time. Not only does working out send more blood and oxygen to the brain, but also concentrating on the next repetition and knowing that he can perform it will, in turn, help your SE form positive mental habits and attitudes in the workout room. This physically grounded optimism can eventually carry over into other aspects of his life on the emotional, mental, and spiritual levels.

For the SE who has always been mentally active, you may be able to help him use this mental determination to access the physical. A small number of older people, usually under 75 years of age, simply decide to start working out because they have heard that it's good for them. Someone like this uses his will power and focus to keep going until, after a few weeks, he begins to feel the positive effects of strenuous workouts. Then, common sense rather than will power will keep him going. So will feeling good.

Tools for Mental Growth and Recovery

People can remain alert, optimistic, creative, and mentally energetic at any age. Further, your SE can derive great satisfaction from planned cycles of mental challenges and recovery periods. You can encourage him to take up or resume some of the following mental exercises:

- Simple things like crossword puzzles, Monopoly, Scrabble, Jumbles, light reading, arithmetic computations in bridge or Pinochle, and the TV show *Jeopardy*. Based on anecdotal evidence, rest periods for these activities are best accomplished with some light physical activity, such as walking outdoors, non-competitive swimming, or dancing.

- Somewhat more complicated pursuits like studying a foreign language, reading a difficult book, taking an academic course in something he has always wanted to learn, and developing a new skill, such as rapid typing, doing his own taxes, or playing a musical instrument. Again based on anecdotal evidence, rest periods for these more demanding mental activities are best accomplished through somewhat more vigorous physical activities, such as gardening or strength training. However, try to keep your SE coming to the gym even if he doesn't exercise his brain a lot.

Encouraging Creativity

If your SE has worked hard all his life and has never had many chances to develop his creativity, you can encourage him to try some of the things mentioned above or any other interests you think he would enjoy. Tell him it's never too late to start something new. Remind him about Grandma Moses, who first started painting folk art in her mid seventies. Did she know she would live to be 101? Even if an activity lasts only a few months, it can increase his pleasure in life.

Creativity looks a little different in each person. Keep the following ideas in mind when you encourage your SE to take up something new or to resume something he used to enjoy:

- Always assume that he *can* do imaginative, intellectual, inventive work. Never assume he can't.

- Encourage his efforts. Never scoff, criticize, judge, or condescend. If you don't feel comfortable praising his accomplishment, at least praise its completion or the work it took. If you have children or have worked with children, you know how to do this in a supportive way.

- Do as much as you can to smooth the path to his creativity. Never stand in the way of his desire to engage in the activities that interest him.

- Seek out and inform your SE about lifetime learning classes, peer groups, and other activities that may be available in your community.

What does creativity look like in older people? It can be as simple as Dad coming up with a new recipe or Mom learning to program the VCR. At the high end, it can be as complex as being a member of the Retired and Senior Volunteer Program and rescuing a small business from failure. Maybe your SE is the next Grandma Moses.

Chances are, your SE's creative efforts will look quite different from your own, and that's all to the good. Just as you did during your childhood, you may learn something from your Significant Elder if you will just give him a chance. Doing this will go a long way toward improving your relationship with him.

Encouraging Problem-Solving

How old were you when you stopped listening to your parents' advice? Somewhere in your teens? That's typical. In adulthood, you may be able to stimulate your SE's problem-solving ability by asking for his help on some difficulty of your own. It doesn't have to be a huge problem, and you don't have to take his advice, but the simple act of asking for his opinion can give him a mental boost. It can also make him feel needed and useful.

> Asking your SE for advice can strengthen him mentally and emotionally.

If your SE seems unable to resolve one of his own difficult decisions, such as whether to move into a retirement facility, try to refrain from jumping in with what you think is the right answer. Big decisions will probably be more satisfactory if made by the people most affected by them. Encourage your SE to recall some hard choices he made in the past. For example, Joanne recalls a conversation with her father, Basil.

Joanne and Basil

"I know it's hard to decide whether to sell the boat," said Joanne. "But you've made tough calls before. Remember when you got that job offer in Tulsa back in 1962 and didn't know whether to take it or not? You penciled out the financial stuff, and then you asked all of us how we'd feel about the move. Some of us didn't care one way or the other, but you really listened to the ones who didn't want to go and figured that their wishes took priority, so we didn't move. That was a tough decision, but it turned out to be the right one, didn't it?"

Share with your SE the problem-solving skills you rely on for your own major decisions. If he seems reluctant to solve his own problems, express confidence in his ability to do so. Assure him that most decisions can be changed if need be and that you will support whatever decision he makes. Emphasize that he has done well to get this far in life.

Finally, encourage your SE to do something physically challenging and then sleep on it before he tries to solve thorny problems or make big decisions. A physical challenge and a good night's sleep are among the best preparations to make before taking on major difficulties. Exercise and sleep also provide a positive foundation for developing the spiritual or purposeful dimension.

Reaching for the Spiritual Dimension

According to Loehr and Schwartz, the main thing that "fuels spiritual energy is character—the courage and conviction to live life by our values, even when doing so requires personal sacrifice and hardship." Related ideas include "passion, commitment, integrity, and honesty. Spiritual energy is sustained by balancing a commitment to others with adequate self-care." (p. 110)

Our oldest family members are quite familiar with denying themselves for the sake of others, but they may not know how to deny others for their own sakes. Consider the story of a mother and daughter we will call Elizabeth and Betty Ann.

Elizabeth and Betty Ann

Elizabeth, 90-something, loves it when her daughter, Betty Ann, 50-something, comes to town for a visit. The two of them have similar interests and really enjoy each other's company. They like nothing better than spending five or six hours shopping for family members and finding perfect gifts for everyone.

However, as Elizabeth ages, she's becoming more and more aware of how hard these shopping marathons are on her strength and health. When Betty Ann leaves, Elizabeth has to rest for several days before she recovers.

When John realized Elizabeth's pattern of visiting to exhaustion and recovering for several days afterward, he began to customize her workouts to accommodate Betty Ann's visits. When Elizabeth tells him her daughter is coming to town, John begins tapering off their workouts about a week or 10 days in advance—lighter weights, fewer reps, longer walks, but shorter rests between sets. He advises her to sleep a lot and eat nutritiously. The day before Betty Ann arrives, Elizabeth does as little as possible, storing as much of her vitality as she can to achieve her goal—spending quality time with her daughter.

On their lengthy sight-seeing and shopping expeditions, Elizabeth claims to ask Betty Ann to slow down from time to time, but it's doubtful that she puts any force behind these requests. It's likely that she speaks jokingly, which makes it easy for Betty Ann to keep pushing. One of Elizabeth's most deeply held values is to enjoy her daughter and the limited time they can spend together. She feels that wearing herself out is better than missing something by taking a breather.

Tools for Spiritual Growth and Replenishment

As Loehr and Schwartz point out, some pursuits promote "spiritual renewal without demanding significant energy expenditure. These include walking in nature, reading an inspirational book, listening to music, or hearing a great speaker." (p. 113)

Your SE may regularly practice these or other activities with varying degrees of uplifting results. If not, you can certainly encourage him to do so for the express purpose of getting better in touch with his values or philosophy of life. If you initiate a thoughtful conversation, you might be surprised at the insights your SE can offer.

Some spiritual practices, note Loehr and Schwartz, "can be renewing and demanding at the same time. Meditation, for example, requires mobilizing highly focused attention to quiet the mind, but may also prompt a rejuvenating experience of expansive openness, connectedness and even joy." (p. 113)

Although your SE might not be interested in formal training in meditation, you can give him opportunities to experience meditative moments when you make it easy for him to hear children laughing, watch a fountain spray water, view a rainbow, enjoy the sensation of sitting outside on a sunny winter day, or smell fresh bread baking.

If your SE is comfortable with prayer, yoga, Tai Chi, or similar practices, he may already have plenty of spiritual growth and recovery in his life. If not, perhaps you can encourage one or more of these activities as the previous chapter suggests.

A Note on Your Significant Elder's Purpose in Life

Without a career, young children, a home, or a similar interest to give meaning to his life, your SE must either find something else to live for or twiddle his thumbs and wait to die. You may feel that there is little you can do to give your SE a purpose in life, and you would be right.

You can't *give* someone a reason to live. However, you can listen appreciatively when your SE mentions something that provides him satisfaction. Support and encourage whatever it is.

The most important and universal purpose in the lives of the older people who have shared their stories with us is *the connection with family members*. As the caregiver for your SE, you are to be congratulated for providing much of this connection. You can also encourage other family members to phone, write, send pictures, and visit as often as they can. More than one octogenarian has kept going in anticipation of a grandchild's wedding or the birth of a great-grandchild. No one can prove that they postponed death for such a significant event, but many seem to do just that.

In addition to family, your SE may consider almost anything as reason enough to live —adding to a doll collection, taking care of a dog or a house plant, praying for world peace, watching his alma mater's football games, setting an example for others to follow, making jokes, helping a friend, and many, many more.

It really shouldn't matter to you what gives meaning to your SE's life. The point is for him to have some reason to get out of bed in the morning. And the point for you is to *listen* as he shares these things with you even if you don't consider the activities important. They are significant to your Significant Elder, and that's what matters.

Conclusions

People in their 70s, 80s, and 90s are, first of all, people. They are a lot like you, only older and probably less strong and healthy than you are—unless you are a devoted couch potato. All of them have suffered major losses, and many feel they lack power or even relevance in the world.

However, you now have a starter kit of tools to use in re-empowering your SE on the physical, emotional, mental, and spiritual levels. It's a big job, admittedly, but you may not have to do it alone. You will probably need to get things started by accepting responsibility for your SE and nudging him into strength training, but then you can call on the entire community. The more friends and family members you can ask for assistance, the better. Encourage everyone surrounding your SE to give him the time, love, respect, and attention that he needs and deserves.

> Empowering your Significant Elder is the right thing to do.

A Note to Certified Personal Trainers

This chapter goes far beyond the normal boundaries of personal training, but it's for a good reason. Take comfort in knowing that when you conduct strength training sessions for your older clients, you improve not only the physical but also the emotional, mental, and spiritual aspects of their lives in an even more radical way than you do with younger clients.

Your older clients may need you a great deal more than your younger ones do. This certainly makes your job challenging but also potentially more gratifying. Remember:

- Progress is made by encouraging your clients to push just a little beyond their current level of performance and then allowing them adequate recovery time to renew their energy resources.

- Rest and recovery are even more important for your older clients than for your younger ones. Planned-for recovery cycles are as important as the exercises themselves.

- Energy can be increased at the physical, emotional, mental, and spiritual levels.

- Watch for ways to encourage growth in all four areas of your older clients' lives.

Summary of the Main Points

Take these points to heart:

- Your SE has borne a great many losses during his life.

- He may feel powerless, useless, and irrelevant in addition to weak, frail, and ill.

- You can empower him physically with strength training.

- Greater physical energy can lead to greater emotional, mental, and spiritual energy.

- It's possible to start with any of the levels, but physical energy provides the engine for growth in the emotional, mental, and spiritual dimensions.

- Always stress the importance of the recovery cycle after any kind of exertion.

- No matter what it is that keeps your SE going, it's important to encourage and celebrate it with him.

- Your SE deserves the best that you and his support group can provide.

- Helping him is the right thing to do.

What's Next for You and Your Significant Elder?

Becoming the parent to your parent can be the start of a great and positive adventure for both parties. This book provides only the beginning of the enhancements that can occur in their lives and yours. The authors are committed to the adventure and will continue the story by periodically updating our website, www.significantelder.com.

Jayne

When you take care of your SE, you may come to feel as Jayne, 34, did. She spent the better part of a month caring for her gravely ill father, Joel, 72, who lives 2,000 miles away from her home. Fortunately, he recovered and is doing well. Later, Jayne reflected on her experience:

"When I was a kid, I used to wonder how you could tell if you're an adult—I decided it's when your parents don't need to take care of you. Now, I realize it's when they need you to help care for them."

We add one more thought—becoming an adult happens when you are excited to help your SE take back his power and grow stronger, healthier, and happier.

> Best wishes and more power to you and your Significant Elder.

Appendix

The following forms are provided as models for developing your own forms or for comparing with those that your Significant Elder's certified personal trainer uses:

- Physician's referral. Ask your SE's doctor to fill out and sign this form. Then give it to the personal trainer or keep it in your files if you are the Strength Coach.

- Client's medical history. Ask your SE to fill out this form. Then give it to the personal trainer or keep it in your files if you are the Strength Coach.

- Client's informed consent. Compare this form with the one that the certified personal trainer uses. If you are the Strength Coach and want to use this form, ask your SE to sign it and keep it in your files.

- Chart to use in keeping records of your SE's workouts. Modify it if desired.

- Tests to check the flexibility and range of motion for the shoulders.

Physician's Referral

Dear Doctor _____ :

Your patient, _____ , has
contacted me, _____ ,
regarding a program of personal training for strength, cardiovascular endurance, and flexibility with
the participant. It is important to understand that this program is preventive and is not intended to
be rehabilitative in nature. In the interest of your patient, and for our information, please complete
the following:

A. Has this patient has undergone a physical examination within the last year to assess functional
capacity to perform exercise?   Yes_____   No_____

B. I consider this patient (please circle one):

    Class I: Presumably healthy without apparent heart disease.

    Class II: Presumably healthy with one or more risk factors for heart disease.

    Class III: Patient is not eligible for this program.

C. Does this patient have any pre-existing medical or orthopedic conditions requiring continued or
long-term medical treatment or follow-up? Yes_____ No_____
Please explain: _____
_____

D. Are you aware of any medical conditions that this patient may have had that could be worsened
by exercise? YES_____ NO _____

E. Please list any currently prescribed medications: _____
_____
_____

Comments:_____

Client's name:_____Phone:_____

Address: _____
_____

Referring physician's signature: _____Date: _____

Client's name:_____Phone:_____

Address: _____

Referring physician's signature: _____Date:_____

Client's Medical History

Name: _____ Date:_____

Address: _____

_____

Birth date and age:_____ Physician:_____

Home phone:_____ Other phone: _____

Circle Yes or No. Use the space below for additional comments.

1. Yes No   Are you taking prescription medications now?
2. Yes No   Do you have a history of heart trouble? Specify _____
3. Yes No   Do you have a history of high blood pressure?
4. Yes No   Has anyone in your family under age 50 died of heart problems?
5. Yes No   Do you have chest pains?
6. Yes No   Do you frequently feel faint or dizzy?
7. Yes No   Do you have to stop when exercising because of shortness of breath?
8. Yes No   Do you smoke? If so, how many packs per day? _____
9. Yes No   Do you have asthma?
10. Yes No   Have you ever had a concussion?
11. Yes No   Have you ever had any trouble with your kidneys?
12. Yes No   Have you ever had any trouble with hernias?
13. Yes No   Have you ever had seizures (epileptic or other)?
14. Yes No   Have you ever had any trouble with your back?
15. Yes No   Do you have anemia?
16. Yes No   Do you have diabetes?
17. Yes No   Have you ever had any fractures or broken bones?
18. Yes No   Do you have any physical condition that exercise makes worse?
19. Yes No   Is there any reason why you could not exercise if you wanted to?
20. Yes No   Have you had a physical from your doctor in the past year?
21. Yes No   Is there any other significant medical information not mentioned above?

_____

_____

_____

Signed:_____Date:_____

Client's Informed Consent

Your fitness evaluation will include tests in the following areas of physical fitness:

- Cardio-respiratory endurance.

- Muscular strength.

- Flexibility.

The most physically demanding tests are the cardio-respiratory and muscular strength tests. The cardio-respiratory test consists of riding a stationary bicycle or walking on a treadmill. The purpose of this test is to examine your heart rate response to sub-maximal exercise and recovery periods.

The muscular strength test consists of one to five repetitions for the muscle groups of the chest, upper back, and legs.

You may experience muscular fatigue during or after one or both of these tests, especially those of sub-maximal nature. If you do not tolerate the exercise well, we will stop right away.

Complications reported in 1 of 10,000 tests include faintness and irregularities in heart function.

Risk of injury in handling the weights is possible but rare.

The flexibility test consists of various stretching and reaching exercises. It is important that you inform the tester if you start to experience any pain at all with these flexibility tests.
In signing this consent form, you acknowledge that you have read and understood the descriptions of these tests and their possible complications. In addition, you affirm that any questions you have asked about the fitness evaluation have been answered to your satisfaction. The tester will make every effort to ensure your health and safety. You enter into the tests willingly and may withdraw at any time.

Note that a physician's examination is recommended for all participants with any exercise restrictions and for those persons over forty (40) years of age. Fitness evaluation participants in these categories who have not had a physical in the past year hereby acknowledge that they have been informed of its importance and, therefore, accept full responsibility for their health and well-being. Participants understand that no responsibility is assumed by the personal trainer,

_____.

_____   Date: _____
Participant's name (Please print)

_____   _____
Participant's signature   Trainer's signature

Sample Workout Chart to Use in Keeping Good Records

Date								
Exercise	Wt	Reps	Wt	Reps	Wt	Reps	Wt	Reps
Chest								
Wall Press								
Bench Press								
Upper Back								
Seated Band Pull								
Standing Band Pull								
Legs								
Chair Squat								
Heel Raise								
Abductor/Adductor								
Leg Curl/Extension								
Shoulders								
Lat Raise								
Dumbbell Press								
Biceps								
Dumbbell Curl								
Triceps								
Armchair Dip								
Lower Back								
Dead Lift								
Good Morning								
Abs								
Chair Crunch								

Shoulder Tests

Widely disseminated in the strength training community in Austin, Texas, is a set of 18 shoulder rehabilitation exercises that Marc Frazier shares with his clients and fellow personal trainers at Hyde Park Gym. Thank you, Marc.

Although the exercises were designed for rehabilitation after a shoulder injury, specifically a rotator cuff injury, John finds them valuable as a diagnostic tool when he first begins working with a new client. He notes which motions are difficult or painful and determines which exercises to avoid or to use with extra caution. He may also incorporate gentle versions of the difficult motions into his clients' regular workouts until they have sufficiently strengthened and rehabilitated the weak areas. When using these motions, John has the client begin with body weight only. He adds 1- or 2-pound dumbbells only when the client can do the motion 10 times with no discomfort.

Faye is the model for the tests because she is one of the few older clients with enough shoulder strength and flexibility to do all of the motions without pain or stiffness.

Performing the Tests

Before starting the 18 tests, ask your Significant Elder to stand in the universal athletic stance. Then ask her to draw the shoulder blades together and down and keep them in this position throughout the tests.

Make sure she performs each test slowly and as smoothly as possible. Caution her against jerking her arms into position because a sudden sharp motion can cause injury.

If your SE tires easily, give her a couple of breaks during the test. Ask her to sit down and take a sip of water before going on with the remainder of the motions. Demonstrate each motion before asking her to perform it. Using only body weight, ask your SE to perform each of the 18 motions one time.

Using the Results

Write down whether your SE could complete all, most, or some of the motions in each test. Also record whether she winced or reported experiencing any pain. If she had difficulty, then see the notes on exercises to avoid or to use with caution. Repeat the tests every few months to check for progress. Recognize that your SE may or may not recover the full range of motion in her shoulders.

1. **The shrug**. With the arms at the sides, raise the shoulders up toward the ears.

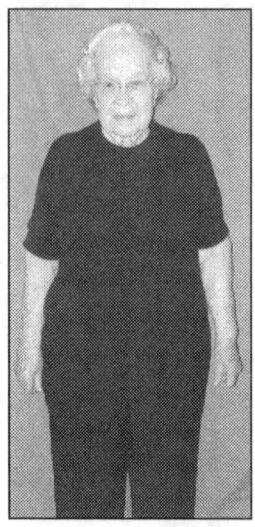

Figure A-1. The ready position

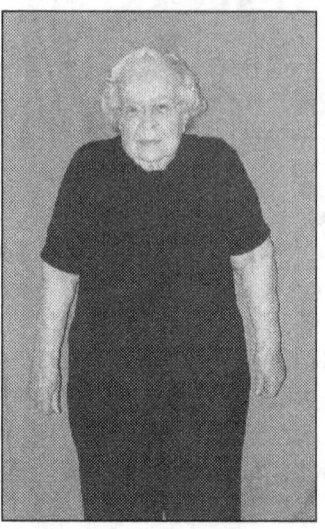

Figure A-2. The shoulder shrug

Virtually everyone can shrug the shoulders. If there is any pain or tightness, ask your SE to perform several low shrugs that don't reach for the ears.

2. **The lateral raise**. Raise the arms out to the sides. Lift the arms as high as possible but no higher than shoulder level.

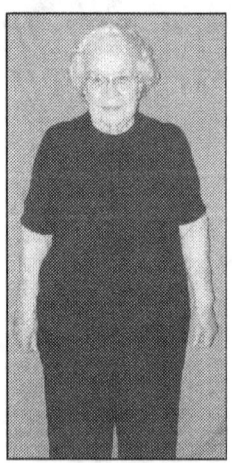

Figure A-3. The ready position

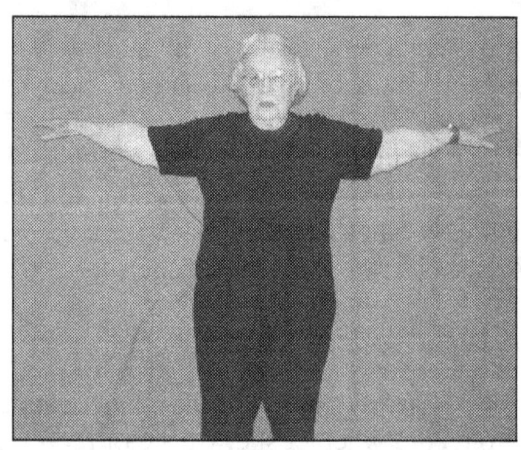

Figure A-4. The lateral raise

If your SE has trouble, avoid the lateral raise exercise or use it with caution. You can substitute the diagonal raise as demonstrated in Figure A-11.

3. **The front raise**. Raise the arms in front of the body as high as possible but no higher than shoulder level.

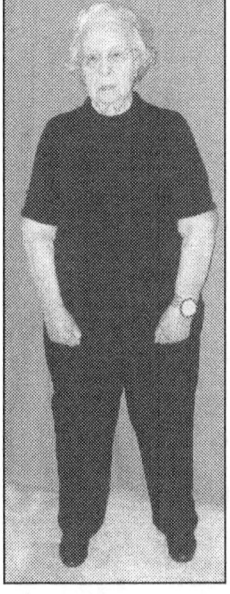

Figure A-5. The ready position

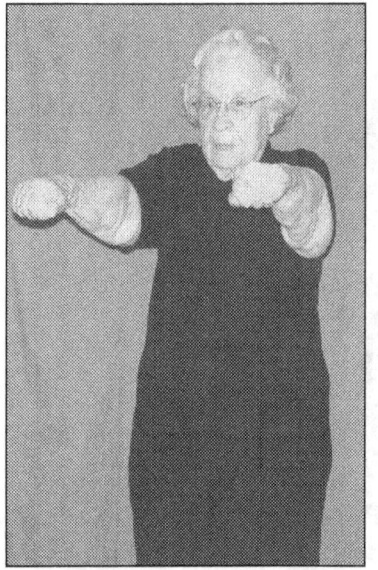

Figure A-6. The front raise

If your SE has trouble, ask her to raise her arms only part of the way. Make sure she pulls her shoulder blades down and together.

4. **The forward shrug roll**. Raise the shoulders up and back. Then roll the shoulders forward and down.

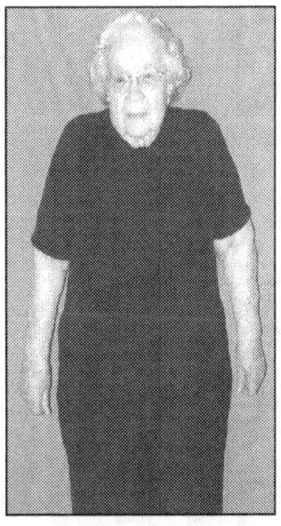

Figure A-7. Shrug Up

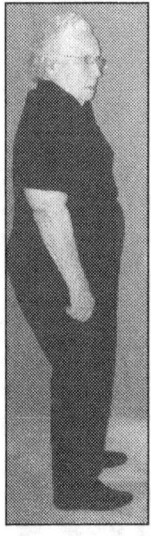

Figure A-8. Back

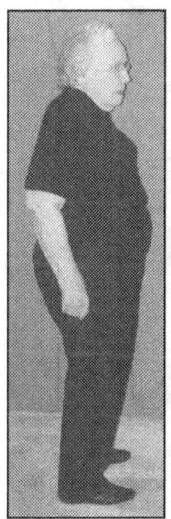

Figure A-9. Forward

Most people can make this motion. If there is any pain or tightness, ask your SE to perform several low shrugs that roll only part of the way to the front and the back.

5. **The diagonal raise**. With the thumbs pointing down, raise the arms to shoulder level at a 45-degree angle—half way between the lateral raise and the front raise.

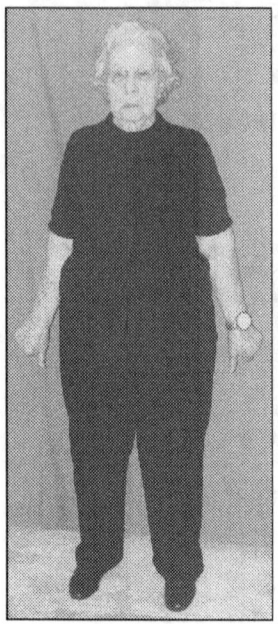

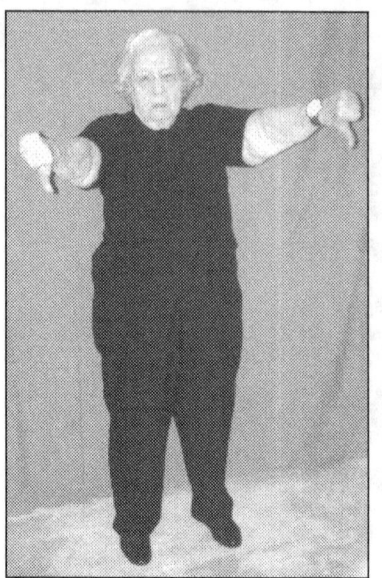

Figure A-11. The diagonal raise

Figure A-10. The ready position

If your SE has pain, avoid the lateral raise, the wall press, and the armchair dip or use them with caution.

6. **The backward shrug roll**. Raise the shoulders up and forward. Then roll the shoulders back and down.

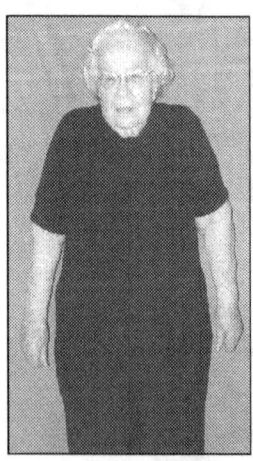

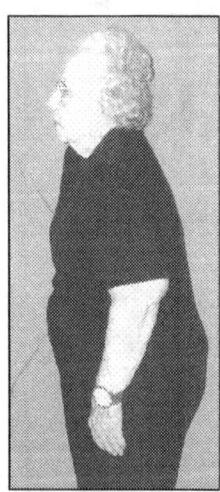

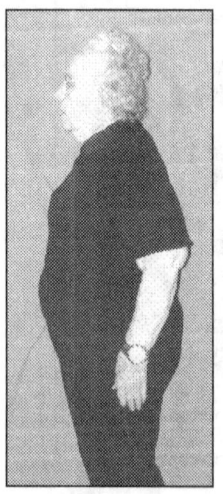

Figure A-12. Shrug Up

Figure A-13. Forward

Figure A-14. Back

Most people can make this motion. If there is any pain or tightness, ask your SE to perform several low shrugs that roll only part of the way to the back.

7. **The lateral rotation raise**. While raising the arms laterally to shoulder level, rotate the palms up.

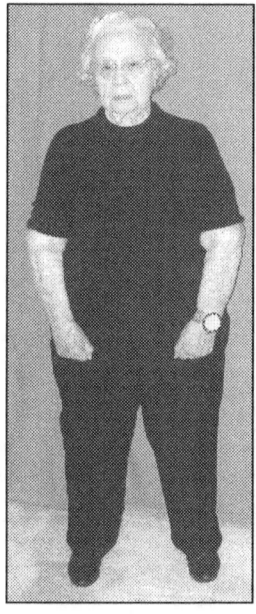

Figure A-15. The ready position

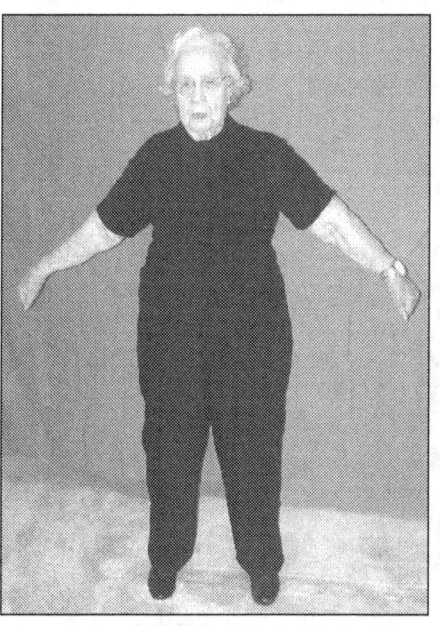

Figure A-16. Part way up

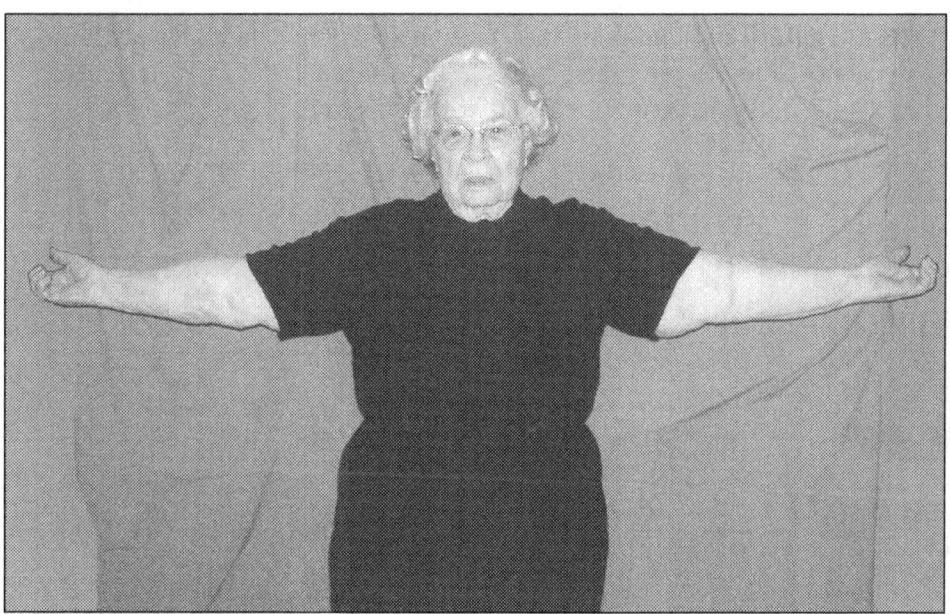

Figure A-17. The lateral rotation raise

If your SE has pain, avoid the lateral raise exercise or use it with caution. You can substitute the diagonal raise in Figure A-11.

8. **The cross-chest raise**. Touch the left shoulder with the right hand, keeping the elbow raised and forward. Extend the right arm in front of the body in a straight line (not shown). Repeat for the left hand.

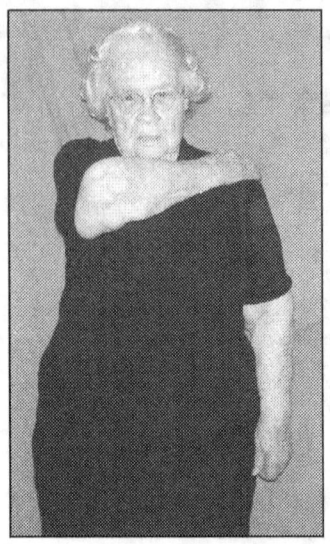

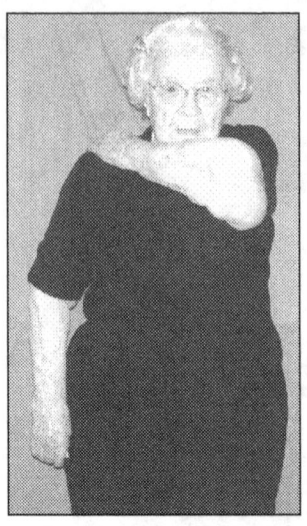

Figure A-18. The right cross chest raise

Figure A-19. The left cross chest raise

If your SE has pain, avoid the dumbbell press and the wall press or use them with caution.

9. **The internal-external rotation**. Bend both arms up in a 45-degree angle. Rotate both arms to the left as far as possible, keeping the elbows at the sides and the forearms parallel to the floor. Do not turn the body. Repeat by rotating both arms to the right.

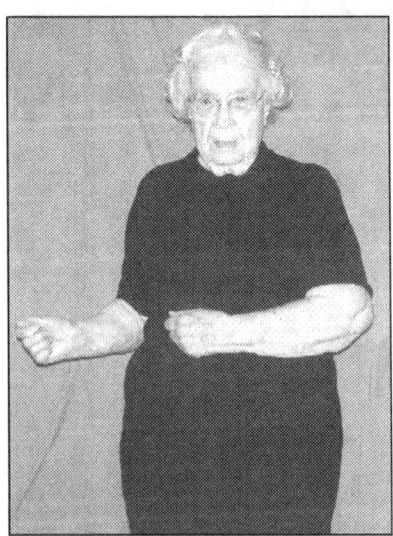

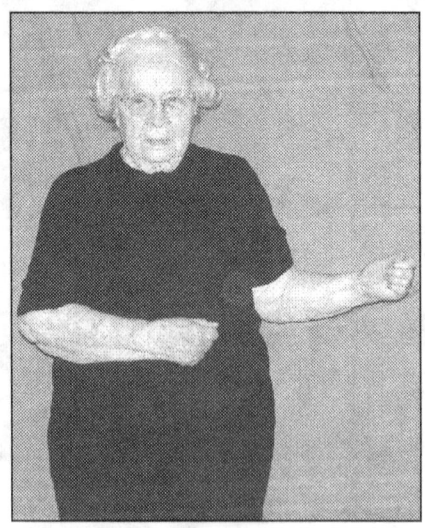

Figure A-20. Rotation to the right

Figure A-21. Rotation to the left

If your SE has pain, use caution with the rotational band pull on page 142.

10. **The horizontal standing flye**. Keeping the arms straight, raise the arms in front of the body to shoulder level. Then move the arms horizontally out to the sides, keeping the palms facing down. Return to the ready position.

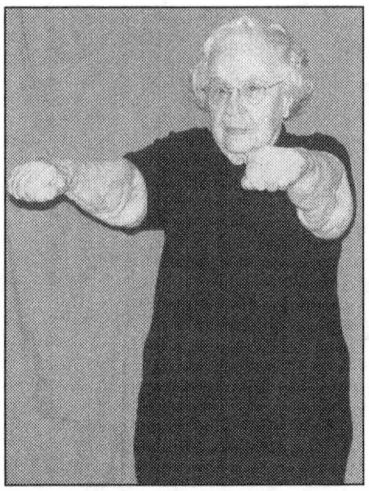

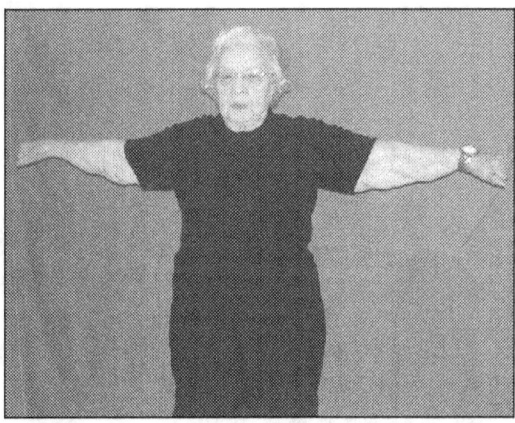

Figure A-23. The horizontal flye

Figure A-22. The ready position

If your SE has pain, avoid the lateral raise or use it with caution.

11. **The horizontal flye with palms rotating from down to up**. While moving the arms up and out to the sides, rotate the palms from facing down to facing up. Return to the ready position.

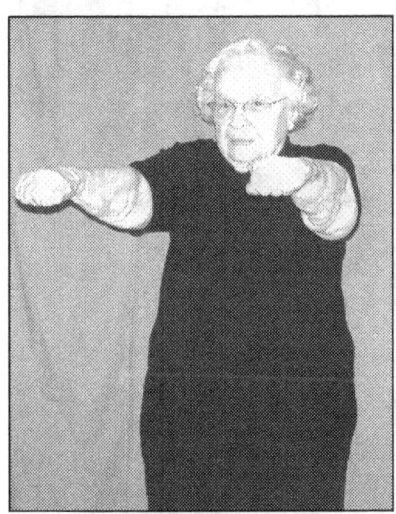

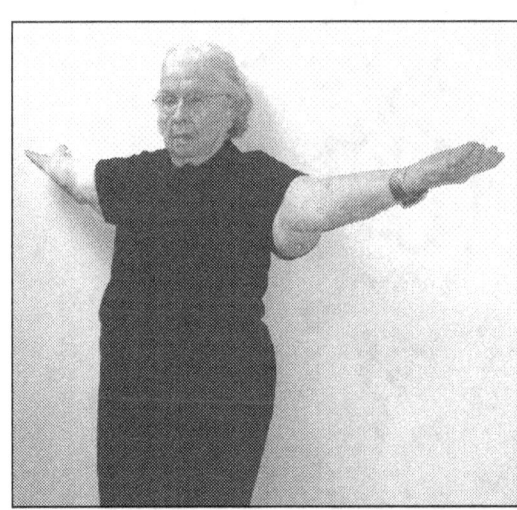

Figure A-24. The ready position

Figure A-25. The flye with palms up

If your SE has pain, avoid the lateral raise or use it with caution.

12. **The horizontal flye with palms rotating from up to down**. Start with the arms in front of the body as in the previous flye but with palms up. Move the arms out to the sides and rotate the palms from facing down to facing up. Return to the ready position.

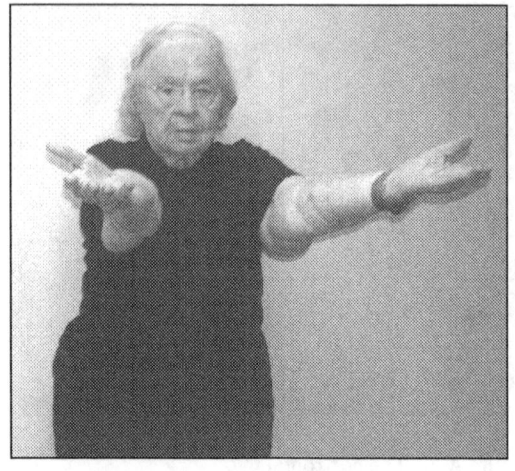

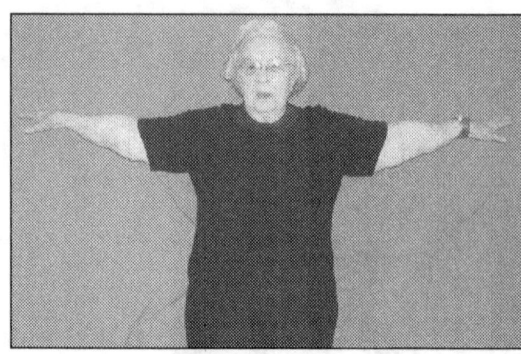

Figure A-27. The flye with palms down

Figure A-26. The ready position

If your SE has pain, avoid the lateral raise or use it with caution.

13. **The side pull-up**. Raise the elbows up laterally to shoulder level.

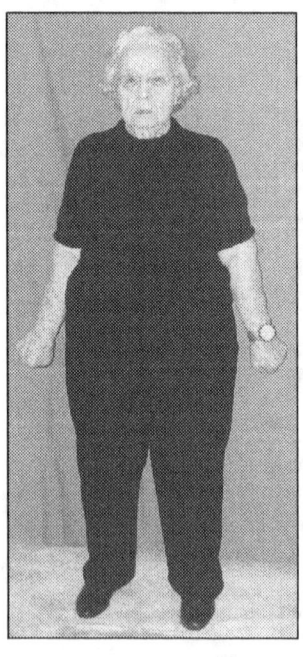

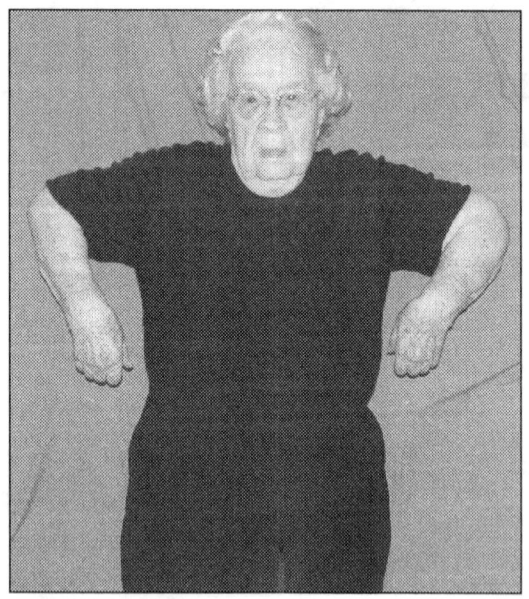

Figure A-29. The side pull-up

Figure A-28. The ready position

If your SE has pain, avoid the wall press and the bench press or use them with caution.

14. **The bent-over row**. Bend the knees, extend the hips back, and bend forward until the back is 30 degrees or less from vertical. It is important not to round the back but to keep it flat. Keep the head up. Then bend the elbows, keeping them close to the sides, and raise the elbows up as high as possible.

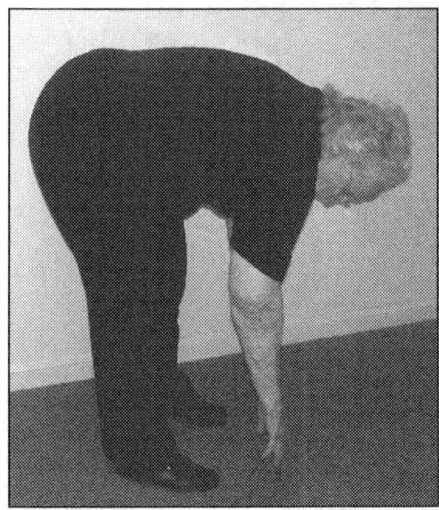

Figure A-30. Ready for the bent row

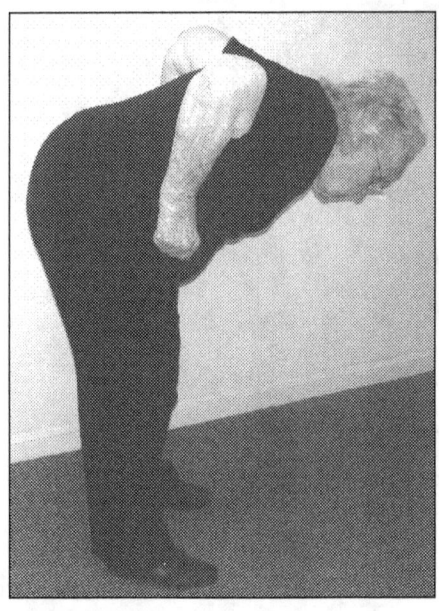

Figure A-31. The bent row

If your SE gets dizzy easily, ask her to pull one arm at the time. Place the other hand on a chair for support.

15. **The side pull-up and press**. Raise the elbows laterally and rotate the hands forward and up. Extend the arms straight overhead or as far up as possible. In reverse order, return to the ready position. Four photographs demonstrate this exercise.

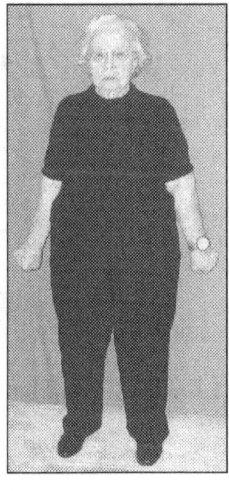

Figure A-32. Ready

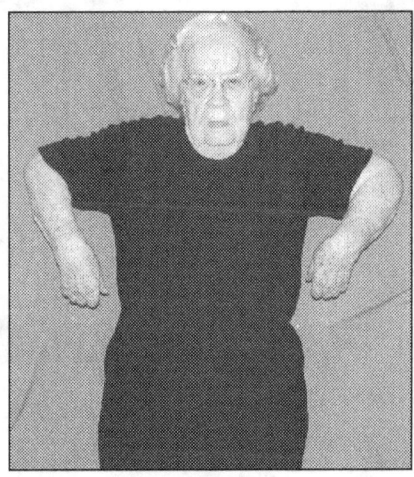

Figure A-33. Elbows up

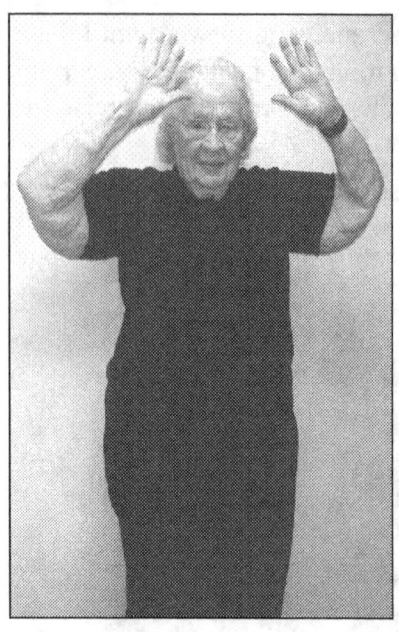

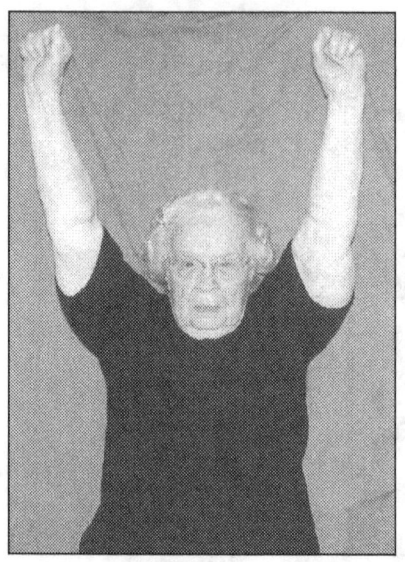

Figure A-35. Overhead press

Figure A-34. Hands up, Mama!

If your SE has pain, avoid the dumbbell press or use it with caution.

16. **The standing overhead lateral press**. Raise the arms. Bring the arms up on the diagonal and move them to the front as high as is comfortable. Keep the elbows close to the ears as in Figure A-38.

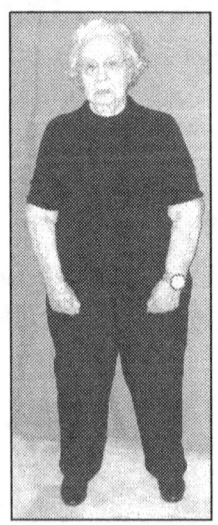

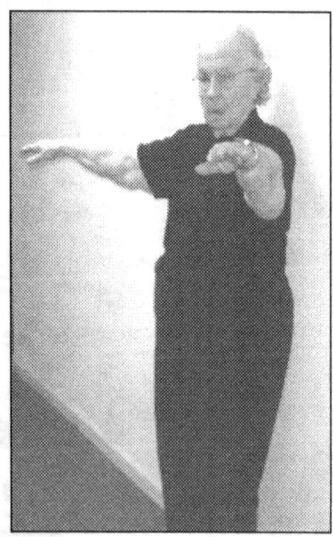

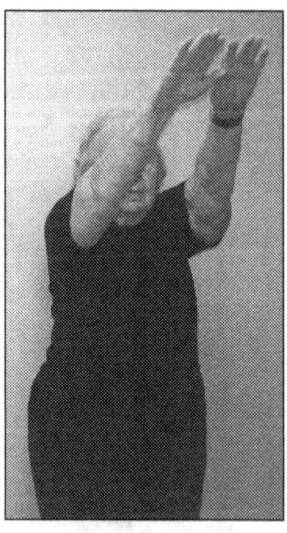

Figure A-36. Ready

Figure A-37. Diagonal

Figure A-38. Overhead

If your SE has pain, avoid the lateral raise and the dumbbell press or use them with caution.

17. **The triceps press**. Bend the elbows, raise them overhead, and let the hands touch the back of the shoulders. Keeping the arms near the head, extend the elbows straight up overhead. Return to the ready position.

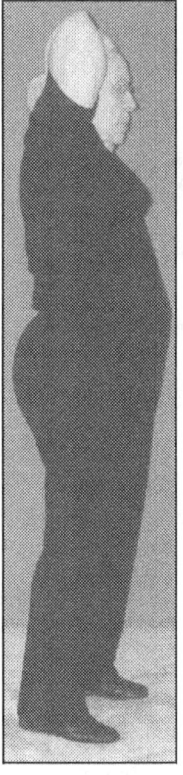

Figure A-39. Ready

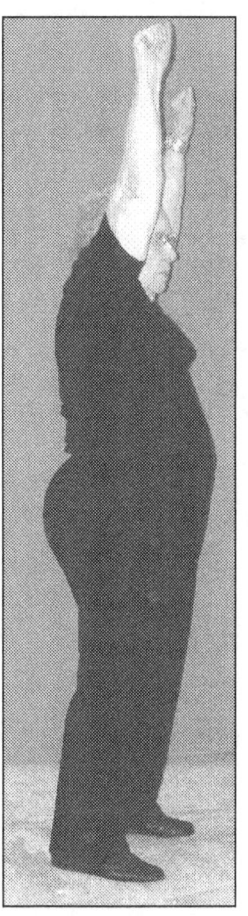

Figure A-40. The triceps press

If your SE has pain, avoid the armchair dip and the dumbbell press or use them with caution.

18. **The biceps curl**. Keeping the elbows close to the waist, bring the hands up to the shoulders.

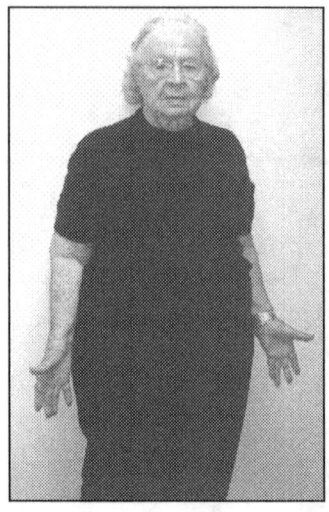

Figure A-41. Ready

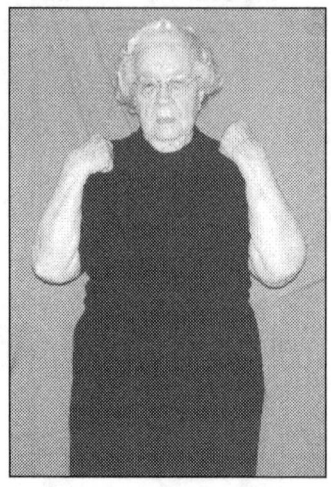

Figure A-42. The biceps curl

If your SE has pain, avoid the biceps curl or use it with caution.

Bibliography

Armstrong, Lance, with Sally Jenkins. *Every Second Counts*. New York: Broadway Books, 2003.

Baum, Ken and Richard Trubo. *The Mental Edge: Maximize Your Sports Potential with the Mind/Body Connection*. New York: Perigee, 1999.

Best-Martini, Elizabeth and Kim A. Botenhagen-DiGenova. *Exercise for Frail Elders*. Chicago: Human Kinetics, 2003.

Biel, Andrew. *Trail Guide to the Body: How to Locate Muscles, Bones, and More*. Boulder, CO: Books of Discovery, 2001.

Bloch, Douglas. *Positive Self-Talk for Children: Teaching Self-Esteem through Affirmations: A Guide for Parents, Teachers, and Counselors*. New York: Bantam, 1993.

Center for Science in the Public Interest. "See More, Eat More." *Nutrition Action Newsletter*. 30 (2003) 8.

Centers for Disease Control and Prevention. "Rate of Perceived Exertion." www.cdc.gov.nccdphp/dmpa/physical/measuring/perceivedexertion.htm.

Chopra, Deepak. *Quantum Healing: Exploring the Frontiers of Mind/Body Medicine*. New York: Bantam, 1990.

_____. *Perfect Health: The Complete Mind-Body Guide*. New York: Crown, 2001.

Connelly, A. Scott, M.D. *Body Rx*. New York: Berkley Books, 2001.

Delavier, Frederic. *Strength Training Anatomy*. Chicago: Human Kinetics, 2001.

Douillard, John, Billie Jean King, and Martina Navratilova. *Body, Mind, and Sport: The Mind-Body Guide to Lifelong Health, Fitness, and Your Personal Best*. New York: Three Rivers Press, 2001.

Dowling, Tim. "Older and Better." *SAGA Magazine*. October (2002) 58-62.

Edelson, Mat. "The Face of Frailty." *Hopkins Medical News*, Spring/Summer (2002). www.hopkinsmedicine.org/hmn/S02/feature.html.

Exercise: A Guide from the National Institute on Aging.
weboflife.ksc.nasa.gov/exerciseandaging/chapter4_balance.html. Printed as
Fitness over 50: An Exercise Guide from the National Institute on Aging. New
York: W. W. Norton, 2003.

Hutchinson, Kathleen M., et al. "Effects of Cardiovascular Fitness and Muscle Strength
on Hearing Sensitivity." *Journal of Strength and Conditioning Research.* 14
(2003) 301-309.

"Injuries in Recreational Adult Fitness Activities." *American Journal of Sports Medicine.*
32 (1993) 461-467.

LeBlanc, Pamela. "Worth the Weight: These Women Prove It's Never Too Late to Pump
Iron." *Austin American-Statesman*, March 28 (2005), E1, E8.

Lichtenstein, Alice. "Forum Explores How and Who to Change Eating Patterns for Better
Health." *Harvard Public Health Now.* October (2003).
www.hsph.harvard.edu/now/oct3/forum.html.

Loehr, Jim and Tony Schwartz. *The Power of Full Engagement: Managing Energy, Not
Time, Is the Key to High Performance and Personal Renewal.* New York: Free
Press, 2003.

McCullough, David. *John Adams.* New York: Touchstone, 2001.

"Miles Away: The MetLife Study of Long-Distance Caregiving."
www.maturemarketinstitute.com.

Milman, Dan. *The Way of the Peaceful Warrior.* New York: H.J. Kramer, 2000.

Moore, K. "The Times of Their Lives." *Runner's World.* 20 (1992): 44-47. Cited in
Spirduso, Waneen W. *Physical Dimensions of Aging.* Chicago: Human Kinetics,
1995.

National Institute of Occupational Safety and Health. "Black Belts: Do They Prevent
Back Injuries?" www.cdc.gov/niosh/blackbelt.html.

National Sleep Foundation. "2003 Sleep in America Poll."
www.sleepfoundation.org/_content/hottopics/2003SleepPollExecSumm.pdf.

Nelson, Miriam E. with Sarah Wernick. *StrongWomen Stay Young.* Rev. ed. New York:
Bantam, 2000.

Peale, Norman Vincent. *The Power of Positive Thinking.* Reissued. New York:
Ballantine Books, 1996.

Perls, Thomas T., Margery Hutter Silver, and John F. Lauerman. *Living to 100: Lessons in Living to Your Maximum Potential at Any Age*. New York: Basic Books, 2000.

Pert, Candace B. *Molecules of Emotion: The Science behind Mind-Body Medicine*. New York: Scribner, 1997.

Pipher, Mary. *Another Country: Navigating the Emotional Terrain of our Elders*. New York: Penguin, 1999.

"Recognizing and Treating Depression." www.ec-online.net/Knowledge/Articles.depressionguide.html.

Richards, Ann with Richard U. Levine. *I'm Not Slowing Down: Winning My Battle with Osteoporosis*. New York: Dutton, 2003.

Rushall, Brent S. *Imagery Training in Sports: A Handbook for Athletes, Coaches, and Sport Psychologists*. New York: Sports Science Association, 1991.

Santana, J. C. *Band Training*. www.performbetter.com.

Sarno, John E, M.D. *The Mindbody Prescription: Healing the Body, Healing the Pain*. New York: Warner Books, 1998.

"Signs of Dehydration." www.aging-parents-and-eldercare.com/Pages/Signs_of_Dehydration.html.

Stanford University. "Geriatric Depression Scale." www.stanford.edu/~yesavage.GDS.english.long.html.

"Ten Tips for Talking to Your Aging Parents." www.maturemarketinstitute.com.

USDA. 2005 Food Guide Pyramid. www.mypyramid.gov

Westcott, Wayne L. and Thomas R. Baeschle. *Strength Training past 50*. Chicago: Human Kinetics, 1997.

Whitmarsh, Blair. *Mind & Muscle*. Chicago: Human Kinetics, 2001.

Index

About the Authors

John B. Payne, 54, is a personal trainer certified by the National Strength and Conditioning Association.

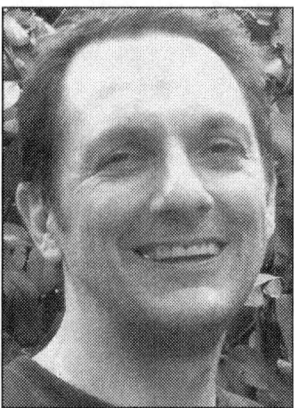

Figure A-43. John B. Payne

John has been a recreational weightlifter since his college days. After careers as a sixth-grade teacher, a petroleum geologist, and a businessman, he has now found the job he always wanted: helping older people stay strong. John is married and has two young adult children.

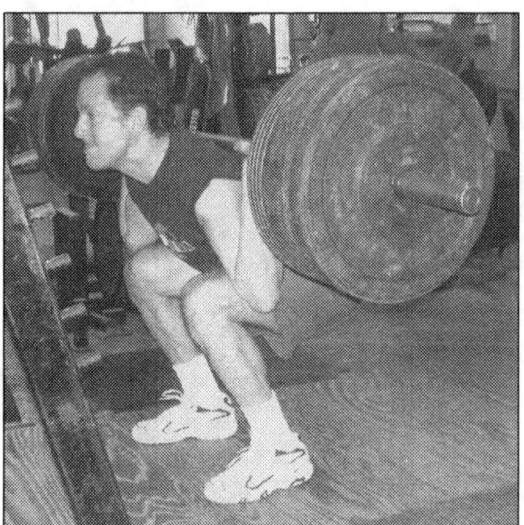

Figure A-44. John squats 286 pounds.

J. Jody Kelly, 68, is a technical writer, non-fiction writer, and instructor of technical, business, and college writing.

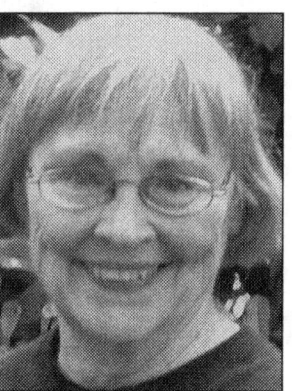

Figure A-45. J. Jody Kelly

For nine years, Jody has trained as a recreational weightlifter with John. Jody recently became a personal trainer certified by the American Council on Exercise. She specializes in helping people over 50 stay strong and healthy. Jody has four adult children and nine grandchildren.

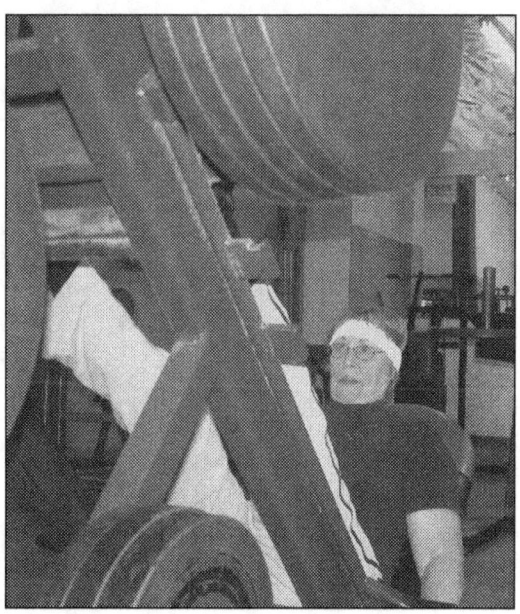

Figure A-46. Jody leg presses 360 pounds.

For more information, see www.significantelder.com.